Contemporary Cardiology

AF147199

Series Editor
Peter P. Toth, Ciccarone Center for the Prevention of Cardiovascular Disease
Johns Hopkins University School of Medicine
Baltimore, MD, USA

For more than a decade, cardiologists have relied on the Contemporary Cardiology series to provide them with forefront medical references on all aspects of cardiology. Each title is carefully crafted by world-renown cardiologists who comprehensively cover the most important topics in this rapidly advancing field. With more than 75 titles in print covering everything from diabetes and cardiovascular disease to the management of acute coronary syndromes, the Contemporary Cardiology series has become the leading reference source for the practice of cardiac care.

Todd J. Cohen • Roger S. Blumenthal
Editors

Surviving and Thriving With Heart Disease

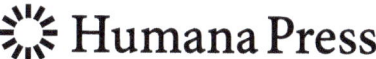 Humana Press

Editors
Todd J. Cohen
NYIT College of Osteopathic Medicine
New York, NY, USA

Roger S. Blumenthal
Johns Hopkins School of Medicine
Baltimore, MD, USA

ISSN 2196-8969   ISSN 2196-8977 (electronic)
Contemporary Cardiology
ISBN 978-3-032-00578-6   ISBN 978-3-032-00579-3 (eBook)
https://doi.org/10.1007/978-3-032-00579-3

This Humana imprint is published by the registered company Springer Nature Switzerland AG
The registered company address is: Gewerbestrasse 11, 6330 Cham, Switzerland

If disposing of this product, please recycle the paper.

Foreword

Heart disease presents as a spectrum from the minor condition to be monitored to the catastrophic event requiring major interventions. When my uncle died at age 76 while playing basketball, he had known of his heart disease for many years and been treated with medications allowing him to continue his favorite weekly event with his friends. I remembered as a youngster he played basketball once a week with his friends and that was a time not to disturb him or plan family events if you expected his presence. Good medical management of his disease allowed him to continue what he loved to do for many years. Today a minimally invasive procedure would have extended his life even longer.

Often when we think of heart disease, we imagine someone quietly sitting on a sofa, walking slowly to another room, and resting once again. Nothing could be further from the truth for the vast majority of patients with heart disease! Today's medical treatments, minimally invasive procedures, and imaging capabilities allow most patients to pursue their hobbies and dreams.

One of my triathlon mentors finished an ironman triathlon after bypass surgery, and one of my family members is enjoying life after a heart transplant! As a physician who has treated patients for over 30 years, I have seen the evolution of this incredible heart care. Giving patients, and their families and friends, their life back is what this is all about.

Dr. Cohen's subject knowledge and his access to specialists give this book the depth it needs, while his understanding of patient care and patients' needs add the important aspects of relevance and readability.

Use this book not only as a resource to expand your knowledge but also as an inspiration to follow your path and your dreams.

Jerry Balentine
President and Chief Executive Officer
New York Institute of Technology,
New York, NY, USA

Preface by Todd J. Cohen

This book is the logical expansion and update to my 2010 Johns Hopkins Health book entitled "A Patient's Guide to Heart Rhythm Problems." It updates and expands on the mission of empowering those with *heart rhythm problems* to help all patients (including their families and friends) *survive and thrive with heart disease*. It does this by not only including broader heart disease related topics, and including the traditional diet, exercise, and lifestyle modifications, but by being more holistic, and giving the reader tips on how to survive, and more importantly thrive! I really appreciated the help of the many healthcare contributors (see Book Contributors) who provided a fresh perspective on heart disease and its current management.

I dedicate this book to all patients with heart disease that need treatment. Various sources of information have been available to you over the years, including magazine articles, pamphlets (often provided by the manufacturers of drugs or implantable devices), and information your physician has provided in discussing your condition and treatment. This book is another source of information. The original "Patient's Guide…" I used in this manner, often giving it to doctors and patients as an educational resource. This newer and expanded book is even more important in this regard.

How does the new book differ from its predecessor? It presents basic concepts of how the normal heart functions, and then expands on these concepts to discuss abnormalities in heart (heart disease) along with their consequences. It discusses tests and studies used in diagnosing heart disease and teaches the reader to know their numbers so they can understand the importance of their heart rate, blood pressure, weight, cholesterol, blood sugar, and their ejection fraction (EF). This is a recurrent theme throughout the book, and Appendix I gives the reader the opportunity to write down and track their numbers and visually see how they change. Finally, the book describes the treatments and prevention measures. In other words, how to survive and more importantly *thrive* with heart disease!

In order to take advantage of the latter, this book pulls in the expertise of some of my wisest and most skilled colleagues that I have turned to help and assist my patients. This book not only will help the reader understand the basic heart tests and treatments but will also expose them to a wider array of treatments including lifestyle modifications, mindfulness, osteopathic as well as allopathic medicine, and alternative therapies.

I have learned from the thousands of patients that I have had the privilege of treating over the years that the ability to adapt to life's changes is a very important factor in order to thrive. One of my patients (referred to in this book) wrote a song that reflects on a method of this flexibility, called "Plan B." It is featured in this book and should be taken to heart (pun intended). The idea of always having alternative plans, when things change or don't work out, has given this patient (and many others) the ability to go with the flow and find even better ways to continue successfully down the pathway of life.

My intention in this book is to provide background to help patients understand their diagnosis, any tests they may undergo, and how doctors might treat the problem. Illustrations and tables are provided to clarify the concepts.

Always ask questions. There is usually an opportunity before any procedure for your doctor and his or her team to answer all your questions and to make sure you are entirely comfortable before proceeding. What is best for you must be considered individually. It is with all these factors in mind that I wrote this book, as a resource for patients, their families, and their loved ones. I hope it helps you gain further understanding of your condition, and not to be redundant, I hope it helps you survive and thrive!

Todd J. Cohen
New York, NY, USA

Preface by Roger S. Blumenthal

Cardiovascular disease or CVD (heart attack, stroke, heart failure, peripheral arterial disease, and arrhythmias such as atrial fibrillation) is the leading cause of death in North America and Europe. Nearly all of the persons who develop CVD have at least one major traditional risk factor and very few have optimal lifestyle habits that are the foundation of prevention. All of us should strive to consume a healthy diet that emphasizes the intake of fruits, vegetables, nuts, whole grains, and fish and engage in at least 150 minutes per week of moderate-intensity physical activity. It is best to minimize trans fats, processed meats, refined carbohydrates, and sweetened beverages. One should also try to replace saturated fats with monounsaturated and polyunsaturated fats and reduce dietary cholesterol and sodium.

Healthcare professionals should identify individuals who are overweight or obese and provide counseling (or refer to other specialists) on comprehensive lifestyle interventions such as caloric restriction and better exercise habits. Individuals who use tobacco products should be assisted and strongly urged to quit. Cardiovascular prevention takes a village, and this great book is a great way to lower your risk of a future cardiovascular event. It was a pleasure to work with my college classmate Dr. Todd Cohen on this project.

Roger S. Blumenthal
Baltimore, MD, USA

Acknowledgments

First, I want to thank all of my patients who made a contribution in one way or another to this book. Some of you added to my experience, such as "Plan B." Others wrote personal cases, which emphasize key points, like how to not only survive but to thrive. Second, I want to thank my coauthor, Dr. Roger S. Blumenthal, Professor of Medicine and Director of the Johns Hopkins Ciccarone Center for the Prevention of Cardiovascular Disease at the Johns Hopkins Hospital for his helpful insights into the field of cardiology and preventive health. He helped pull this book together and make it a useful tool for all patients and their families and friends. Third, I give a special thanks to all those practicing physicians and healthcare workers who contributed significantly to this broad layperson's heart book (listed below; Book Contributors). Fourth, I want to thank Michael Zierler, Science Writer/Editor, for his helpful comments and edits. Fifth, I also want to thank the many great New York Institute of Technology College of Medicine faculty and medical students (who are now physicians) who helped organize the illustrations, permissions, and a myriad of other tasks. I want to thank Dr. Ermin Tale, as well as fourth-year medical student Demetra Menoudakos, for their assistance with the book's final update and editing. Sixth, thanks to my engineering team for developing the "Create your Surviving and Thriving Card" button on my practice's website: www.liheartrhythmceneter.com. Seventh, I wish to acknowledge with gratitude the contributions of Terri Sepalla and Jeffrey Mizel, whose involvement was completed prior to their passing. Lastly, thanks to our Provost and Executive Vice President, Dr. Jerry Balentine, for his encouragement and support during this process. New York Tech is a wonderful place, and he sets an inspirational example for the rest of us at the medical school.

Sincerely,

Todd J. Cohen MD, Distinguished Professor – Clinical Specialties, Chief of Cardiology, Director of Medical Device Innovations, New York Institute of Technology College of Osteopathic Medicine

Introduction

Case 1: Surviving and Thriving

I was taking a stress test at the Hofstra Health Dome in 1987. I had lost 80 pounds and needed clearance to begin a workout regimen. I passed with flying colors; 15 minutes later, my life changed forever. I had a massive MI and "coded" on the way to the hospital. Did I mention I was 35 years old, with two little boys and a beautiful wife? Luck was on my side and I survived. It changed my life, but I went on.

I did fine until 1997, maybe too fine. My weight ballooned to 360 pounds. My legs hurt and I couldn't breathe. Heart failure was now my enemy. More than anything else, I wanted not to die.

I lost 170 pounds and my face was on cereal boxes in supermarkets (Fig. 1, actual Kashi Cereal box showing a leaner meaner me—Jeffrey Mizel). I loved life and my family. Not a chance I would not survive. Did I mention I developed Diabetes? Oh, I also was diagnosed with a heart rhythm problem (arrhythmia), and a pacemaker/ defibrillator was a new improvement.

While seeing an endocrinologist, thyroid nodules were found. Of course, they were malignant, and surgery was next.

To this day, after several rounds of thyroid cancer (not to mention cancer of my left kidney that required part of that kidney to be removed), my wife and I never skipped a beat. We would just say it was another adventure. We would just deal with it and go on. By the way, I found time for four melanoma skin cancer surgeries on my back as well as spine surgeries on my neck and lower back. Somehow a bout with septic shock happened as well. Good news is I am learning to walk again and getting better at it.

Although I have had many adventures to date, I am alive and loving every second. I live for my beautiful wife who has supported all my adventures, two sons, two beautiful daughters-in-law and the highlight of my world, four awesome grandchildren. Not to be forgotten, I have a team of doctors who are always there for me.

Life is awesome!

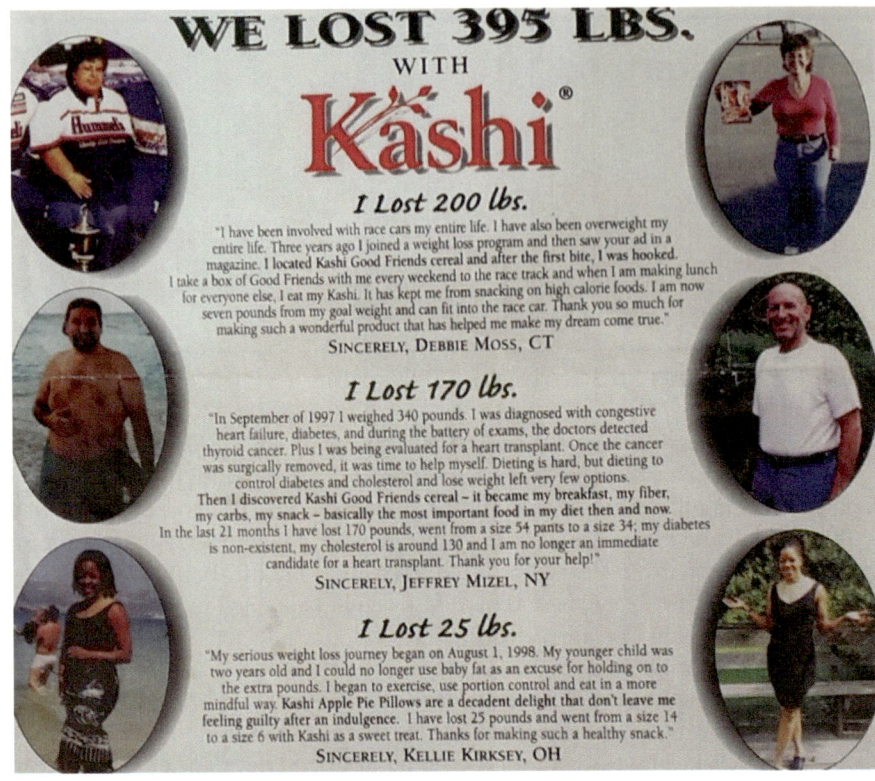

Fig. 1 The actual cereal box that capitalized on my weight loss, a means to surviving and thriving with my heart disease

Contents

Editors and Contributors

About the Editors

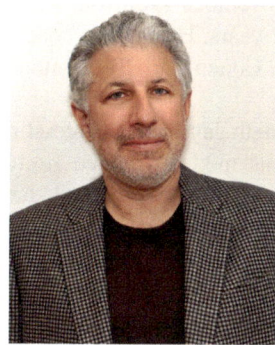

Todd J. Cohen, MD is a triple-boarded (Johns Hopkins, Stanford, and UCSF trained) inspirational cardiologist, inventor, entrepreneur, and educator. After witnessing his grandfather suffering a heart attack, receiving a pacemaker implant, and eventually succumbing to heart disease, he dedicated his life to advancing the field of cardiology.

With over 300 publications, his articles have appeared in journals such as the *New England Journal of Medicine*, *JAMA*, and *Circulation*; his books include a Library Journal Best Consumer Health Book entitled *A Patient's Guide to Heart Rhythm Problems* (Johns Hopkins Press, 2010), a trade book entitled *Practical Electrophysiology, Third Edition* (HMP Communications, LLC, 2016), and a fictional novel entitled *Pollock No. 5* (Black Opal Books, 2021). He has 38 issued U.S. patents and has licensed and/or sold inventions to several leading companies in the field of electrophysiology, catheter ablation, implantable devices, and robotics.

Dr. Cohen built and directed two of the busiest EP programs on Long Island (North Shore Univ. and Winthrop Univ. Hospitals). He is currently the Chief of Cardiology, Director of Medical Device Innovation, and a Distinguished Professor at NYIT in Old Westbury, New York. He is the Director and Founder of the Long Island Heart Rhythm Center (www.liheartrhythmcenter.com) and an attending physician at Mt. Sinai Morningside in New York City. He recieved the AOA Innovations Research Award twice, the NYSOMS Distinguished Service Award, and is a Fellow in the

National Academy of Inventors. He has a passion for art and is the President of the Board of Trustees and Chairman of the Art and Exhibition Committee at the Nassau County Museum of Art, in Roslyn, New York.

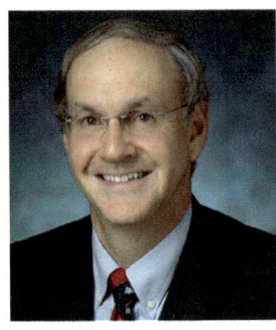

Roger S. Blumenthal, MD is the principal developer and Director of The Johns Hopkins Ciccarone Center for the Prevention of Cardiovascular Disease. The comprehensive clinical and translational research program is named after former Johns Hopkins Lacrosse Coach Henry Ciccarone, who guided the Hopkins Blue Jays to a record seven straight NCAA championship games and three straight national titles. Coach Ciccarone died of sudden cardiac arrest in November 1988 following two heart attacks in the prior 2 years. He was the coach of Johns Hopkins when Drs. Cohen and Blumenthal attended the university.

Dr. Blumenthal is the Kenneth Jay Pollin Professor of Cardiology. He received his medical degree from Cornell Medical College, where he was awarded the Weiss Prize for Excellence in Clinical Medicine. He then did his Internal Medicine and Cardiology Fellowship training at Johns Hopkins before joining the faculty. He received the 2019 Society of Cardiovascular Computed Tomography (SCCT) Arthur S. Agatston Cardiovascular Disease Prevention Award.

Together with Dr. Mariell Jessup, he was co-chair of the American College of Cardiology/American Heart Association (ACC/AHA) subcommittee that oversaw the updates of all the Prevention-related guidelines (Blood Pressure, Cholesterol, Risk Assessment). Dr. Donna Arnett and he were co-chairs of the 2019 ACC/AHA Primary Prevention of Cardiovascular Disease Guideline.

In *Surviving and Thriving with Heart Disease*, Drs. Cohen and Blumenthal utilize their passion for healing and put together a "one-of-a-kind" empowering book that can help all patients and their friends and families learn how to "survive and thrive" with heart disease.

Contributors

Jean Aronoff Yoga Instructor at Om Sweet Om, Port Washington, NY, USA

Jerry Balentine, DO President of New York Institute of Technology, Old Westbury, NY, USA

Thomas Chan, DO Associate Dean-Academic Affairs, New York Institute of Technology College of Osteopathic Medicine, Old Westbury, NY, USA

Marilyn Chengot, MD Department of Cardiology, Amityville Heart Center, Amityville, NY, USA

Thomas Chengot, DO Department of Cardiology, Amityville Heart Center, Amityville, NY, USA

Brittany Cohen Electrical Engineer at ARC by ChargeItSpot, Philadelphia, NY, USA

Zachary Coopee, DO Department of Anesthesiology, Yale School of Medicine, New Haven, CT, USA

Alyssa Curcio, DO Department of Dermatology, St John's Episcopal Hospital, Far Rockaway, NY, USA

Emily Dries, DO Department of Pediatrics, The Children's Hospital at Montefiore, Bronx, NY, USA

Slava Gitelman, DO Department of Osteopathic Manipulative Medicine, St. Barnabas Hospital, Bronx, NY, USA

Robert Hubley, DO Department of Internal Medicine, Walter Reed National Military Medical Center, Bethesda, MD, USA

Nicole Hunzeker, DO Department of Internal Medicine, NYU Langone Hospital, Brooklyn, Brooklyn, NY, USA

Jerry Jose, DO Department of Primary Care Internal Medicine, SUNY Downstate Health Sciences University, Brooklyn, NY, USA

Daniel Kersten, DO Department of Cardiology, NYU Langone Hospital – Long Island, Mineola, NY, USA

Roger Kersten, DO (Retired) Department of Cardiology, St. Francis Hospital & Heart Center, Roslyn, NY, USA

Davendra Mehta, MD, PhD Icahn School of Medicine at Mount Sinai, New York, NY, USA

Demetra Menoudakos, Medical Student, New York Institute of Technology College of Osteopathic Medicine, Old Westbury, NY, USA

Jeffrey Mizel Sales Consultant at RF Industries East LTD (Patient), Island Park, NY, USA

Sarah Jane Muder, DO Department of Obstetrics and Gynecology, St. Luke's University Health Network, Bethlehem,PA, USA

Srihari Naidu, MD Department of Cardiology, Westchester Medical Center, Valhalla, NY, USA

Jillian Nostro, DO Department of Family Medicine, Plainview Hospital, Plainview, NY, USA

Anu Raj, PsyD Department of Family Medicine, New York Institute of Technology College of Osteopathic Medicine, Old Westbury, NY, USA

Bernadette Riley, DO Department of Family Medicine, New York Institute of Technology College of Osteopathic Medicine, Old Westbury, NY, USA

Amer Sayed, MD Department of Cardiology, Adams County Regional Medical Center, Cincinnati, OH, USA

John Seppala Director at Telehealth Associates (Patient), East Setauket, NY, USA

Terri Seppala CEO and President of Telehealth Associates, East Setauket, NY, USA

Ermin Tale, DO Department of Internal Medicine, Jacobi Medical Center – Albert Einstein College of Medicine, Bronx, NY, USA

Matthew Tarrash, DO Department of Anesthesiology, Hackensack University Medical Center, Hackensack, NJ, USA

Sheldon Yao, DO Department of Osteopathic Manipulative Medicine, New York Institute of Technology College of Osteopathic Medicine, Old Westbury, NY, USA

Jeffrey Mizel (1951–2022) contributed to this book before his passing
Terri Sepalla (1947–2024) contributed to this book before her passing

Part I

The Basics

This part of the book will provide you and those you care about with the information needed to understand how the heart works. Read it and ask questions when you see your doctor. The more you know, the better you will understand why certain tests are being ordered or what treatments are being suggested. This book is intended to give you the tools so that you are empowered and can take control of your own heart health.

Overview: Your Heart

Todd J. Cohen

In order to understand heart disease, you first need a basic understanding of your heart. Your heart is a muscular structure, located in the middle of your chest, that pumps blood throughout your body. It is a vital organ with both electrical and mechanical components. The electrical system produces the rhythm, and the mechanical components provide the pumping. Mechanically, the heart has four chambers and four valves, as shown in Fig. 1.1. The heart consists of two upper chambers and two lower chambers. Each upper chamber is called an *atrium* (right atrium and left atrium). Together, these chambers are called the *atria*. They *receive* blood, which is then pumped into the lower chambers. The lower chambers, called the *ventricles, pump* blood to the lungs (right ventricle) and to the rest of the body (left ventricle).

The electrical system (which is also called the conduction system) tells the heart (and its chambers) when and in what sequence it should contract and relax to pump blood to the rest of the body (Fig. 1.2). The electrical impulses begin high up in the right atrium, in a structure called the *sinus,* or *sinoatrial, node* (SA node). A node is defined as a beginning structure or a point for electrical signals to come together and then be redirected to another region in the heart. There are two nodes in the heart:

T. J. Cohen (✉)
NYIT College of Osteopathic Medicine, New York, NY, USA
e-mail: tcohen03@nyit.edu

© The Author(s), under exclusive license to Springer Nature Switzerland AG 2025
T. J. Cohen, R. S. Blumenthal (eds.), *Surviving and Thriving With Heart Disease*,
Contemporary Cardiology, https://doi.org/10.1007/978-3-032-00579-3_1

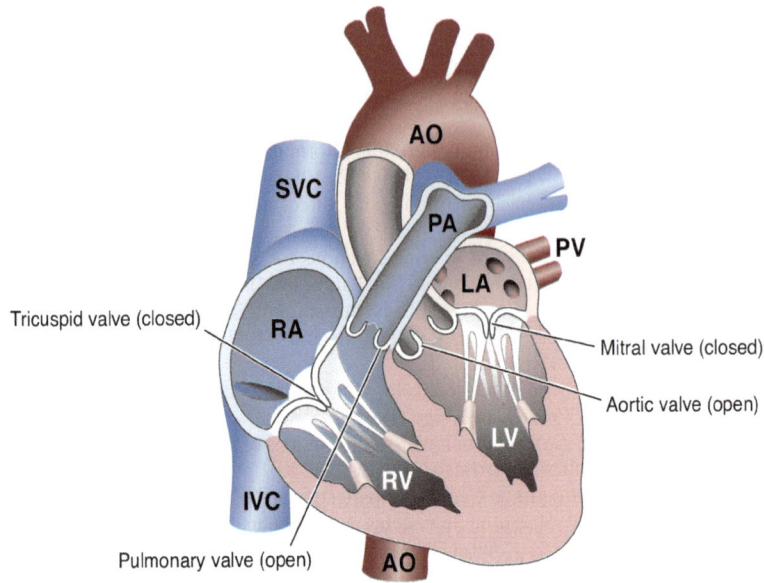

Fig. 1.1 The structure of the heart—its chambers, valves, and great vessels. AO aorta, IVC inferior vena cava, LA left atrium, LV left ventricle, PA pulmonary artery, PV pulmonary veins, RA right atrium, RV right ventricle, SVC superior vena cava. (See also color version.)

the SA node and the *atrioventricular node* (AV node). Impulses move from the SA node across the atrial structures to the AV node (located in the middle of the heart, between the atria and ventricles). A small delay in the electrical signal typically occurs in the AV node before the impulse travels to a specialized conduction bundle (called the *His bundle*); it then moves down through the right and left bundles to specialized *Purkinje fibers* before activating the ventricles.

The presence of disease in any of the specialized electrical conducting tissues may disrupt the flow of electricity through the heart, slowing or pausing the heart rate. When the heart rate is too slow, a person may develop symptoms and may need to have a pacemaker surgically implanted to correct the problem. Disease inside or outside the specialized cardiac conduction tissue can also result in fast heart rhythm problems that might require treatment with medications, catheter ablation (a procedure that identifies the heart rhythm abnormality and destroys specific tissue to cure the rhythm problem), or an implantable device such as a defibrillator (see Part V).

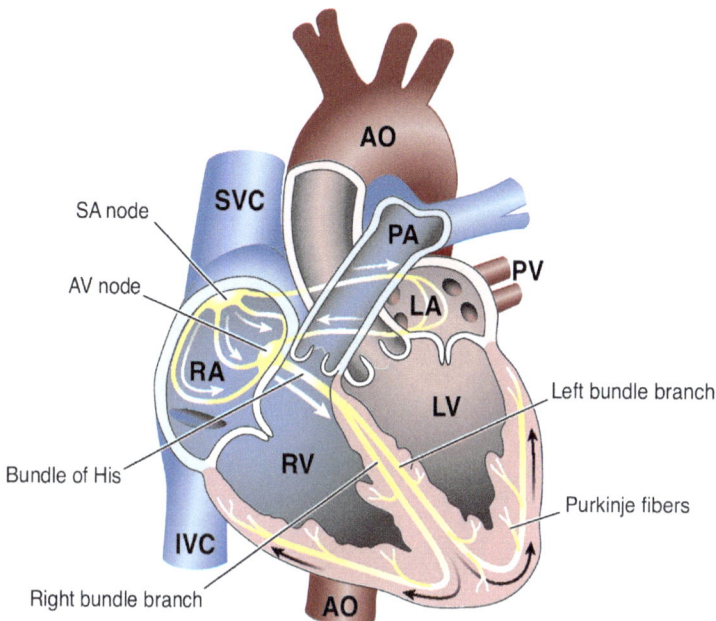

Fig. 1.2 The conduction system of the heart. The arrows show the electrical impulses, which begin in the sinus node and travel through the atria to the atrioventricular node. After a slight delay there, these impulses are conducted through the His bundle and through the right and left bundle branches to the Purkinje fibers, which carry the impulses into the ventricles. AO aorta, AV node atrioventricular node, IVC inferior vena cava, LA left atrium, LV left ventricle, PA pulmonary artery, PV pulmonary veins, RA right atrium, RV right ventricle, SA node sinus node, SVC superior vena cava. (See also color version.)

Blood Movement Through the Heart

Blood flow through the healthy heart's chambers should be smooth and rhythmic. The right side of the heart receives deoxygenated blood (devoid of oxygen) from the rest of the body via two large veins, called the *superior vena cava* and *inferior vena cava* (Fig. 1.3). Blood enters the right atrium and travels through the tricuspid valve to the right ventricle. Then it is pumped out the pulmonary valve through the pulmonary artery into the lungs, where oxygen is put into the blood. Oxygenated blood returns through pulmonary veins to the left side of the heart and into the left atrium. The blood then travels across the mitral valve into the left ventricle and is pumped out through the aortic valve into the aorta and then to the rest of the body.

The heart itself is nourished through the coronary arteries, which arise from the proximal (first part of the) aorta. The coronary arteries consist of a left coronary artery (which branches into the left anterior descending and the left circumflex

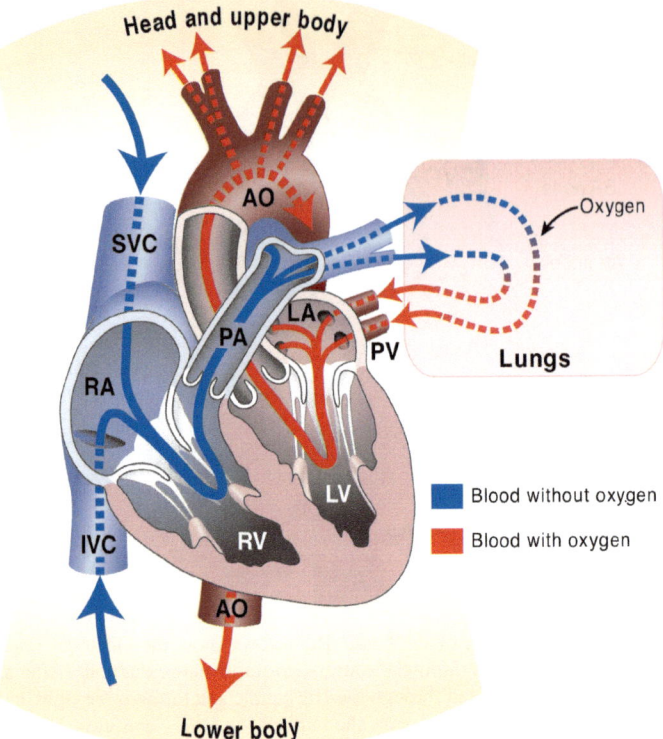

Fig. 1.3 The sequence of circulation. The blue arrows show blood deprived of oxygen (deoxygenated blood) returning to the right side of the heart. The blood is then pumped to the lungs to receive oxygen. Oxygenated blood, indicated by red arrows, returns to the heart via the pulmonary veins and is then pumped from the left side of the heart to the rest of the body. AO aorta, IVC inferior vena cava, LA left atrium, LV left ventricle, PA pulmonary artery, PV pulmonary veins, RA right atrium, RV right ventricle, SVC superior vena cava. (See also color version.)

Table 1.1 Heart facts

The heart is a four-chambered muscular structure.
It is about the size of your fist but can get much larger with disease.
It pumps 1,500 gallons of blood each day.
It normally beats at a rate of 60 to 100 times per minute (your heart rate).
It beats about 100,000 times per day and 36 million times per year.
Heart muscle does not usually regenerate.

coronary arteries) and a right coronary artery. Blockages (or moderate narrowings) in these arteries (or in their branches) may lead to a lack of blood flow and oxygenation of heart tissue (called *ischemia*). When the blockage is severe and lasts long enough (usually following plaque rupture), the person may have a heart attack (also called a *myocardial infarction*; see Chap. 11). For a summary of basic facts about the heart, see Table 1.1.

Talking to Your Heart Doctor

2

Todd J. Cohen

Heart disease is often discovered when your primary care provider (PCP) detects an abnormality. This individual may be an internist, family physician, or nurse practitioner. Alternatively, acute heart conditions, such as heart rhythm problems and heart attacks, may involve emergency room physicians. In both cases, an initial assessment is performed, including a history, physical examination, and an electrocardiogram (see Chap. 16). After the assessment, the doctor will make a referral to a cardiologist to help manage and treat your heart-related condition. A cardiologist is a *heart doctor* who specializes in the care of patients who have (or are suspected of having) heart disease. This referral is best performed by a "handoff," in which your important medical information regarding your condition, along with an electrocardiogram, is provided to a cardiologist. In essence, the handoff is the transfer of care from the PCP to the specialist, who will treat the patient and eventually "handoff" the patient back to the PCP.

It is very important to talk to your cardiologist and have him or her explain to you, in terms you can understand, your heart problems (heart disease).

- Remember: Don't be shy. Feel free to ask your questions until you have a full understanding.
- It is very helpful to take notes.
- Do not accept complicated or fancy terms you do not understand. Ask him or her to explain these terms in a way that you can appreciate.

T. J. Cohen (✉)
NYIT College of Osteopathic Medicine, New York, NY, USA
e-mail: tcohen03@nyit.edu

Table 2.1 Tips on talking to your cardiologist

Don't be shy; remember to ask your questions.

Bring paper and pen, or use your smartphone to take notes.

Bring a list of what medications you are taking, both prescription drugs and any supplements.

Ask your healthcare provider why a test, procedure, or treatment is being recommended.

Tell your healthcare provider when you don't understand them.

Ask your healthcare provider to repeat and/or clarify anything that you don't understand.

Make sure you understand the risks, benefits, and alternatives to any test, procedure, or treatment.

Ask your cardiologist to share test results and other details about your treatment with all the other doctors and healthcare practitioners who take care of you. That way, everyone will be on the same page.

- If a test or procedure is recommended, ask your doctor why it is being recommended and how it would change your management. Are there potential risks to the procedure and how frequently do they occur?
- How much will the test cost you?
- What are the risks and benefits of the test? Are there any alternatives?
- Do you need to have the test done now or at a later date?
- Ask your cardiologist to share test results and other details about your treatment with all the other doctors and health care practitioners who take care of you. That way, everyone will be on the same page.

There is no such thing as a stupid question. This book will help guide you on what to ask your cardiologist before undergoing any tests or invasive procedures. You can refer to Table 2.1 for tips on things to remember when talking to your healthcare provider.

Cardiology Specialists

There are different types of cardiologists that you might see, depending on your problem. A *general cardiologist* specializes in a wide range of heart-related problems. In addition to medical school training, cardiologists have three years of internal medicine preparation and at least three years in cardiology. Subspecialists such as those described below often have training beyond that of general cardiologists.

A *cardiac imaging cardiologist* specializes in noninvasive imaging studies that help diagnose structural and functional abnormalities of the heart. Studies include echocardiography, computer tomography angiography (CT angiography) with contrast dye, cardiac magnetic resonance imaging (cardiac MRI), and nuclear cardiology (Part IV).

A *cardiac electrophysiologist* specializes in diagnosing and treating heart rhythm problems by invasive and noninvasive means and typically has at least one additional year of training beyond general cardiology training. One invasive procedure that electrophysiologists perform is called an *electrophysiology study*. This test

Fig. 2.1 This figure shows a cardiac electrophysiologist (Dr. Todd Cohen) and his physician assistant (Alexandru Mitrache) hard at work in an electrophysiology laboratory control room

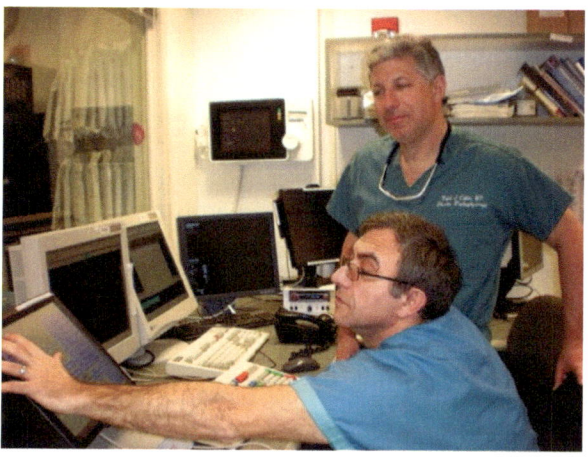

helps diagnose a particular rhythm problem (Chap. 21). Once the rhythm abnormality is identified, it can be treated with a special tube (called a *catheter*) that maps and ablates (gets rid of) the problem (Chap. 29). In addition, these doctors can treat heart rhythm abnormalities with devices such as implantable cardiac monitors, pacemakers, and defibrillators (Chap. 30). They also can insert a device called "the Watchman," which can help prevent a stroke from atrial fibrillation in those who require, but cannot take, blood thinners (Chap. 32). Figure 2.1 shows a cardiac electrophysiologist (this book's coauthor, Dr. Todd Cohen) with his former physician assistant (Alexandru Mitrache) in an electrophysiology laboratory control room.

An *interventional cardiologist* specializes in the diagnosis and treatment of heart-related problems by inserting catheters into blood vessels and then injecting contrast dye into the catheters to visualize abnormalities. One of the invasive procedures these specialists perform is a percutaneous coronary intervention (PCI), in which coronary artery blockages are opened via a balloon (angioplasty), and one or more stents (small metal mesh tubes) are placed to keep the vessels open (Chap. 24). Interventional cardiologists can also insert and/or repair artificial valves without having to open the chest and undergo heart surgery. Procedures such as TAVR (transcutaneous aortic valve replacement) and the mitral clip are just some of the ways your interventional cardiologist can repair the diseased heart (Chap. 27). This specialty typically requires at least one year of additional training beyond general cardiology.

A *cardiac rehabilitation cardiologist* is a general cardiologist who helps patients recover from heart surgery and other heart interventions using a graduated and monitored exercise program. These doctors often educate patients and coach them on healthy diet, exercise, and lifestyle modifications.

A *heart failure specialist* is a cardiologist who specializes in the treatment of congestive heart failure and helps patients maintain an optimal diet and lifestyle. These specialists also prescribe and monitor patients' medications and strive to provide optimal medical therapy (Chap. 25).

A *cardiothoracic surgeon* performs open-heart surgery to bypass blocked arteries and to treat valvular heart disease (Chap. 33). The cardiac surgeon may also perform procedures to treat heart rhythm abnormalities and has the advantage of directly visualizing the heart. The cardiac surgeon may work together with the electrophysiologist and/or interventional cardiologist in order to assist and/or back up procedures such as pacemaker or defibrillator lead extraction, perform cardiac ablation of atrial fibrillation and other arrhythmias, and implant a TAVR-type device (to name a few). Cardiothoracic surgery encompasses different training than is required in general cardiology and its subspecialties.

Monitor Your Pulse: Heartbeat and Rhythm

3

Todd J. Cohen

When the heart muscle contracts, it pumps blood throughout the body via a series of pipes called arteries. This blood, full of oxygen and nutrients, travels to the brain and the rest of the body's vital organs, delivers the nutrients and oxygen to these organs, and then returns to the heart via another series of blood vessels called veins. With each contraction of the heart, the blood being propelled can be felt as a series of pulsations known as the arterial pulse. The pulse is a reflection of the pumping of blood from your heart through the arterial blood system throughout the body. Your heart's pulsation may be felt (or palpated) in various places, including over the chest near where the heart is located, as well as at the wrist (radial pulse), the groin (femoral pulse), and the neck (carotid pulse). Each heart pulsation is a single heartbeat.

The quality of the pulse and the rate of your heart rhythm can be measured by taking your pulse. You or a family member should use the radial pulse location, at the thumb side of the wrist, because this is the most practical place to feel a pulse consistently. To take your pulse, with your palm up, place the first and second fingers of your other hand (do not use your thumb) over the radial side (Fig. 3.1). This is where your radial pulse can be found. You should be able to feel the quality of the pulse itself.

Is it strong, indicating adequate blood pressure (or perfusion)?
Or is it weak, indicating a lack of adequate blood pressure?
Is it fast or slow?

T. J. Cohen (✉)
NYIT College of Osteopathic Medicine, New York, NY, USA
e-mail: tcohen03@nyit.edu

© The Author(s), under exclusive license to Springer Nature Switzerland AG 2025
T. J. Cohen, R. S. Blumenthal (eds.), *Surviving and Thriving With Heart Disease*,
Contemporary Cardiology, https://doi.org/10.1007/978-3-032-00579-3_3

Fig. 3.1 The proper way to take your pulse. With your palm up, place two fingers of your other hand on the thumb side of the wrist to feel the pulse. The heart rate can be calculated by counting the number of palpated beats over 15 s and then multiplying that number by 4. For example, if 20 beats are counted over a 15 s period, that number multiplied by 4 gives a heart rate of 80 beats per minute

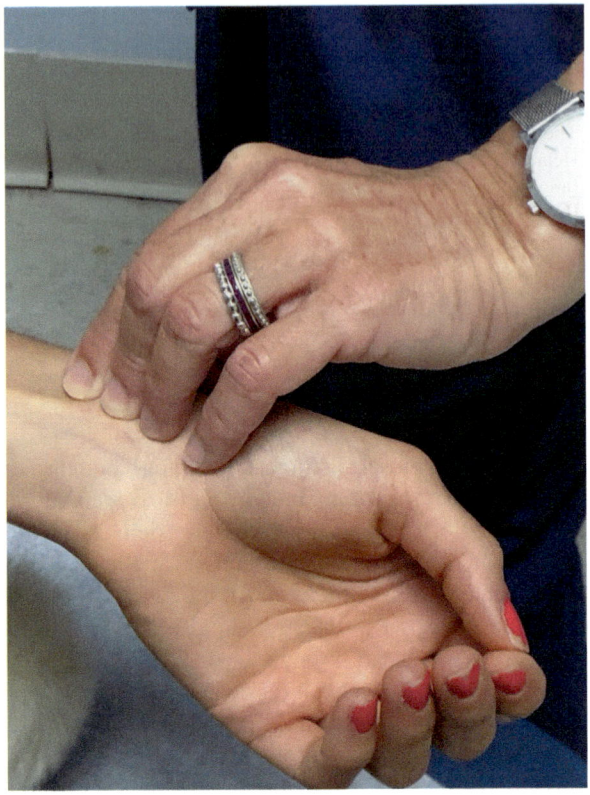

By counting the number of pulsations (heartbeats) over a 15-s interval and multiplying that number by four, you can calculate your heart rate (in beats per minute).

Example If 20 pulsations (heartbeats) are counted over 15 s; multiply the pulsations by 4 to get your heart rate. 20 pulsations × 4 = 80 beats per minute

A normal adult heart rate is generally regarded to be between 60 and 100 beats per minute. Heart rates as low as 40 beats per minute in asymptomatic adults may still be physiologically normal and not a sign of illness. Some devices, such as Apple Watches, track your heart rate. So do some exercise machines, such as rowers, stationary bikes, ellipticals, and so on.

Just because your pulse is below or above these numbers does not mean that you have heart disease. If your resting heart rate is slow (in the 40s, for example) and you feel well, this may not require treatment. Similarly, if your heart rate is fast (above 100 beats per minute) from stress or exertion, and you have no symptoms, no intervention may be needed. Is your pulse regular, like a clock, or irregular or

Table 3.1 Pulse facts

Take your pulse with your first and second fingers, not your thumb.

Count the number of heartbeats that occur in 15 s and multiply that number by 4 to get the heart rate in beats per minute.

The normal heart rate is 60–100 beats per minute.

Heart rates slower than 60 beats per minute can be normal if you don't have symptoms such as fatigue, shortness of breath, light-headedness, or dizziness.

Rapid heart rates (greater than 100 beats per minute) may be normal or abnormal, depending on circumstances.

Note: Some devices, such as at-home blood pressure machines, Apple watches, and other technologies can track your heart rate. It's important to get a doctor to check out any irregularities as these devices are not always accurate.

erratic? An erratic pulse is commonly found in a condition called *atrial fibrillation* (or Afib, for short; see Chap. 9). Your cardiologist should determine whether your rhythm is normal *for you* and correlate any of your symptoms to your heart rate and its rhythm. Pulse facts helpful to heart disease patients and their families and friends are shown in Table 3.1.

Your pulse and heartbeat can be a guide to whether you have a heart rhythm problem or abnormality. Just about everyone will face a heart rhythm abnormality at some time during their life.

The Normal Heart Rhythm

The normal pulse and heartbeat are regular, with typical rates between 60 and 100 beats per minute. The flow of electrical impulses is sequential, beginning in the SA node (see Fig. 3.2) and traveling through atrial tissue, which causes the atrial muscle to contract. Electrical impulses continue through the AV node, His bundle, and Purkinje fibers, and then to the ventricles, causing the muscles in the ventricles to contract. This flow of electrical impulses from the atria to the ventricles helps to propel blood from the heart to the rest of the body. The cycle typically repeats well over two billion times in the course of a lifetime. The pulse should be easily palpable at the outside of the wrist (radial pulse) and should beat in a regular, rhythmic fashion.

An arrhythmia is a heart rhythm that is irregular or in other ways abnormal. Arrhythmias may come from the atria or the ventricles. People may or may not have symptoms, such as a pounding heartbeat (fluttering), heaviness in their chest, shortness of breath, sweating, dizziness, passing out, or a feeling of impending doom (feeling of death). Cardiac arrest is the complete collapse of the patient's circulatory system and, unfortunately, is the first symptom for some people. The different kinds of heart rate abnormalities are discussed below and in more detail in the chapters ahead.

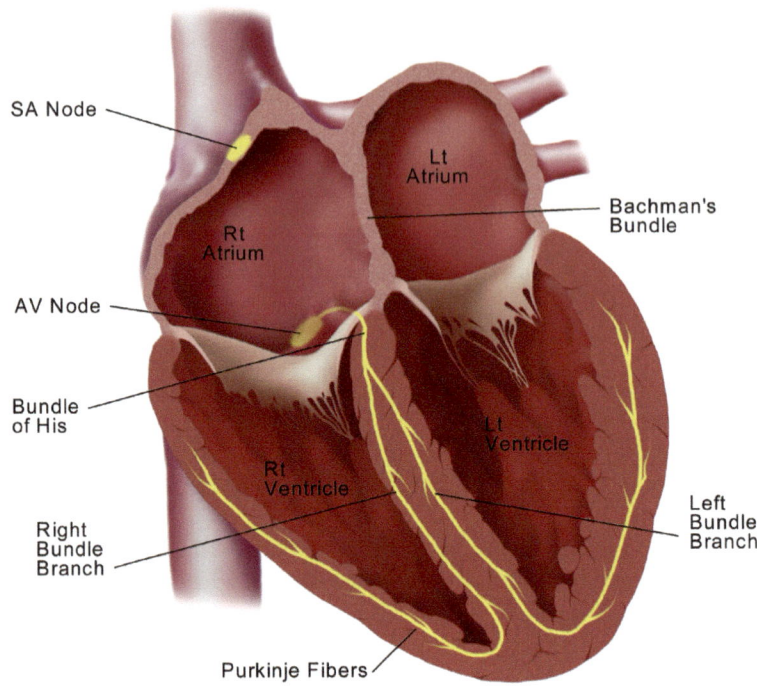

Fig. 3.2 This figure shows the main parts of the electrical wiring system of the heart. Impulses begin in the SA node (or pacemaker of the heart) and travel through atrial tissue to the AV node (which delays these impulses slightly). Then impulses normally travel through the Bundle of His to specialized His-Purkinje fibers, which become the bundle branches that supply impulses to the right and left ventricles. The yellow color highlights these specialized wiring structures within the heart

Abnormal Heart Rhythms (Arrhythmias)

Disease in the heart and/or its conduction system may result in a slow or fast heart rate or an irregular heartbeat. Blocked electrical impulses from the atria to the ventricles are termed *heart block*. Problems can occur anywhere in the electrical system and interfere with the pumping mechanism of the heart. In addition, problems can occur outside the conduction system, possibly as a result of disease within the heart muscle itself.

Rapid Heart Rhythms (Tachycardias)

Rapid heart rhythms, called *tachycardias*, have heart rates greater than 100 beats per minute and possibly much faster. The faster the heart rate, the greater the chance that delivery of oxygen and other nutrients to the brain and other organs will be impaired. With very fast heart rhythms (greater than 200 beats per minute), the person will likely become light-headed and dizzy, and may even faint (syncopize). Sudden cardiac arrest is a condition often caused by a rapid heartbeat or rhythm from the lower chambers of the heart. This rapid rhythm is called *ventricular tachycardia* or *ventricular fibrillation*, in which the lower chambers of the heart beat too fast to effectively pump blood to the rest of the body. This is because when the heart is beating too fast, the heart chambers do not have enough time between beats to fill and therefore they have too little blood to squeeze out (see Chap. 7).

If the person loses consciousness, his or her pulse may feel weak or may even be impossible to feel. If the rhythm is not treated immediately or does not revert to a normal or slower rhythm on its own, the person will not survive. If, however, the patient is treated immediately with cardiopulmonary resuscitation (CPR; Chap. 47) or advanced cardiac life support measures, including defibrillation (a shock administered to the chest using a defibrillator; see Chap. 26), or if the rapid rhythm breaks on its own accord, a palpable pulse may be restored (indicating the return of adequate circulation), and the person will usually survive. Other forms of tachycardia may originate in the upper chamber of the heart (supraventricular) and may be treated using less aggressive means (medications, cardioversion, and/or ablation). You will learn more about these rhythms in the chapters ahead.

Slow Heart Rhythms (Bradycardias)

The heart may also beat too slowly (called *bradycardia*), with heart rates below 60 beats per minute. The slow rate is significant, especially if correlated with symptoms. Even though the heart muscle may be contracting adequately, if the rate of contraction is too slow (less than 40 beats per minute), there may not be sufficient blood being sent to vital organs, especially the brain. If your pulse and heart rate are very slow and you feel weak, fatigued, short of breath, lightheaded, dizzy, or lose consciousness, a pacemaker may be required. The latter is very useful if the condition is not easily reversible.

Did you know that a slow heart rate is not always a sign of a problem? Many athletes have a slow heartbeat because their bodies have adapted to intense exercise routines. Bradycardia may be a normal physiologic finding and usually is only of concern if associated with significant signs and symptoms.

Irregular Heart Rhythms

An irregular pulse and heartbeat might indicate early beats, called premature contractions (coming from either the atria or the ventricles), or may be an indicator of a rhythm problem called *atrial fibrillation or atrial flutter*, in which the atria beat at very rapid rates and your overall heart rate might be fast (see Chap. 9). The latter conditions are important to diagnose since they may place you at higher risk for a stroke and possibly weaken your heart.

Appendix I: Know your numbers lists the numbers that you should track in order to lower your risk of heart disease. Alongside the recording of your blood pressure and weight or body mass index (BMI), you should record your heart rate. This is because your heart rate has some relationship to blood pressure and is affected by blood pressure medications such as beta-blockers and calcium channel blockers.

Your Heart Pump: One Muscle, One Life

4

Todd J. Cohen

You have one heart muscle (or heart pump) to go with your one life. I say that, because it is a rarity to get a second heart (heart transplant), and even when that occurs successfully, your life is no bed of roses. Knowing that, you should treat your heart wisely. Take care of it. Do whatever you can to keep it, and the rest of your body, fit. That means don't abuse your body. Things like too much alcohol and fatty foods can wreak havoc on your heart. Alcohol in moderation may be okay, but in excess it can cause arrhythmias such as atrial fibrillation and even cause a weakened heart muscle (cardiomyopathy). A fatty diet of fried foods and sweets most of the time can cause a progressive buildup of fat deposits or plaque over time (a process known as atherosclerosis) in the coronary arteries and lead to coronary artery disease, ischemia (lack of blood flow to the heart muscle), and even a heart attack.

The Heart as a Pump

The heart is, in fact, a pump. The right side of the heart receives blood deprived of oxygen (which is consumed by all body organs and tissues) via the veins. Although the blood in your veins appears blue (when looking at your arms or legs), that's not true. All blood (in humans, at least) is red; the blue color is an optical illusion. The heart then pumps the low-oxygen blood to the lungs, where oxygen from the freshly breathed air is added and carbon dioxide, a waste product formed by the body's organs and tissues, is removed. The freshly oxygenated blood then returns to the left side of the heart, which then pumps the blood to the rest of the body via the arteries. Each heartbeat pumps blood returning from the body to the lungs, as well as blood returning from the lungs to the rest of the body.

T. J. Cohen (✉)
NYIT College of Osteopathic Medicine, New York, NY, USA
e-mail: tcohen03@nyit.edu

T. J. Cohen, R. S. Blumenthal (eds.), *Surviving and Thriving With Heart Disease*,
Contemporary Cardiology, https://doi.org/10.1007/978-3-032-00579-3_4

A strong heart muscle and proper timing of the opening and closing of the heart valves ensure adequate delivery of oxygenated blood to the body's vital organs and tissues. Certain heart valves must open at specific times to allow the forward flow of blood and must close at other times to prevent backflow (blood flowing back into the chambers rather than out to the body). The timing of the opening and closing of the valves is controlled by the heart's conduction system. If the valves are incompetent or are unable to handle a large volume of fluid because of ineffective pumping from the heart, fluid will back up and accumulate in the lungs and other tissues, resulting in *congestive heart failure*, symptoms of which include shortness of breath, leg swelling, and fatigue.

Ejection Fraction

Your doctor may describe the strength of your heart using terms such as cardiac output and ejection fraction. *Cardiac output* is a measure of how much blood your heart can pump out in liters per minute. A normal cardiac output is greater than 4 liters per minute. *Ejection fraction* (EF) is a more commonly used term than cardiac output; it represents the *percentage* of blood that is ejected from the heart. EF can be measured using various imaging modalities, including echocardiography, angiography, and cardiac MRI, or as part of a nuclear study. These studies approximate the EF by calculating the difference between the amount of blood contained within the left ventricle during a complete relaxation and the amount of blood contained during a complete contraction, divided by the amount of blood in a complete relaxation phase; this number is then multiplied by 100 to give the EF as a percentage. When EF is used alone, it typically refers to the left ventricular EF. If the right ventricular function is specified, it would include an additional descriptor such as "right ventricular" EF. For a summary of key ejection fraction facts, see Table 4.1.

Table 4.1 Ejection fraction facts

Ejection fraction (EF) measures the percentage of blood that is ejected from the heart (and when used alone specifically refers to left ventricular EF). If targeting the right ventricle, the additional descriptor of "right ventricular" EF is used.

The EF can be calculated through various tests by determining the difference between the volume of blood in the left ventricle at the end of a full contraction and the volume of blood in the left ventricle at the end of a full relaxation. That number is then divided by the volume of blood at the end of full relaxation, and the result is multiplied by 100 to define the EF as a percentage.

If your EF is less than 35%, talk to your doctor about whether you might benefit from an implantable cardioverter defibrillator.

If your EF is greater than 50%, you are less likely to need an implantable defibrillator. An exception is hypertrophic cardiomyopathy, a condition in which the heart muscle is thickened and its contraction is very strong. The EF in this condition may be greater than 70 percent (hyperdynamic). If you have hypertrophic cardiomyopathy, you may be at risk for sudden death from ventricular arrhythmias, especially if your heart muscle is very thick or your family has a history of sudden death, ventricular tachycardia, or syncope (sudden loss of consciousness).

Know Your EF

First and foremost, every heart patient should know his or her EF. A normal EF is between 50% and 70%. Keep in mind that people with a seemingly normal EF can have a condition called *hypertrophic cardiomyopathy* (see Chaps. 13 and 36). People with this condition have a thickened heart muscle and often have a very strong heart contraction—the EF is typically well above 50% and may even be greater than 70%, called hyperdynamic. This condition may put a person at risk for sudden death from ventricular arrhythmias, especially if the heart muscle is very thick or if the patient has a family history of sudden death, ventricular tachycardia, or syncope (sudden loss of consciousness).

An EF of less than 50% is *low* and *abnormal*. A low EF may be associated with signs and symptoms of heart failure (see Chap. 14) and risks life-threatening heart rhythm problems, resulting in sudden loss of consciousness or sudden cardiac arrest and potentially death if not promptly treated. Depending on your symptoms and medical history, and whether you have ventricular tachycardia, an EF between 35% and 50% may benefit from an ICD. Discuss your EF number with your cardiologist, who may advise you to see an electrophysiologist (heart rhythm specialist), who can assist in the decision process.

If your EF is 35% or less, ask your doctor if you are on the key medications that are recommended for persons with low EF. If so, you should suggest an implantable cardioverter defibrillator (ICD). This device is typically implanted in the chest and can detect heart rhythm abnormalities (fast and slow) and treat them accordingly (see Chap. 30: Pacemakers and Implantable Defibrillators). The EF table (Table 4.2) can help you assess the strength of your heart. For more information related to heart failure, see Chap. 14.

Table 4.2 What does your ejection fraction (EF) mean?

EF (%)	Severity of heart weakness
50 or greater	Normal
40 to 49	Mild heart weakness
30 to 39	Moderate heart weakness
Less than 30	Severe heart weakness
Greater than 70	Hyperdynamic

Lifestyle Modifications: Eat Right, Exercise, and Reduce Stress

5

Roger Kersten and Todd J. Cohen

This book focuses on how you can survive and thrive with heart disease. Figure 5.1 shows five key components: high cholesterol, high blood pressure, obesity, smoking, and diabetes. These risk factors are covered in Chaps. 37, 38, 39, 40, and 41 in detail. This chapter provides information on diet, exercise, and coping with emotional stress. These topics are so important that you'll find more information throughout the book, including in Chaps. 37, 38, 39, 40, and 41 and in the appendices (at the end of the book).

R. Kersten (Retired)
Department of Cardiology, St. Francis Hospital & Heart Center, Roslyn, NY, USA

T. J. Cohen (✉)
NYIT College of Osteopathic Medicine, New York, NY, USA
e-mail: tcohen03@nyit.edu

5 RISK FACTORS FOR
HEART DISEASE & STROKE

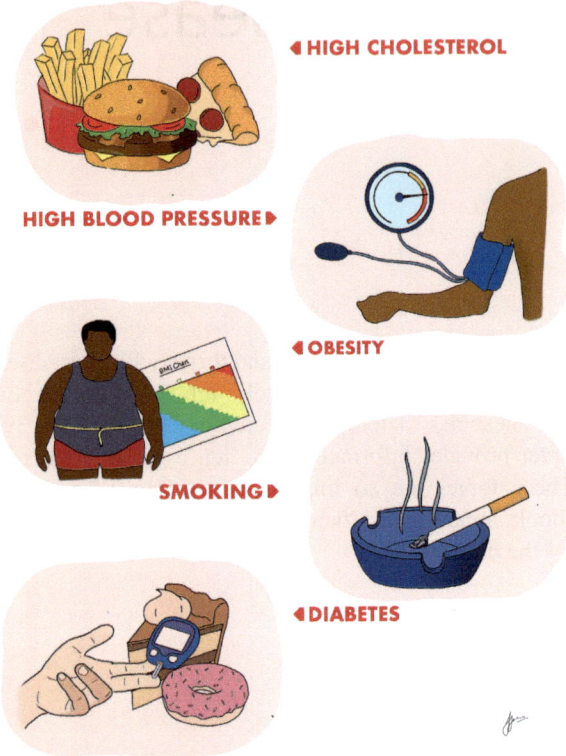

Fig. 5.1 This illustration (by Jerry Jose, DO) shows the five risk factors for heart disease and stroke. They are each featured in Chaps. 37, 38, 39, 40, and 41. The first figure shows a typical American diet of processed foods high in saturated fats and salt. Many Americans grab a slice of pizza or stop at the local hamburger joint for a burger and fries. They do not eat the appropriate amounts of fruits and vegetables that should be part of their daily diet. The second figure shows blood pressure which is elevated in many Americans. The third is weight. Can you imagine that nearly 70% of adult Americans are overweight or obese? This is a BIG problem (no pun intended). Each of the chapters that focus on these first three risks reinforce the centerpiece concepts of this book, which are (1) diet, (2) exercise, and (3) know your numbers (that is your cholesterol, blood pressure, and weight (body mass index or BMI)). Smoking is a bad habit that needs to be more than addressed. It is a modifiable risk factor that can make a dent in worldwide mortality. Lastly, sugar intake and weight management all impact your blood sugar and risk for developing pre-diabetes or diabetes. There are things we can all do to improve our cholesterol, blood pressure, weight, exposure to smoke and smoking, as well as the risk of developing diabetes. So to quote NIKE, "Just Do It!"

Diet

What you eat is a key component of health and illness. While we tend to think about diet in terms of weight management, it is also a way to keep your heart healthy and improve your overall health.

Our choices of foods play an important role in both nutrition and reducing inflammation (the latter plays a key role in the development of plaque, rupture, and clot formation within coronary arteries). Importantly, maintaining a healthy weight is associated with less inflammation than obesity. Obesity and diet have been linked to certain types of cancers, in addition to some types of heart disease. How our bodies use energy from food is complicated. *Generally, processed and fast foods should be minimized*, as these foods tend to be high in saturated fat, salt, sugar, and additives, such as preservatives. While there is no one perfect diet for everyone, low simple carbohydrate diets seem to be beneficial in a wide range of people for weight control and reducing blood sugars in persons with diabetes. It is important to realize that fat in our diet is not necessarily bad; one should try to restrict saturated fat, but not mono- or polyunsaturated fats.

Choosing a diet should be based on one's specific medical needs, tolerability, and the ability to remain compliant with the eating plan through a variety of real-life situations. There is no shortage of diets from which to choose. Clinical trials are often difficult to analyze, as many of them depend on patients accurately reporting their intake. The DASH diet (Dietary Approaches to Stop Hypertension), Mediterranean diet, Atkins diet, Sugar Busters diet, Ornish diet, Weight Watchers, Vegan lifestyle, and Nutrisystem eating plans are among the most popular. Most diets will cause weight loss if they are followed because they help adults reduce daily caloric intake. The dieting plan needs to be flexible to allow commonly encountered situations, such as dining out. Some plans may become too expensive if one needs to purchase food from the plan.

Vegan and Mediterranean diets are known to lower inflammation of heart arteries, which helps reduce the risk of atherosclerosis (hardening of the arteries). Vegan diets have no animal nutrition sources. The Mediterranean diet has mostly fish, fowl (such as chicken), and small amounts of red meat as primary protein sources. Both diets are rich in vegetables. Both diets use mostly olive oil as the fat source and are rich in fruits, vegetables, nuts, and whole grains.

For people who need to lose weight and have cardiovascular disease, a low simple carbohydrate version of the Mediterranean diet is a great combination. Low carbohydrate diets may also help diabetic patients control their blood sugars, which may result in the ability to lower the doses and number of their medications. Simple carbohydrates are easily digested and absorbed in the intestinal tract and lead to a rapid increase in blood glucose levels; examples include cookies, corn syrup, fruit juice, sugar-sweetened beverages, sugary cereals, and candy.

Some specific foods and supplements seem to be beneficial in reducing inflammation, such as curcumin (an element found in turmeric), spirulina, ginger, and green tea. However, consumption of these foods has not been shown to reduce cardiovascular disease. Caution is advised before loading up on vitamins and herbs, since the best way to take them, or even the quantity, may not be standardized; it is much better to simply increase one's consumption of fruits and vegetables. There are also possible adverse interactions with some prescription medications, and impurities in the preparation of some supplements can be harmful.

Red yeast rice supplements may interact with certain prescription drugs, causing them to have worse side effects or be less effective. If you are taking a medication to thin your blood, such as warfarin (Coumadin), intermittently eating large amounts of leafy green vegetables can cause interactions with your meds too; regular consumption of green vegetables does not affect the use of warfarin and is strongly preferred.

Exercise

If exercise were a drug, everyone would want to take it. Exercise increases a sense of well-being, helps with weight management, decreases inflammation, improves physical conditioning, improves sleep, and reduces stress. Speak with your healthcare provider about specific recommendations for exercise in your specific situation. There are monitored cardiac rehab programs that may be covered by medical insurance in some circumstances.

Aerobic exercise such as taking a brisk walk, jogging on a treadmill, riding a bike, using an elliptical machine, and rowing for only 30 min per day, five or more days per week, is all that it takes. Using light weights in addition to aerobic exercise is ideal. Weights and aerobic exercise can be used on alternate days. It is better to do indoor exercise in your home, if possible, to avoid interruption and falling out of a routine due to bad weather or not being able to get to a gym. *I recommend that the intensity of the exercise program be gradually increased to improve physical conditioning.* Often with exercise programs, people notice they no longer get short of breath going upstairs and that other chores seem easier.

Information about specific exercise plans and other details is beyond the scope of this book. One recommended source for additional information, including step-by-step instructions for different types of exercises as well as all kinds of tips, visit the website of the American Heart Association. (https://www.heart.org/en/healthy-living/fitness/fitness-basics/aha-recs-for-physical-activity-in-adults).   Another option is a new book by Johns Hopkins University Press on healthful eating and activity; the book by Drs. Cheskin and Gudzune is called "Weight Loss for Life" and covers various diets, activities, and healthy behaviors.

Emotional Stress

Emotional stress is an underrecognized and undertreated source of inflammation in our bodies. Several studies relate levels of stress hormones to inflammation and heart disease. Emotional stress can cause the release of hormones and chemicals that are designed to make our bodies ready to run or protect ourselves from danger. You may remember learning about the "fight or flight" reaction that helps us escape from or confront dangerous situations. Important hormones are released into our bloodstream during this process, including cortisol, adrenaline (epinephrine), and noradrenaline (norepinephrine). These substances are good things to have when our lives are threatened or when we need to react quickly. When these hormones enter our bloodstream, they cause our heart rates to increase, pupils to dilate, and vision to sharpen. Additionally, glucose becomes more available, and the blood vessels to your muscles dilate to help you run faster and increase your strength.

Your adrenal glands, where these hormones are stored, release these substances when you are threatened by illness as well as emotional stress. You can release stress hormones in response to almost anything if you do not control your reactions to stressful situations. A common example is road rage, where a minor situation provokes a perceived life-and-death battle, with an immense release of these stress hormones.

Each of us needs to control our reactions to stressful circumstances and lower our levels of stress hormones. By reducing our reactions to our triggers, we can decrease the damage to our hearts and blood vessels. The release of stress hormones can be so intense that it rarely can cause the heart muscle to weaken. A weakened heart muscle is referred to as a cardiomyopathy. A stress cardiomyopathy where the heart function is low can be dangerous. Sometimes, this condition can completely reverse when the severe stress passes.

So, what can you do, in addition to eating healthy, being active, and making sure to see a doctor and dentist? You should make an effort to limit stress in your life (as much as possible) and to react to it in better ways. One proven technique to help you deal with stress is called mindfulness. According to the American Psychological Association (APA.org, 2012), mindfulness is:

> …a moment-to-moment awareness of one's experience without judgment. In this sense, mindfulness is a state and not a trait. While it might be promoted by certain practices or activities, such as meditation, it is not equivalent to or synonymous with them.

Incorporating mindfulness into your life can help reduce your brain's reaction to stress, amplify your focus, and improve your problem-solving skills. There are ways that you can lower your heart rate and improve your tolerance to temperatures and physical discomfort.

You can train your brain to allow yourself to change your mental and chemical reactions to different stresses. *Meditation is one mindfulness technique that has been used successfully to help reduce stress and even treat diseases with mental imagery.* There are several different techniques for meditation, though common to each is achieving a very relaxed feeling during which we make ourselves more responsive to suggestions. With meditation, suggestions are coming from within. *For some, guided meditation, counseling, or cognitive behavioral therapy (CBT) may be more effective.* In all three of these processes, there is another person who is trained in these techniques to help you to be able to receive the suggestions.

Another general tip to lower your stress levels is to attempt to see things from another viewpoint, even if you may not agree with it. Heated arguments can be a source of frustration and lead to bad feelings. It is important to keep perspective and remember that so many things that can upset you are not worth the stress that they cause. There are lots of free resources for you to learn more about mindfulness and stress relief, including the National Alliance on Mental Illness (nami.org) and the American Psychological Association (apa.org). For more on mindfulness, see Chap. 43.

Commentary from Dr. Todd Cohen

One trick that I tell my patients is to use controlled breathing to help control their emotions in stressful situations. By using a technique known as square or box breathing technique for as little as three minutes, my patients have been effective in controlling their stress. This involves taking a long slow deep breath in through your nose over four seconds, holding your breath for four seconds, followed by a long slow exhalation over four seconds, and then holding your breath for four seconds. This is repeated over a three-minute interval and will help you gain control of a perceived out-of-control situation. It is important to deal effectively with stress, to prevent rage, control your behavior, and control the effect of stress hormones on your body.

Increased anxiety and stress have also been shown to increase the risk of heart attack and illness in general. Both conditions can be helped with the same techniques that are used to reduce stress, although, at times, medications may also be necessary. Similarly, depression may contribute to heart disease, and when treated, *there is even an improvement in survival.*

In general, there are a number of things that can be done to complement what healthcare providers and medicines offer. Lifestyle modification is a very powerful but often glossed-over part of a treatment plan. Taking medication should be used in combination with a healthy lifestyle and not used as a substitute for lifestyle modification. Whether the objective is to decrease the chance of developing vascular disease or prevent a heart attack or stroke, lifestyle modification is a key component to achieving this goal. Table 5.1 summarizes some key points to focus on with regard to lifestyle modifications. The best approach is a combination of optimal medical therapy and lifestyle modification to improve overall health and to both survive and thrive with heart disease. For more information on lifestyle modifications, please see Part VI of this book.

Table 5.1 Cornerstones of lifestyle modifications

Eat right by avoiding processed foods, red meats, and those high in saturated fats, sugars, salts, and additives.

Maintain a healthy weight (or body mass index, also called BMI); keep your level of belly (abdominal) fat in check. Fat in this part of your body is associated with poorer health outcomes.

Be active; just 30 min of some activity five days a week is all it takes.

Try methods such as Yoga and meditation to reduce stress.

Remember: It's not always what you're eating, but what is eating you.

Learn square breathing.

Part II

Heart Rhythm Problems

This book divides the understanding of heart problems into two areas. In Part II, we discuss heart rhythm problems, and then in Part III, we discuss heart muscle problems. Heart rhythm problems (also called arrhythmias) are common—you could say they are a part of life. This book will help you understand them as well as their severity. Symptoms of fatigue, shortness of breath, lightheadedness and dizziness, and loss of consciousness (syncope) should prompt you to seek medical assistance.

Slow and Fast Rhythms

6

Todd J. Cohen

Slow Rhythms (Bradycardias)

Any abnormality in heart rate and rhythm—whether it is too fast, too slow, "skips" a beat, races, or is irregular—is considered an arrhythmia. There are many different kinds of arrhythmias. A heart rate of fewer than 60 beats per minute may be called a slow rhythm, or bradycardia (*brady* means "slow"). A delay of more than 3 s from one heartbeat to another is called a pause. Such a rhythm may not be clinically significant unless the person is experiencing symptoms such as fatigue, shortness of breath, light-headedness, dizziness, or loss of consciousness (also called *syncope*).

Causes of Bradycardia

Slow rhythms are sometimes caused by medications. For example, beta blockers, calcium channel blockers, and digitalis might slow down the heart rate and cause bradycardia (Table 6.1). Some antiarrhythmic drugs, such as sotalol and amiodarone, which have properties similar to beta blockers and calcium channel blockers, can also cause bradycardia.

These slow rhythms may also be caused by an underactive thyroid gland (hypothyroidism) or an infection such as Lyme disease. They may also be caused by intrinsic disease of the heart's conduction system, caused by lack of blood flow, long-standing hypertension, scarring, calcification, fibrosis, or some other condition. Bradycardia caused by hypothyroidism and Lyme disease may be treated with

T. J. Cohen (✉)
NYIT College of Osteopathic Medicine, New York, NY, USA
e-mail: tcohen03@nyit.edu

© The Author(s), under exclusive license to Springer Nature Switzerland AG 2025
T. J. Cohen, R. S. Blumenthal (eds.), *Surviving and Thriving With Heart Disease*,
Contemporary Cardiology, https://doi.org/10.1007/978-3-032-00579-3_6

29

Table 6.1 Medications that may cause bradycardia

Beta-blockers
Calcium channel blockers
Digitalis
Antiarrhythmic drugs[1]

[1]E.g. antiarrhythmic drugs sotalol has beta-blocker properties and amiodarone has both betablocker and calcium channel blocker properties.

Table 6.2 Reversible causes of bradycardia

Nonessential medications
Lyme disease
Hypothyroidism
Electrolyte abnormality
Drug toxicity

Table 6.3 Common types of slow heart rhythms

Sinus bradycardia
Second-degree heart block, Mobitz type I (block typically occurs in the AV node)
Second-degree heart block, Mobitz type II (block typically occurs in the His bundle or below)
Third-degree heart block or complete heart block
Asystole

Table 6.4 Symptoms of slow and fast heart rhythm problems

Tiredness and fatigue
Shortness of breath
Palpitations (more for fast heart rhythm problems)
Lightheadedness and dizziness; loss of consciousness (syncope)

medications that address the underlying condition (thyroid hormone replacement for hypothyroidism and antibiotics for Lyme disease). Occasionally, the person's heart needs to be supplemented with temporary artificial pacing (stimulation) until the medications adequately treat the underlying problem.

Some causes of bradycardia are reversible (see Table 6.2). Examples include drug toxicity and electrolyte abnormalities. Correcting drug toxicity and electrolyte abnormalities can restore a more normal rhythm. For common types of slow heart rhythms, see Table 6.3. Table 6.4 shows common symptoms of slow heart rhythm problems (as well as fast heart rhythm problems).

Common Bradycardic Rhythms

One of the most common slow rhythms is sinus bradycardia, in which the SA node is sluggish in initiating electrical impulses to the heart. Second-degree heart block means that some of the impulses from the atria do not arrive at the ventricles. In Mobitz type I second-degree AV block, there is a progressive delay in the AV node, and the doctor can recognize a clear pattern of grouped beating on an electrical recording of the heart rhythm called an electrocardiogram (ECG or EKG; see Chap. 16). This condition may not be significant, especially if the patient has no symptoms.

In Mobitz type II second-degree heart block, the loss of conduction of an atrial beat to the ventricle occurs suddenly, without any ECG pattern of delay (again, however, the doctor can recognize it). In third-degree heart block, also called *complete heart block*, none of the impulses from the atria conduct to the ventricles. Conduction disease in Mobitz type II second-degree heart block and third-degree heart block are usually at the level of the His bundle or lower. These represent much more serious conditions than a Mobitz type I second-degree AV block, and will usually require treatment (see below). Finally, no heart contraction at all for a prolonged period is called *asystole,* regardless of what is causing it.

Diagnosing and Treating Bradycardia

The ECG is a simple, noninvasive test used to record and identify various heart rhythm abnormalities (see Chap. 16). The ECG tracing shown in Fig. 6.1 is of a normal heart rhythm, also known as *normal sinus rhythm*. Normal sinus rhythm begins in the sinus, or SA node, in the right atrium and has a heart rate between 60 and 100 beats per minute. Figure 6.2 shows sinus bradycardia, in which the heart

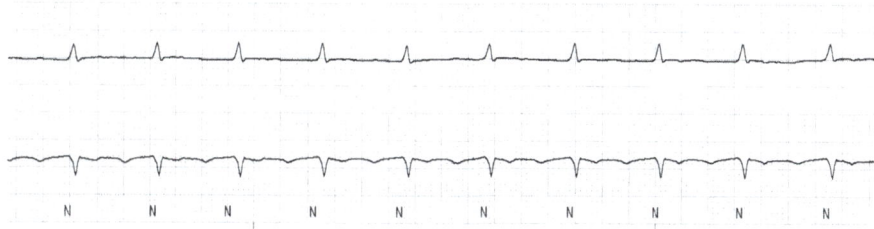

Fig. 6.1 An electrical recording of the heart is called an electrocardiogram (ECG or EKG; see Chap. 16 for more information). This ECG tracing shows a normal heart rhythm, also called normal sinus rhythm. The heart rate for normal sinus rhythm is between 60 and 100 beats per minute. (Adapted from T.J. Cohen, *A Patient's Guide to Heart Rhythm Problems* (Baltimore, MD: The Johns Hopkins University Press, 2010), p. 25)

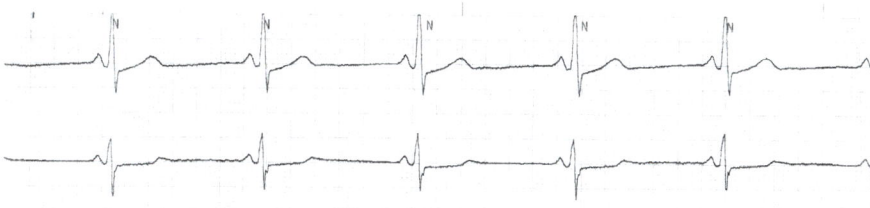

Fig. 6.2 An ECG tracing demonstrating sinus bradycardia (slow heart rhythm) in which the heart is beating at approximately 46 beats per minute (normal is 60–100 beats per minute). (Adapted from T.J. Cohen, *A Patient's Guide to Heart Rhythm Problems* (Baltimore, MD: The Johns Hopkins University Press, 2010), p. 26)

rate is 46 beats per minute. This may be a normal phenomenon based on one's overall health, an effect of medications, or what is known as vagal tone (as occurs during sleep). This is not a profound slow heart rhythm and, if there are no symptoms, may require no treatment.

Significant bradycardia due to intrinsic conduction disease or essential medications, in which the heart rate is lower than 40 beats per minute or pauses are greater than 3 s, may require implantation of a permanent pacemaker if you have significant symptoms such as tiredness and fatigue, shortness of breath, lightheadedness and dizziness, or loss of consciousness (see Table 6.4). Bradycardia occurring as the result of high-grade heart block (Mobitz type II second-degree AV block or third-degree AV block) may also require treatment with a permanent pacemaker, especially if irreversible and symptomatic. If asystole is not due to a reversible cause, a permanent pacemaker will likely be required. If you have a slow rhythm and your doctor does not suggest that you get a pacemaker, ask your doctor whether you need one and find out why or why not. By doing so, you are communicating about a treatment that you may need now, later, or never.

Fast Rhythms (Tachycardias)

If you take your pulse while exercising, you will find that your heart rate is higher than it is at rest. If you take your pulse a few minutes after exercising, you will find that your heart rate has returned to a normal rate (though it might stay elevated for a while after exertion). At rest (when you are resting or being still), your heart rate should be no greater than 100 beats per minute; while exercising, your heart rate may increase well above 100 beats per minute. In normal rhythm, impulses originate in the SA node, which is located in the top part of the right atrial chamber. When the SA node fires at rates greater than 100 beats per minute, this is known as *tachycardia* (*tachy* means "fast"). An increase in heart rate during exertion is a normal response and is called *appropriate sinus tachycardia*. There are target heart rates based on age, which also provide a guide for how hard you should exercise. These are discussed in Appendix K.

Signs and symptoms of fast heart rhythms are similar to those of slow heart rhythms and include fatigue, lightheadedness, dizziness, shortness of breath, and loss of consciousness (syncope). Palpitations (the sensation of the heart beating heavy, fast, or irregular) are much more common with fast heart rhythm problems. The overlap in the symptoms of slow and fast heart rhythm problems occurs because both conditions can cause hypoperfusion (lack of oxygen delivery) to the brain, heart, and other organs (see Table 6.4). An abnormally fast rhythm can lead to a life-threatening situation. If you experience any of these symptoms, *contact your doctor immediately or call 911.*

Table 6.5 Common types of fast heart rhythms

Sinus tachycardia (often benign)
Atrial fibrillation
Atrial flutter
Atrial tachycardia
Paroxysmal supraventricular tachycardia (PSVT)
Ventricular tachycardia
Ventricular fibrillation

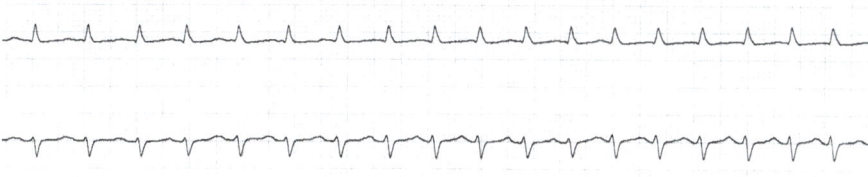

Fig. 6.3 An ECG tracing of an abnormal heart rhythm called supraventricular tachycardia, when the heart is beating at greater than 100 beats per minute. This patient's heart is beating regularly at 188 beats per minute. The precise type of supraventricular tachycardia may be difficult to discern with only one or two ECG leads. (Adapted from T.J. Cohen, *A Patient's Guide to Heart Rhythm Problems* (Baltimore, MD: The Johns Hopkins University Press, 2010), p. 26)

Common Tachycardic Rhythms

Some common types of fast heart rhythms are listed in Table 6.5. The first five tachycardias on the list are *supraventricular* in location (occurring above the ventricles). Sinus tachycardia, probably the most common problem, originates in the SA node, is often benign and does not require treatment. Rarely, this condition is considered *inappropriate sinus tachycardia*, especially when it is not due to a physiological condition or situation (such as an infection, low blood count, or anemia).

Some fast heart rhythms may originate above the ventricles (supraventricular tachycardia). Supraventricular arrhythmias include premature atrial complexes (PACs; early atrial beats), atrial fibrillation (a common rapid, chaotic atrial rhythm), atrial flutter (a more organized, rapid atrial rhythm), atrial tachycardia (a rapid atrial rhythm coming from a point source in the atrium), and paroxysmal supraventricular tachycardia (PSVT; a rapid rhythm that typically involves extra connection(s) between the atria(s) and the ventricle(s). An ECG strip of supraventricular tachycardia is shown in Fig. 6.3. The specific type of supraventricular tachycardia may be difficult to discern (though this could be atrial flutter, see Chap. 9) and would be better defined if a more complete twelve-lead ECG is performed.

Other arrhythmias originate in the ventricles. These include premature ventricular complexes (PVCs; early beats from the ventricles), ventricular tachycardia, and/or ventricular fibrillation. The latter two may be associated with sudden cardiac arrest and death. For more details on supraventricular tachycardias and ventricular tachycardias see Chaps. 8 and 7, respectively.

Ventricular Tachycardia, Ventricular Fibrillation, and Sudden Cardiac Arrest

Todd J. Cohen

Death from sudden cardiac arrest is usually caused by an arrhythmia. Most people who die from sudden cardiac arrest experience a fast heart rhythm from the lower chamber of the heart known as *ventricular tachycardia*. Many of them have heart disease as the result of coronary artery disease and have possibly had a previous heart attack. Others have a weakening or thickening of the heart muscle from some other cause, such as a failing heart structure (valve disease) or long-standing high blood pressure. Some people have a genetic condition (see Chap. 15) in which ventricular arrhythmias occur even though the person has a structurally normal heart.

Premature ventricular complexes (PVCs) are early beats that originate in the ventricle. They can be benign if they are infrequent and/or originate in some common areas such as the right or left ventricular outflow tracts. PVCs have characteristic ECG findings that can help distinguish whether they are benign or more serious (malignant), and are treated (1) if patients are symptomatic, (2) if they occur frequently (and make up a high percentage of heartbeats, typically a burden of greater than 10%), and/or (3) if they have specific ECG patterns that indicate they are not benign. Treatments can include medications such as beta-blockers and calcium channel blockers (see Chap. 25) and/or catheter ablation (Chap. 29).

Ventricular tachycardia and *ventricular fibrillation*, in which the lower chambers of the heart beat very rapidly, are the leading causes of sudden cardiac arrest. If a person has ventricular tachycardia or fibrillation and becomes unconscious, his or

T. J. Cohen (✉)
NYIT College of Osteopathic Medicine, New York, NY, USA
e-mail: tcohen03@nyit.edu

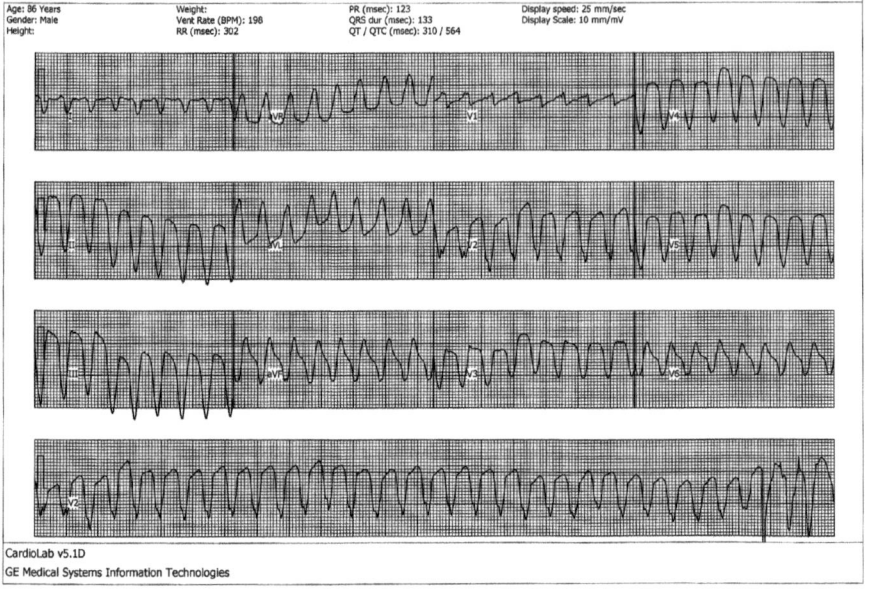

Fig. 7.1 This figure shows a characteristic 12-lead ECG from a patient who was in ventricular tachycardia. This is a rapid wide complex rhythm that originates in the left ventricle (Reproduced with permission from HMP Communications LLC from Practical Electrophysiology, Third Edition)

her condition should be treated very quickly by defibrillation. People who are at continued risk for this condition should be considered for an implantable defibrillator. Sometimes medications and catheter ablation can help treat this condition as well.

Ventricular tachycardia is a rapid rhythm from the lower chamber of the heart (see Fig. 7.1). This figure shows a 12-lead ECG with a fast or rapid wide complex rhythm arising from the ventricle. Wide complex refers to the width of the ventricular complexes on the ECG. A wide complex rhythm may indicate ventricular origin; however, supraventricular rhythms with a conduction delay may also show this abnormality. Figure 7.2 shows an illustration of ventricular tachycardia, which typically originates in the left ventricle and less frequently in the right ventricle.

When the rhythm is less organized and the lower chamber of the heart is quivering instead of contracting and pumping, the rhythm is termed *ventricular fibrillation*. The most effective way to treat this abnormal rhythm is with a defibrillator. This device delivers a shock to the patient to break the ventricular tachycardia or

Fig. 7.2 Ventricular tachycardia, originating from the lower chamber of the heart (the ventricle). The arrows demonstrate the starting point of this rapid rhythm (in this figure, the ventricular tachycardia originates in the left ventricle). LA, left atrium; LV, left ventricle; RA, right atrium; RV, right ventricle

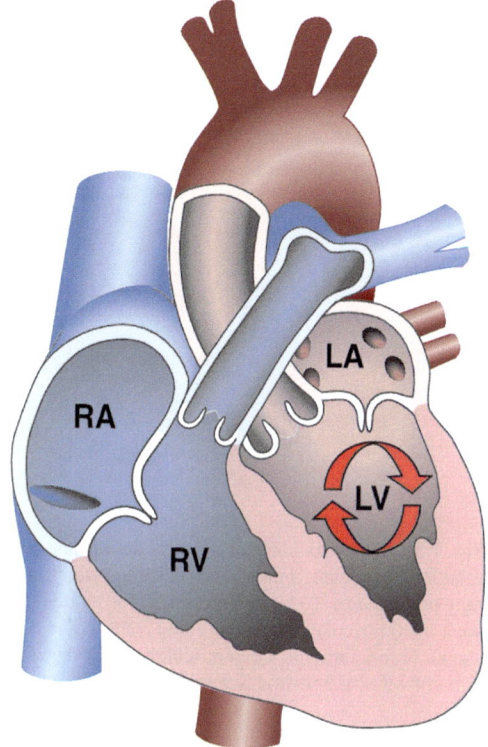

fibrillation and restore a normal heart rhythm. An external version of the defibrillator is commonly seen on TV and in movies, in which paddles are placed on the chest and a shock is delivered to stop the arrhythmia and restore a more normal rhythm. The version that you may see in airports, schools, churches, and stadiums is called an *automatic external defibrillator* or *AED*. It is an important first line of treatment for those who experience sudden cardiac arrest and is used by paramedics and emergency medical technicians (EMTs).

An internal version called an *implantable cardioverter defibrillator* (ICD) can perform the same task and improve survival in high-risk patients. An ICD generator is shown in Fig. 7.3. This device is connected to wires (or leads) and inserted in a vein into the heart. The version shown is called a biventricular defibrillator and is intended to provide cardiac resynchronization therapy to treat heart failure. The wires are typically placed in the right atrium and right ventricle and through the coronary sinus vein to the left ventricle.

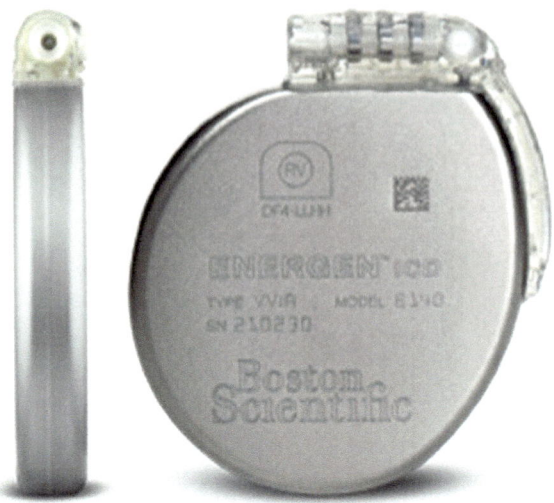

Fig. 7.3 An implantable cardioverter defibrillator (ICD) pulse generator. This device is connected to at least one wire, which is typically inserted through a blood vessel into the heart. Your doctor may prescribe an ICD if you are at risk for sudden cardiac death. It helps to treat lethal arrhythmias such as ventricular tachycardia and ventricular fibrillation. Note that the specific type of ICD shown in this figure is a biventricular device (see Chap. 31). (Image provided courtesy of Boston Scientific. ©2020 Boston Scientific Corporation or its affiliates. All rights reserved)

Sudden Cardiac Arrest

Sudden cardiac arrest is a condition in which a patient collapses suddenly due to a heart rhythm abnormality. In the United States, sudden cardiac arrest takes a life every 2 min—nearly 1000 individuals each day. Unfortunately, this all-too-common problem may account for more deaths than cancer and acquired immunodeficiency syndrome (AIDS) combined.

Heart rhythm problems that may cause sudden cardiac arrest are listed in Table 7.1. The event is most often associated with rapid rhythms from the lower chamber, called ventricular tachycardia or ventricular fibrillation. The heart rhythm problems that cause sudden cardiac arrest most often affect people who have heart disease (an abnormal heart) caused by a heart attack, blockages of the coronary arteries, a weak heart muscle, thick heart muscles, or other problems.

The best initial treatment for sudden cardiac arrest from ventricular tachycardia or ventricular fibrillation is rapid defibrillation (electrical shock therapy). Defibrillation is a procedure in which electrical energy (direct current energy) is delivered to terminate the tachycardia or fibrillation and restore a normal rhythm. Defibrillation is often applied in the field by paramedics, emergency medical technicians, and lay personnel using a device called an automatic external defibrillator (AED). When the cause of ventricular tachycardia or fibrillation cannot be

Table 7.1 Heart rhythm causes of sudden cardiac arrest

Ventricular tachycardia
Ventricular fibrillation
Supraventricular tachycardia (rarely)
Complete or high-grade heart block
Asystole
Slow heart rhythms (bradycardias, rarely)

Table 7.2 Reversible causes of sudden cardiac arrest

Cause	Treatment
Drug toxicity[a]	Remove toxic drug
Electrolyte abnormalities[b]	Correct electrolyte abnormality
Blocked coronary artery	Remove blockage (stent) or bypass blockage (surgery)

Note: These conditions don't necessarily require an ICD
[a]Common drugs that can cause cardiac arrest include some commonly prescribed medications, including some antidepressants and neuroleptics, along with other illicit drugs
[b]Common electrolyte abnormalities that can cause cardiac arrest include low potassium, calcium, and/or magnesium

permanently reversed, an implantable cardioverter defibrillator (ICD) may be the best treatment (see Chap. 6). Catheter ablation and medications may also serve an important role in the treatment of this life-threatening arrhythmia.

Sudden cardiac arrest can also be caused (though less often) by supraventricular tachycardia (rhythm problems from the upper chambers of the heart) and slow heart rhythms (bradycardias), as a result of either a severe blockage in the electrical wiring system between the upper and lower heart chambers or the cessation of electrical impulses altogether (a condition called asystole). These two types of bradycardias are typically treated with an implantable device called a *permanent pacemaker*, which delivers electrical impulses to the heart (see Chap. 30).

The reversible causes of sudden cardiac arrest are listed in Table 7.2. Reversible causes include drug toxicity, electrolyte abnormalities, or a blocked coronary artery depriving the heart of oxygen from its blood supply. These reversible causes can be treated by discontinuing the drug, restoring electrolyte balances, or opening or bypassing the blocked coronary artery. Treating these causes of sudden cardiac arrest often does not require an ICD, especially if the treatments just mentioned successfully reverse the problem.

Coronary artery disease develops as the result of a complex process involving damage to the arterial wall and then fat and calcium deposits forming plaques, a process called *atherosclerosis*. It takes many years for atherosclerosis to lead to significant plaque formation. The link between atherosclerosis and sudden cardiac arrest is described in Table 7.3. The plaques that build up can rupture within the artery, blocking the heart muscle's supply of blood and oxygen. When blood and oxygen are cut off, ventricular tachycardia or ventricular fibrillation may result. After the patient is successfully resuscitated and defibrillated, the doctor may find

Table 7.3 The link between atherosclerosis and sudden cardiac arrest

Atherosclerosis: a buildup of calcium and fatty deposits in the arterial walls following an insult to an artery.

Consequences: coronary artery disease (CAD), which may manifest itself as chest pain (angina), heart attack, arrhythmias, or sudden cardiac arrest. When blood supply to the brain and limbs is impaired, atherosclerosis can cause mini-strokes, strokes, and peripheral arterial disease.

Links to sudden cardiac arrest:

Two-thirds of Americans (approximately 2 million) have some plaque buildup (CAD) by age 35.

Each year, approximately 800,000 Americans have their first heart attack and 500,000 Americans will have a recurring attack (according to the American Heart Association).

CAD with a prior heart attack is a leading risk factor for sudden cardiac arrest.

Sudden cardiac arrest kills nearly 300,000 Americans each year.

Source: Derived from the Sudden Cardiac Arrest Association, "Fact Sheet: Atherosclerosis and SCA."

changes in the ECG suggesting that the patient has had an acute myocardial infarction or has unstable angina or acute coronary artery syndrome. A test called a *coronary angiogram* can show the location of this newly blocked coronary artery. A percutaneous coronary intervention (PCI), such as an angioplasty or stenting, may be performed to open the blockage.

An angioplasty involves placing a balloon catheter into a coronary artery to open the blood vessel. A thin wire is placed across the blockage and a balloon catheter is fed over that wire. When the balloon catheter is inflated, it can open up the occluded blood vessel. A stent (an expandable piece of metal similar to the spring inside a pen) may be inserted across the opened blockage to keep the coronary artery open. Stents may be made of bare metal or coated with drugs to prevent blood clotting (also called drug-eluting stents or DES), depending on what the physician believes is best for the patient. Coronary artery bypass surgery may be required when the coronary artery disease is extensive or too dangerous to be treated by a PCI.

Treatment following coronary artery revascularization procedures -such as stent placement or bypass surgery- includes preventive measures such as an American Heart Association diet, lifestyle changes (exercise and smoking cessation), and medications (aspirin, other antiplatelet agents, beta-blockers, statins to prevent the progression of coronary artery disease) and avoiding re-occlusion of the stent (see Chaps. 5 and 25). An ICD may be required if revascularization is not complete or if a heart attack damages a significant amount of the heart muscle (especially if this damage persists beyond 90 days). An ICD may not be required in patients who have suffered sudden cardiac arrest due to a blocked coronary artery, especially if the heart function is not impaired and the blockage is corrected.

My recommendation, however, is that the patient's household be trained in cardiopulmonary resuscitation (CPR) and consider purchasing an automatic external defibrillator (AED) in case of emergency. These devices are expensive and may not be covered by your health insurance. The American Heart Association has helpful information to review before buying a defibrillator. You may need some training (or

Table 7.4 Preventing and treating sudden cardiac arrest

Know your risk factors for heart disease. These include family history, age, high blood pressure, high cholesterol, diabetes, obesity, smoking, poor diet, and sedentary lifestyle.

Know how to treat risk factors: Take care of your health through diet, exercise, stress reduction, and medications (as prescribed by your doctor). For more information, see Chaps. 37, 38, 39, 40, and 41

Know your EF (ejection fraction). If your EF is 35% or less, ask your doctor if you can benefit from an ICD.

Know how to get help in an emergency: call 911.

Know how to perform CPR (see Chap. 47).

Know how to use an automatic external defibrillator (see Chap. 47).

at least a familiarity with the device) to understand its maintenance and charging, patch application and placement, and AED usage. In general, these devices were designed to be easily used by laypeople, with minimal training.

The limited availability of AEDs throughout the community is a problem. Outside the hospital setting, most people who experience sudden cardiac arrest will die before emergency help arrives. This situation has raised awareness in communities and has led to grassroots efforts to provide cities, suburbs, and rural areas with AEDs. Find out where in your local community AEDs are located. They are now found in many public places, such as airports, sports arenas, and community sports playing fields.

Patients who are at risk for heart disease in general are also at risk for heart rhythm problems, including ventricular tachycardia and ventricular fibrillation (and sudden cardiac arrest). There are a few things you should know if you or a loved one is at risk for sudden cardiac arrest (Table 7.4). Anyone at risk must work with his or her doctor(s) to prevent and treat risk factors. Steps include stopping smoking, treating high blood pressure, treating high cholesterol, treating diabetes, eating healthfully, losing weight, being active, controlling the amount of alcohol you drink, and limiting emotional stress. Patients and their friends and family members should learn resuscitation methods such as CPR and the proper use of an AED. In addition, people at risk for heart disease should know how and when to get help, and they or their loved ones should call 911 if they have symptoms of sudden cardiac arrest and related critical conditions.

Some early warning signs of sudden cardiac arrest, in particular, include chest pain (pressure and/or discomfort), rapid heart palpitations, significant lightheadedness or dizziness, blueness (cyanosis), sudden shortness of breath, and loss of consciousness/collapse.

It is important to understand the similarities between a heart attack and a stroke. Family history, smoking, high blood pressure, diabetes, and high cholesterol are risk factors for both conditions. When a blockage occurs in a coronary artery, the heart muscle can be injured and a heart attack may ensue. A similar process occurs with the occlusion of blood vessels that supply blood and oxygen to the brain. Early signs of stroke including slurred speech, definable weakness or paralysis, facial droop, and abrupt vision change should also prompt emergency care. Always engage emergency services and/or 911 care when sudden cardiac arrest warning signs are

Table 7.5 When to call your healthcare provider and 911

Suspect stroke, seizure, heart attack, sudden cardiac arrest, respiratory difficulty, or significant heart rhythm problem? Call 911 if you experience:
  New or different chest pain or discomfort
  Difficulty breathing
  Turning blue (cyanotic)
  Shaking and/or having a seizure
  Sudden collapse
  Lightheaded/dizzy and/or loss of consciousness (syncope)
  Sudden change in mentation, vision, slurred speech, weakness or paralysis
  Defibrillator fires (once call your doctor; twice call 911)

present, but be aware that other conditions may look similar to sudden cardiac arrest (see Table 7.5 for when to engage your healthcare provider and 911). These include suspected heart attack, stroke, seizure disorder, acute respiratory failure (from a myriad of causes including asthma, heart failure, and pulmonary embolism), and when ICD patients experience a shock. *When in doubt, call 911 early to get the help you need!*

People at risk for sudden cardiac arrest should know their ejection fraction (EF; see Chap. 4). If their EF is reduced (35% or lower), they should talk to their doctor about whether they need an ICD.

If you or a family member is at risk for sudden cardiac arrest, all family members should be trained in CPR. Read the patient's story at the end of this chapter to appreciate why learning CPR is so important. Classes are available through the American Heart Association (AHA), the American Red Cross, and many local hospitals. For more information, contact AHA toll-free at 800-242-8721 or visit www.heart.org.

Support groups have been established to provide educational and emotional support for people affected by sudden cardiac arrest (see Chap. 51). In addition, the Sudden Cardiac Arrest Association hosts a website with an extensive library of resources, including a patient discussion forum. You can contact this group at www.suddencardiacarrest.org.

Case 2: Sudden Cardiac Arrest

I was fortunate, at age 56, to be active enough to play in a 40-and-over softball league. In the 10 years that I had been playing in the league, not one single player ever sustained any on-the-field injury more serious than a pulled muscle, although that happened quite frequently.

One evening while playing at Oceanside High School, the last thing I remember is taking my position at third base in the fourth inning and talking with a friend of mine on the other team. I have since been told that I returned to the dugout, sat down, and keeled over. Fortunately, one of my friends called 911, and another friend, who had CPR training but had never had to use it on a real person, started to bang away at my chest. It turns out that they had followed the recommended guidelines by immediately calling 911 and by starting CPR. My friend who had started the CPR has since told me that he really didn't know what he was doing, but he had been taught that doing something was better than doing nothing.

The high school was conducting a review course that evening, and just as my incident occurred, the students were being let out of the school. Two of them saw what had happened and ran to their mothers, who immediately came to my rescue. One of them was a nurse, and the other was a former EMT worker. I have come to think of them as angels who were sent by God to save me. I will be forever grateful to them. The police and the emergency medical team arrived within 3 min, and they successfully defibrillated me. I had several burn marks on my skin to prove that.

The next thing I remember is being in some confined space and someone whom I had never met telling me that I was a lucky guy. I had a very hard time comprehending what was happening to me, but I knew that I was still alive. My initial thoughts were to ask the people around me to tell my wife that I was OK, and from that point on, my foremost thoughts have been for her and not for myself. I next recall being wheeled into the emergency room and seeing my wife and children and my brother and his family.

I had visited numerous friends and family members in the hospital over the years, and it was very unusual and uncomfortable to be the one in the hospital bed. I had always been the one bringing the flowers. I thought back a few years, when I had seen my father in a cardiac care unit in Florida after he had undergone a mitral valve replacement, and I recalled how sorry I had felt for him and how helpless he had looked. I felt just as helpless now. I had always been the rock of my family, their provider and protector, and here I was, the subject of their fear and concern. I had to first reassure them, and then myself, that I would be fine and that we'd get through this together.

The next few days were a blur. After meeting some wonderful nurses that night, I met my doctor, a fine, warm, and caring cardiologist who discussed my medical care with me as a new cardiac patient. I could not believe that he was actually talking to me about the necessity of undergoing a cardiac catheterization the next morning to determine the cause of my cardiac arrest. As he explained to me that he might need to place stents in me or, if my case was more serious, that I might need cardiac bypass surgery, it seemed as if he was talking about someone else. I was still having trouble believing that he was talking about me.

The procedure itself went quickly, and I remember the doctor's reassuring words. He had found two major blockages in the left anterior descending artery, which he had been able to treat with stents. I would not need bypass grafts, and I had not sustained any heart damage. He was the first of hundreds of people to tell me how lucky I was. I have since learned that a blockage in the left anterior descending artery is called "the widowmaker" and that sudden cardiac arrest victims have a 93% fatality rate. I started to struggle with the concept of why this had happened to me and why I had been saved.

The days and months following my cardiac arrest have been filled with thoughts about what happened and about what almost happened. Although I have come to understand that I would be fine physically, I initially felt older and less capable. I *began to wonder why this happened to me and not to the thousands of other people who, I suddenly noticed, were terribly overweight and were eating things that I never would have eaten even before my event. I felt as if my world had been turned upside down, and I realized that the psychological effects on me could be greater than the physical effects.*

I have come to learn much more about coronary artery disease than I ever thought I would. Before this incident, unfortunately, I took my health for granted. After working with several doctors, nurses, and nutritionists, I now understand that there are several risk factors everyone can control or modify. I also understand why most people don't pay much attention to this. They just don't give any thought to the idea that it could happen to them. Unfortunately, it took my incident for me to understand the importance of taking steps to become healthier in general.

Supraventricular Tachycardia

8

Todd J. Cohen

Many fast rhythms fall into a larger category that generally occur above the ventricles and are known as *supraventricular tachycardias*. The specific categories were introduced in Chap. 6 in the section on Fast Rhythms (Tachycardias). In that chapter, the terms premature atrial complexes, atrial fibrillation, atrial flutter, atrial tachycardias, and paroxysmal supraventricular tachycardia are introduced. This chapter gives more details on these arrhythmias that may be helpful to those who suffer from these conditions.

Premature atrial complexes (PACs) are early beats that originate in the upper chamber of the heart. They are quite common and may trigger supraventricular tachycardias. Typically, PACs are not treated unless patients are symptomatic.

Atrial fibrillation is a common type of arrhythmia (supraventricular tachycardia) in which the atria move very chaotically and rapidly. It often originates from the pulmonary veins in the left atrium but may originate in other locations and occur transiently following open heart surgery. Atrial fibrillation is often referred to as an irregular rhythm. The rhythm may be associated with an increased risk of stroke, and if the heart rate is not controlled, patients may develop a weakened heart muscle (tachycardia-induced cardiomyopathy). Medications can help reduce stroke incidence in high-risk patients (blood thinners or anticoagulants), control the heart rate (with medications such as digitalis, beta-blockers, or calcium channel blockers), and even suppress the arrhythmia altogether (see Chap. 25). The latter is not without risks, including proarrhythmia (the production of an even worse rhythm), and therefore, more definitive catheter ablation may be beneficial and often curative (see Chap. 29).

T. J. Cohen (✉)
NYIT College of Osteopathic Medicine, New York, NY, USA
e-mail: tcohen03@nyit.edu

In general, the longer a patient has been in atrial fibrillation, the harder this condition is to cure. Relatively new-onset atrial fibrillation, which comes and goes (called "paroxysmal"), is easier to cure than long-standing (chronic or persistent) atrial fibrillation, where the atrium has remodeled and fibrosed, making it harder to cure.

Atrial fibrillation can lead to clot formation in the left atrium (typically a part called the left atrial appendage), which might increase a person's risk for a stroke. Anticoagulants (blood thinners) are often prescribed for this condition, depending on the person's medical history. People with this condition who are older than 65 years and have heart failure, diabetes, hypertension, or a prior stroke may also benefit from anticoagulants. A single episode of atrial fibrillation in a patient with a structurally normal heart and no other medical abnormalities might be treated with aspirin alone.

Atrial flutter is a more regularized supraventricular tachycardia with some similarities to atrial fibrillation. Typical atrial flutter can be easily cured by catheter ablation, but atrial fibrillation requires a more invasive ablative approach. These arrhythmias may also predispose to stroke and may require blood thinners. Rate control and drug suppression are options in symptomatic patients, but ablation is often curative. Atrial fibrillation and atrial flutter are so common among rhythmic heart problems that Chap. 9 is entirely dedicated to those disorders, and Chap. 29 focuses on catheter ablation.

Atrial tachycardia is often the result of a focus, or spot, within the atrium (right or left) firing at a rapid rate (but typically slower than atrial flutter or fibrillation). Although medications may be helpful, catheter ablation can be curative. Figure 8.1 shows the mapping of atrial tachycardia in the right atrium with a non-fluoroscopic

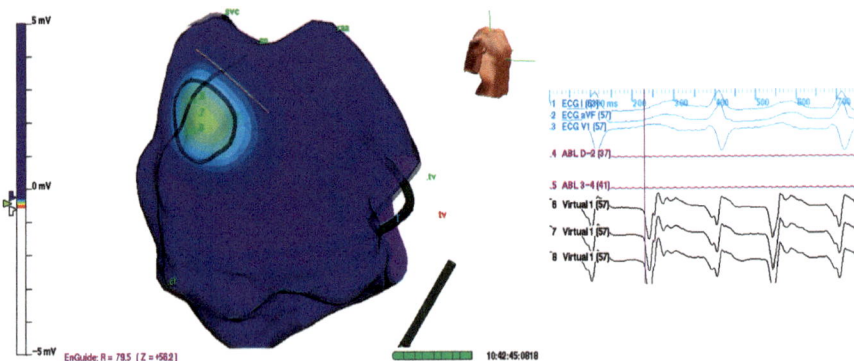

Fig. 8.1 This figure demonstrates the utility of nonfluoroscopic three-dimensional mapping in order to find the origin of an atrial tachycardia. The right atrium is purple, and the tachycardia is mapped precisely to the small green area. Catheter ablation can then be delivered to terminate and eliminate the source of this tachycardia. (Reproduced with permission from HMP Communication LLC from Practical Electrophysiology, Third Edition). In essence, the atrial tachycardia is a focus in the atrium that fires rapidly. Catheter ablation is capable of eliminating this focus and curing this tachycardia

three-dimensional mapping system that works much like GPS. Once mapped (green spot), the origin of the tachycardia can undergo catheter ablation to treat the problem.

Paroxysmal supraventricular tachycardia (PSVT) involves an extra connection between the atria(s) and the ventricle(s). When the extra connection falls within the AV node, the arrhythmia is called *AV node reentrant tachycardia*. The AV node normally has one pathway, but in this case, two pathways are present (typically a fast one and a slow one). To treat this condition, catheter ablation can be highly effective at destroying the slow pathway of the AV node and leaving a fast pathway for normal conduction.

Accessory Pathway: Wolff-Parkinson-White Syndrome

An extra connection can also be present between the atria and ventricles but outside the AV node and is called an *accessory pathway*. These pathways can be located on the right and/or left side of the heart, as well as near the middle (septum). People experiencing symptoms of a fast rhythm (see Chap. 6) who also have evidence of this pathway on their ECG have a condition known as *Wolff-Parkinson-White syndrome* (WPW). This disorder can lead to loss of consciousness and sudden cardiac arrest. Occasionally, people can have more than one accessory pathway. Right-sided pathways are easy to reach through a leg vein (typically a femoral vein). Left-sided pathways typically require a transseptal puncture procedure to place a catheter from the right atrium into the left side of the heart. Blood thinners are required during left-sided procedures to prevent clot formation on the catheters and minimize the risk of stroke during the procedure. Catheter ablation is very helpful in eliminating the extra pathway(s) and curing this disorder in a high percentage of patients.

In summary, many of these arrhythmias can be managed initially with medications; however, the majority can be cured by catheter ablation with a high success rate and low complication rate (see Chap. 29). Table 8.1 shows some key features of supraventricular tachycardias.

Table 8.1 Supraventricular tachycardia (SVT)

SVT is a fast heartbeat originating in the upper chamber of the heart.
Often diagnosed by a heart monitor or implantable device.
If symptomatic, it can be treated with medications or ablation.
AV node reentrant tachycardia (AVNRT) is a form of SVT in which there are two pathways in the AV node. This can be treated with medications, but more typically cured by catheter ablation.
Wolff Parkinson-White Syndrome is a condition in which an extra connection (accessory pathway) is present connecting the upper to lower heart chambers, bypassing the normal wiring system of the heart. It usually can be cured by catheter ablation.
Atrial fibrillation and flutter are common types of SVT, and rate control medications plus a blood thinner (anticoagulant) may reduce your risk of stroke. If symptomatic and recurrent despite medications, catheter ablation can be considered.

Atrial Fibrillation and Atrial Flutter

9

Todd J. Cohen

One of the most common abnormal heart rhythms, atrial fibrillation (commonly referred to as Afib), occurs when the upper chambers (atria) of the heart contract and relax very quickly. This common rhythm disorder occurs more often in older than younger people and may be a result of long-standing high blood pressure or other heart disease. Obesity, sleep apnea, and alcohol intake have also been associated with the development of atrial fibrillation. These risk factors can be modified, which may help reduce the frequency and severity of atrial fibrillation. The location of the atria quivering in atrial fibrillation is illustrated in Fig. 9.1. Figure 9.2 shows an electrical recording from the heart and body surface (ECG) during an electrophysiology study (Chap. 21), which shows the rapid and chaotic nature of atrial fibrillation. The problem typically originates in the left atrium.

A heart rate that is poorly controlled (too fast and irregular in cadence) may stretch or weaken the heart muscle and cause shortness of breath, fatigue, lightheadedness, and dizziness. Therefore, controlling the heart rate with medications is important. Another effect of atrial fibrillation is an increased risk of stroke or ministroke (especially in people with congestive heart failure, high blood pressure, diabetes, or advanced age).

Risk factors for atrial fibrillation are listed in Table 9.1. People who have these risk factors are more likely to develop the condition. Early treatment of atrial fibrillation and aggressive treatment of these risk factors may help to prevent atrial fibrosis (scarring), which may result in persistent atrial fibrillation.

For a summary of important facts about atrial fibrillation, see Table 9.2. In this table, "atrial fibrillation begets atrial fibrillation" means that the longer you are in

T. J. Cohen (✉)
NYIT College of Osteopathic Medicine, New York, NY, USA
e-mail: tcohen03@nyit.edu

Fig. 9.1 Atrial fibrillation is a fast rhythm that originates in the upper chambers of the heart, or atria. In many cases, atrial fibrillation may be caused by triggers that start from the pulmonary veins and then proceed into the left atrium. Catheter ablation, in which the pulmonary veins are isolated from the left atrium, can help treat some forms of atrial fibrillation. The arrows depict the fibrillation of the top chambers. LA left atrium, LV left ventricle, RA right atrium, RV right ventricle

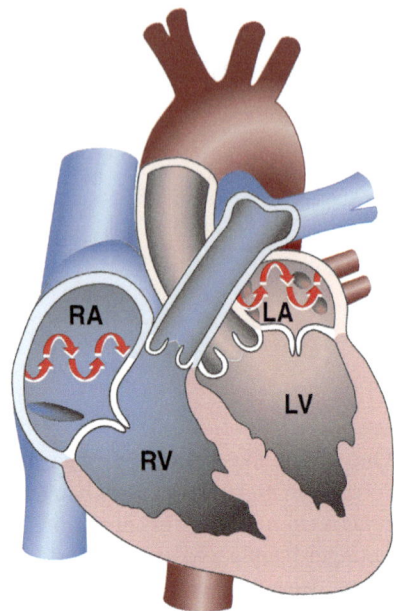

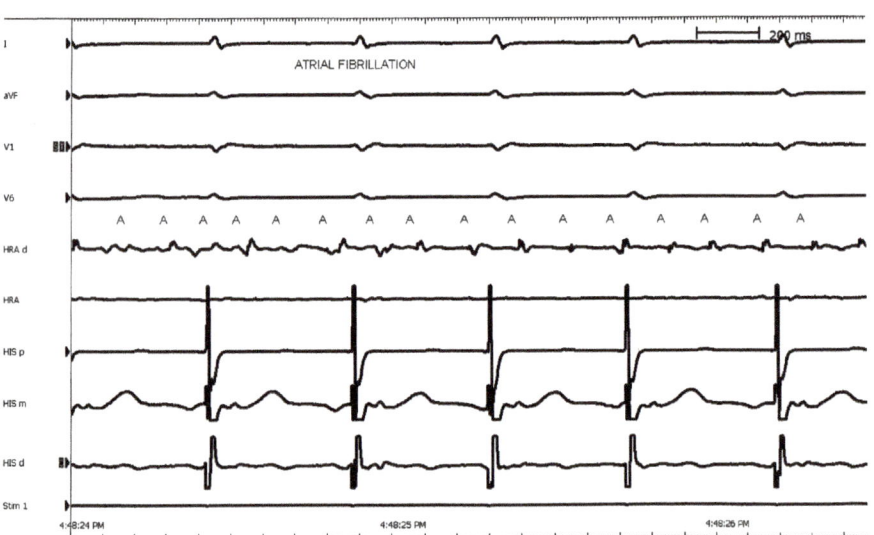

Fig. 9.2 Atrial fibrillation recorded during an electrophysiology study is present. This is a very regular and rapid arrhythmia typically originating in the left atrium. (Reproduced with permission from HMP Communications LLC from Practical Electrophysiology, Third Edition)

atrial fibrillation, the longer you are likely to stay in atrial fibrillation. Long-standing atrial fibrillation can lead to scarring of the atrial heart muscle tissue. It may be possible to prevent or slow down this scarring process with early and aggressive

Table 9.1 Risk factors for atrial fibrillation

High blood pressure (hypertension)
Diabetes
Congestive heart failure
Coronary artery disease
Myocardial infarction
Thyroid disease
Open heart surgery
Chronic obstructive lung disease
Sleep apnea
Obesity
Increased age

Table 9.2 Atrial fibrillation facts

Atrial fibrillation is a very common heart rhythm problem.
It is known as an "irregular rhythm".
The chance of developing atrial fibrillation increases with age; according to recent statistics from the American Heart Association, atrial fibrillation may be found in 3–5% of people over the age of 65 (see Table 9.1 for other atrial fibrillation risk factors).
Atrial fibrillation begets atrial fibrillation (i.e., the longer you are in atrial fibrillation, the longer you stay in atrial fibrillation).
Early treatment may help slow down the progression to persistent atrial fibrillation.
Blood thinners (anticoagulants) are recommended in patients with congestive heart failure, hypertension, age greater than 75 years, diabetes, or history of stroke.
First-line treatment is medication, including antiarrhythmic drugs.
If antiarrhythmic drug therapy fails, catheter ablation should be considered.
Inciting causes should also be treated such as excess alcohol consumption, ischemia, hypertension, stimulant use, and thyroid disorders.
Can be helpful to treat obesity and obstructive sleep apnea.

treatment of atrial fibrillation and its risk factors (as noted above, treatment may include statin therapy and possibly an ACE inhibitor).

Stroke Prevention

Blood thinners (anticoagulants) help prevent stroke, especially if the person has risk factors for stroke. The CHA2DS2-VASc score is shown in Table 9.3. The American Heart Association, the American College of Cardiology, and the Heart Rhythm Society all recommend using the CHA2S2-VASc score as a stroke risk assessment score. The CHA2DS2-VASc scoring considers everything in the simpler CHADS2 score (one point for congestive heart failure, hypertension, and diabetes and two points for stroke or mini-stroke; but instead of just giving a point for age above 65 years, CHA2DS2-VASc gives a point for age 65 to 74 years and two points for age 75 years or greater). CHA2DS2-VASc also includes an additional point for vascular disease (such as peripheral arterial disease, aortic plaque, or prior myocardial infarction) and an additional point for the female sex category (Sc). The range of this

Table 9.3 CHA2DS2-VASc score

	Points
Congestive heart failure	1
Hypertension (high blood pressure)	1
Age of 65 to 74 years	1
Age of 75 years or greater	2
Diabetes	1
Stroke or TIA (mini-stroke)	2
VAscular disease (MI, PVD, aortic plaque)	1
Sex category (women)	1

Score is 0–9: Anticoagulation recommended for men with 1 point and women with 2 points)
MI myocardial infarction, *PVD* peripheral vascular disease, *TIA* transient ischemic attack

scoring system is from 0 to 9 (with annual stroke risk increasing from 0 to about 15%).

If the CHA2DS2-VASc score is low, 0 for men and 1 for women, no anticoagulation therapy may be recommended. Anticoagulation should be considered for anyone with a score higher than those values. My recommendations are as follows: anticoagulation should be considered to reduce the risk of stroke from atrial fibrillation *in men with a score of 1 or more and in women with a score of 2 or more*. The greater the score, the greater the importance of being on anticoagulants. See Chap. 25 to learn more about anticoagulants, including coumadin (warfarin) and the newer novel oral anticoagulants (NOACs). Additionally, when patients cannot take anticoagulants, a Watchman-type procedure can be performed to occlude the left atrial appendage and minimize the risk of stroke without oral anticoagulants. To learn more about this procedure, see Chap. 32.

Lifestyle modifications and medications are typically first-line treatment for atrial fibrillation. Risk factors such as excess alcohol consumption, high blood pressure (hypertension), obesity, and sleep apnea should be addressed to minimize their role in this disorder. Other factors to consider may include thyroid or heart valve disease, use of stimulants, and myocardial ischemia (lack of blood flow to the heart). Treatment of those conditions may reduce the frequency and severity of atrial fibrillation. If you continue to experience atrial fibrillation despite lifestyle changes, heart rhythm drugs (antiarrhythmic drugs) may be used to help suppress this rhythm, along with anticoagulants if indicated. If you remain symptomatic and fail to respond to antiarrhythmic medications, your cardiologist may recommend catheter ablation (see Chap. 29). Catheter ablation may be considered as a first-line therapy for symptomatic atrial fibrillation patients who prefer not to take medications.

Atrial fibrillation ablation is an invasive procedure, which typically involves a transseptal puncture to permit catheter placement from the right side of the heart through the septum (the tissue that separates the atria) to the left side of the heart. Ablation is typically performed in the left atrium around the outside of pulmonary vein openings (the veins that attach to the left atrium) to prevent electrical triggers, which occur within the veins, from escaping into the left atrium and triggering atrial fibrillation. Once these veins are isolated, the electrical triggers within the veins are unable to travel into the atrium, and atrial fibrillation cannot occur through this route. This form of atrial fibrillation ablation is called a pulmonary vein isolation (PVI) procedure.

Typically, all four pulmonary veins are isolated as part of this procedure and can be mapped, along with the left atrium, using non-fluoroscopic three-dimensional mapping. In addition, the doctor may ablate other areas in the left atrium by creating lines or ablating areas of continuous electrical activity. Ablation may be necessary in the right atrium as well. This procedure is one of the most invasive that electrophysiologists perform. Unfortunately, more than one procedure may be necessary to completely suppress atrial fibrillation (because of either an incomplete ablation or recurrence).

The best outcomes occur in patients who have relatively normal hearts and who go in and out of atrial fibrillation on their own (called *paroxysmal atrial fibrillation*). People who are elderly or have significantly abnormal heart structures and who have been in atrial fibrillation for a long time (also called *persistent*, or *chronic*, atrial fibrillation) are less likely to be cured by an ablation than people with paroxysmal atrial fibrillation. Complications from this procedure include bleeding, blood clots, vascular damage, damage to heart structures, perforation of the heart or blood vessels, heart attack, stroke, occlusion of the pulmonary vein or veins (causing shortness of breath), development of a connection between the atrium and the esophagus, and death.

Occasionally, surgery can provide a useful adjunctive approach to treating atrial fibrillation, especially if it can be done while another heart surgery, such as mitral valve repair or replacement, is being performed. One such procedure is called the *maze procedure*, in which a "maze" is created within the left atrium to prevent the perpetuation of atrial fibrillation. Surgical procedures, even minimally invasive surgical procedures, usually have even more significant risks compared with catheter-based electrophysiology procedures such as catheter ablation.

The success rate for these procedures continues to improve as we learn more about atrial fibrillation, as newer techniques are developed, and gain additional clinical experience. Your physician should be willing to fully discuss the risks and treatment options with you. It is worth emphasizing that the use of catheter ablation should be limited to symptomatic patients who have failed to improve with or who cannot tolerate heart rhythm (antiarrhythmic) medications.

A simpler, less invasive procedure called an *AV junction ablation* (or AVJ ablation) can be performed in people whose heart rates fail to be controlled despite multiple medications (typically three or more drugs). By ablating the AV node or junction, it is possible to prevent the electrical signals from the upper chambers (atria) from conducting to the lower chambers (ventricles). After AVJ ablation, the person requires a permanent pacemaker to maintain an adequate heart rate and regularize the rhythm. This procedure is much simpler to perform than atrial fibrillation ablation and may be useful in elderly people and in those with multiple medical problems who may not be good candidates for the atrial fibrillation ablation procedure.

People who receive an AVJ ablation and pacemaker should be aware, however, that they will likely become dependent on the pacemaker to provide every beat to the heart. Further, the AVJ ablation does not cure atrial fibrillation, which means that these patients will still have to take anticoagulants. In contrast, patients may be cured by the more invasive and more complicated atrial fibrillation ablation and may be able to discontinue anticoagulants after prolonged monitoring and conclusive evidence of cure.

Atrial Flutter

Atrial flutter is similar to atrial fibrillation in that the atrium beats very rapidly. However, the atrial rhythm seen with atrial flutter usually has a more organized pattern than that of atrial fibrillation. Atrial flutter arising from the right atrium of the heart is depicted in Fig. 9.3. An ECG tracing of atrial flutter (Fig. 9.4) demonstrates jagged, or sawtooth, waves (regularized atrial activity, or P waves) between the ventricular events (QRS complexes; see Chap. 16).

The electrical waves causing atrial flutter move in a circular rhythm through a funnel-like structure called the *isthmus*. If an ablation line is created by catheter ablation across this critical area, the rhythm can easily be cured (see Chap. 29 for a thorough discussion of catheter ablation). This type of ablation is usually simpler to perform when compared to an atrial fibrillation ablation procedure. In typical atrial flutter, which occurs in the right atrium, there is usually no need to perform a more invasive transseptal puncture to get to the left side of the heart (as is true for atrial fibrillation ablation).

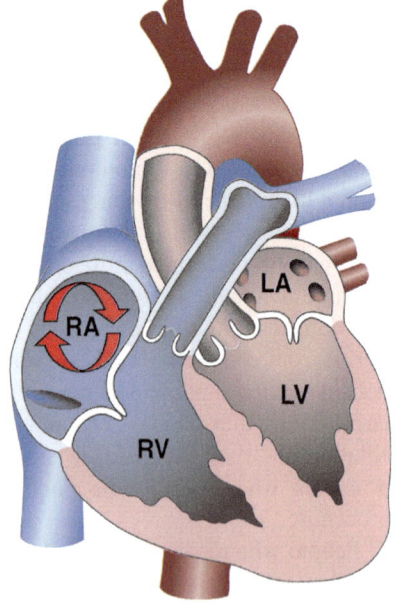

Fig. 9.3 Atrial flutter is a rapid abnormal heart rhythm that originates from the upper chambers (atria). This figure illustrates typical atrial flutter, which originates in the right atrium. The arrows depict a larger, more organized rhythm than found in atrial fibrillation (see Fig. 10.1). LA left atrium, LV left ventricle, RA right atrium, RV right ventricle

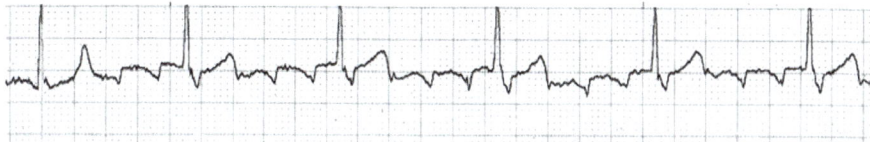

Fig. 9.4 Atrial flutter is similar to atrial fibrillation; however, the atrial rhythm is more regular and organized. This ECG strip shows rapid, regular, jagged (or sawtooth) waves coming from the atrium before each ventricular event. (Adapted from T.J. Cohen, *A Patient's Guide to Heart Rhythm Problems* (Baltimore, MD: The Johns Hopkins University Press, 2010), p. 38.)

Table 9.4   Atrial flutter facts

Atrial flutter is more organized than atrial fibrillation.
Atrial flutter should be treated like atrial fibrillation with respect to medications, including blood thinners (anticoagulants).
Atrial flutter is much easier to cure with catheter ablation than atrial fibrillation is. Catheter ablation can be considered a first-line therapy for symptomatic atrial flutter.
Catheter ablation success rates for the typical forms of atrial flutter are higher than those achieved with atrial fibrillation.

Catheter ablation of typical atrial flutter can be performed by placing a catheter across the tricuspid valve and ablating down to the inferior vena cava. The clinician's experience often dictates how long this procedure will take and how effective it will be.

Alternatively, medications can be used to treat and control this arrhythmia. People who require cardioversion (breaking of the rhythm) and people with risk factors for stroke (see CHA2DS2-VASc score above, which applies to both atrial fibrillation and flutter) may need to take anticoagulants (blood thinners). Some key facts about atrial flutter are presented in Table 9.4.

Case 3: My Afib Experience

My first experience with atrial fibrillation ("Afib") was in 2003 at the age of 60, when I woke up one morning with a strange lightheaded feeling and a racing pulse. I thought perhaps I was having a heart attack, though the symptoms were nothing like what I had experienced 5 years earlier when I had a mild MI. This was also my first-ever ambulance ride to the emergency room. At the hospital, they told me I had Afib, something that I was predisposed to, since I was over 60 with a previous heart history.

Over the years, my Afib attacks were few and far between; when I reached my early 70s, I began having attacks more frequently. Looking more closely at my Afib experience, I noticed that symptoms usually occurred when I drank alcohol, sometimes even as little as a glass or two of wine. As I looked more closely at my experiences, I noticed that when I drank alcohol, my heart rate tended to speed up. If it accelerates far enough, it often triggers an Afib episode.

Some people who have Afib are asymptomatic. That is, they don't feel it and are totally unaware they have it. My father-in-law was in Afib for the last 10 years of his life, and it didn't affect him at all. I don't like Afib. Even though in most cases symptoms only last 24 to 36 hours or so, it pretty much ruins my day. My blood pressure drops so I get dizzy and lightheaded, I get winded easily, and my normally good mood turns sour. Therefore, I do whatever I can to avoid it. In my case, this pretty much translates into staying away from alcohol, which is harder than it sounds as my wife and I have been wine enthusiasts for decades.

At one point, my doctor put me on beta-blockers (propranolol) as a possible prophylaxis. I didn't tolerate them well. They did regulate my heart rate, and I was able to drink wine with less risk, but there were other unwelcome side effects: my normally low blood pressure got even lower causing me to feel lightheaded and dizzy all day. They also caused me to feel fatigued and tired. Long-term beta-blocker use was out of the question for me.

I've always been an experimenter. I decided to try using one dose of propranolol prior to alcohol consumption (my own idea). My reasoning was that if alcohol caused my heart rate to accelerate, I could get in front of the problem by using propranolol to regulate it in advance. The strategy worked! I found that I could drink wine in moderation with much less risk of triggering an Afib episode. I don't do it often because I believe that alcohol use over time has a cumulative effect, but I can enjoy it occasionally in social situations, which is all I really want. I still have to deal with a moderate beta-blocker "hangover," but, if the wine is good enough, it's worth it.

The above patient is also a musician and has composed a song entitled "Plan B," which he plays on his guitar. The song provides an important lesson in life.

"Plan B" – written by the above patient John Seppala (you can view and listen to the song by copying the following web address into your browser and clicking play). Follow the lyrics below.

https://drive.google.com/file/d/10xmG2AQUyOf24ssvFqNFyhBk--kNpYjqQ/view?usp=sharing

When I was a young man
Full of vigor and vim
My dad said, Son, you gotta
Sink or swim

Life's gonna hand you
Some lousy breaks
The thing that's gonna get you
Through the heartaches
Is Plan B

You gotta try again
Plan B
Give it another spin
Plan B
You don't wanna give in
When Plan A fails
Don't sit in and wail
You gotta keep keepin on

Now Dad said, you don't have to take it from me
History's loaded with examples, you see
Nobody's succeeded right from the top
Everybody sometime took a great big flop

They told Colonel Sanders to take a hike
1005 times, or some such like
He went back again to another door
Now we're eating fried chicken
Forever and more

Plan B
He tried and tried again
Plan B
Gave it another spin
Plan B
He just wouldn't give in
When Plan A failed
He didn't sit in and wail
He just kept keepin on
Tom Edison tried to make a lightbulb glow
And when he failed, he didn't get low
They said, Tom, why don't you just get over
He said, version ten thousand and one might put me in Clover

Plan B
He tried and tried again
Plan B
Gave it another spin
Plan B
He just wouldn't give in
When Plan A, B, C, D, et cetera failed

He didn't sit and wail
He just kept keepin on

So that's how I roll
Through all of my life
Even though I've had my share of strife
When I get rejected or turned away
My best girl left, or my plans went astray
I went for a drive and my tires went flat
I tried to go camping and my tent collapsed
My job disappeared and I got downsized
I always was able to realize

Plan B...

Now you might have wondered
How things worked out
And I turned my plans
All inside out
Well let's just say that I'm a happy guy
Because I know there's always something to try

Plan B
Gonna try again
Plan B
Give it another spin
Plan B
I don't wanna give in
When Plan A fails
You won't hear me wail
I'll just keep on keepin on

Plan B: Commentary by Dr. Todd Cohen

The song Plan B written by my patient aptly describes the importance of being flexible. In other words, and I know that it sounds cliché, but if life throws you a lemon, you need to make lemonade. So, let's talk about flexibility. If you are rigid, and things change in your life (such as a close friend of family dies, you lose your job, or come down with heart disease), you have two choices. Either you can fight the concept, and say why me! And go into a severe depression, and flail. Or you can adapt and realize that these events are beyond your control and go on with your life by following an alternative pathway. In other words, Plan B. The ability to have a myriad of backup plans, should you lose your job, or a loved one, or even lose some faction of your health, is an important tool to continue to thrive in your new reality.

When I was asked to write about this book, I immediately thought of one of my patients who was always cheery and optimistic, even though he was constantly dealing with adversity. His ability to adapt to changes in his health, and accept these changes, and go down a Plan B, helped make him a happier and healthier person.

Plan B was also the alternative title of this book originally. Why? Because it is an important theme of life, and at the end of the day, this book gives you the tools to empower your heart health during all sorts of conditions. This includes access to your medical information. Normally, you would have access to your medical records and critical medical information using your portal through your electronic medical records. But what if you forget your password, can't get access, are traveling, or just forget? This book provides you with a bifold "Surviving and Thriving" card to let you have your critical medical information with you (the "Plan B" side of the card) as well as track your blood pressure, weight/BMI, cholesterol, and other important heart health numbers (the "Know Your Numbers" side of the card). Plan B is a critical part of your "Surviving and Thriving" card, and you can also cut out a copy of the card in Appendix J of this book and fill in your information.

You should also have a copy of your ECG attached inside your bifold card. Just put a copy of your "Surviving and Thriving" card (together with your ECG) in your wallet, purse, or glove compartment of your car. Keep a copy anywhere that you think you might need it as a backup. You can also create and print out as many copies of your "Surviving and Thriving" card by going to my practice's website, www.liheartrhythmcenter.com, and printing it out. This makes it easy to have your medical information always with you, even when there is a power outage, or you're lost and out of your home country. So, always have a Plan B, no matter what you do!

Syncope

10

Todd J. Cohen

Loss of consciousness—passing out or fainting—is called *syncope* in medical terms. Although brief periods of syncope are often dismissed or self-diagnosed as "nothing to worry about," you should be sure to report any incident to your doctor. Repeated episodes of syncope should prompt you to see your doctor. In fact, fainting is one of the most common reasons people are brought to the emergency room or admitted to the hospital.

The workup for these patients (as with any heart rhythm patient) begins with a history, a physical examination, and an ECG performed by the medical team. If the history and physical exam fail to identify any signs of a heart problem or any clinical clues that would lead to a specific diagnosis, a tilt table test may be useful (this is a noninvasive test in which the patient, on a table, is stood nearly erect and the heart rate and blood pressure are monitored; see Chap. 22). If, on the other hand, the initial workup identifies a heart rhythm-related risk factor or abnormality, the doctor will probably consider doing an electrophysiology study (an invasive test of the patient's heart rhythm and heart wiring system).

T. J. Cohen (✉)
NYIT College of Osteopathic Medicine, New York, NY, USA
e-mail: tcohen03@nyit.edu

Table 10.1 Causes of syncope

Neurocardiogenic syncope or vasovagal syncope
Dehydration
Postural orthostatic tachycardia syndrome
Valve problems (aortic stenosis or mitral stenosis)
Seizure disorder or stroke
Heart rhythm problems

Vasovagal

Common causes of syncope are listed in Table 10.1. One is a condition called *neurocardiogenic syncope* or *vasovagal syncope*, which may be triggered by standing still for a long time. Under this circumstance, the body may release a hormone called *adrenaline*, which triggers the nervous system to respond. Sometimes, this response leads to an overactivation of the vagus nerve (a nerve that originates in the brain and affects many structures, including the heart), which may cause the heart rate to slow and blood pressure to drop. The result of these physiological changes is a feeling of dizziness, and sometimes people syncopize.

Your doctor may prescribe a simple noninvasive test called a tilt table test to help determine whether vasovagal syncope is present. During this test, the patient is strapped to a mechanical table, which is utilized to bring the patient from a supine position to standing (typically at 70–80 degrees) while the blood pressure and electrocardiogram are recorded. If clinical symptoms are reproduced and/or a significant change in vital signs occurs during the test, treatment may be prescribed, which can include salting, hydration with electrolyte solutions, support stockings, medications, and/or education.

Dehydration

Another common cause of syncope is dehydration. In this case, the body is deprived of fluid and nutrients, and one can become symptomatic when changing position, such as going from lying down (supine) to sitting or standing. Typically, the blood pressure drops (hypotension), and the heart rate increases (tachycardic). The condition is a form of orthostatic intolerance (inability to tolerate standing up for a prolonged period). The treatment is often hydration with electrolyte solutions.

Postural Orthostatic Tachycardia Syndrome (POTS)

POTS is a common cause of orthostatic intolerance. People with this condition have dysfunction of the autonomic nervous system (dysautonomia) and experience palpitations when changing position (similar to dehydration). Typically upon standing, those with this condition experience a heart rate increase of at least 30 beats per minute over 10 min or a heart rate of greater than 120 beats per minute. The condition may be associated with presyncope (lightheadedness and dizziness) and syncope. POTS is frequently observed in patients with Ehlers-Danlos syndrome (see Chap. 45), and can be exacerbated by stress or infections like COVID-19. These patients, similar to those with dehydration, benefit from hydration with electrolyte solutions, along with high-compression support stockings. Additionally, medications may be needed in those who remain symptomatic despite hydration and support stockings.

Identifying Other Causes of Syncope

It is important to note that syncope may also occur, though rarely, during some other neurologic conditions such as a stroke or seizure.

Heart rhythm problems as well as heart valve disease, such as aortic or mitral stenosis, can also cause syncope. People with these cardiac causes of syncope have the worst prognosis if left untreated. When a heart rhythm problem is suspected, but not observed, extended monitoring with either an external or implantable loop recorder may be helpful. Sometimes, based on the cardiac history and/or electrocardiogram, an electrophysiology study (EP study) may help to define the heart's conduction and propensity to heart rhythm abnormalities. Importantly, once diagnosed, many heart-related causes of syncope can be effectively treated with medications, catheter ablation, heart surgery, or an implantable device (pacemaker or implantable defibrillator).

A thorough medical workup may help identify your problem and resolve the condition. If a complete workup fails to uncover the cause of syncope, then a wearable or implantable cardiac monitor may be useful in elucidating a heart rhythm problem that could be causing the syncope (Chap. 19 describes implantable and wearable cardiac monitors). An implantable cardiac monitor can help find the cause of infrequent syncope. In many people, slow heart rhythm problems (bradycardias) are uncovered, and a pacemaker is then recommended. Figure 10.1 shows a rhythm recorded from a patient with syncope of unknown cause who received an

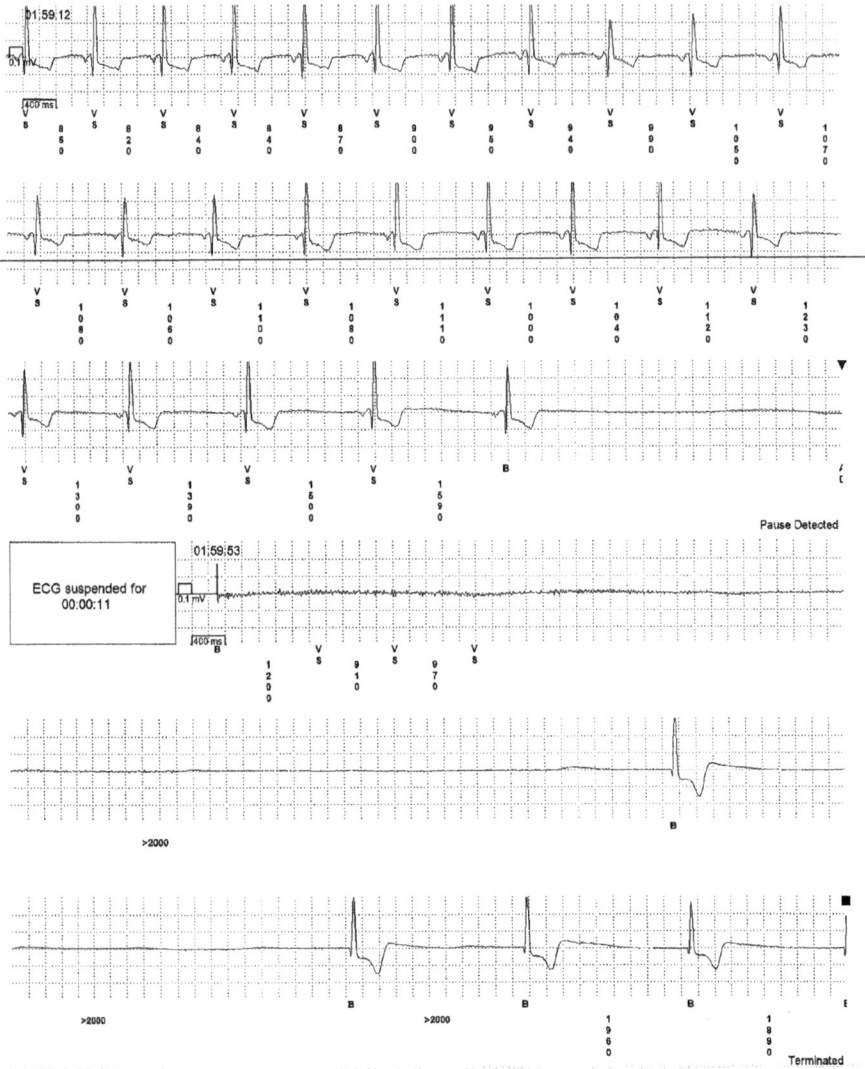

Fig. 10.1 This figure shows severe sinus arrest leading to a long pause (asystole). The pause was detected by an implantable loop recorder and almost lasted 30 seconds except for one heart-beat and the patient eventually required a permanent pacemaker. (Courtesy of HMP Communications LLC from Practical Electrophysiology, Third Edition)

Table 10.2 Syncope facts

Syncope is one of the most common reasons a person visits the emergency room.

Syncope from heart problems is often more serious (there is a higher chance of dying) than syncope from non-heart-related problems.

Heart-related syncope is often readily treatable.

A tilt table test can be used to assess syncope, especially if the history, physical exam, and ECG fail to elucidate any significant cardiac findings.

An electrophysiology study (invasive heart rhythm test) is useful, especially when heart rhythm–related abnormalities are discovered in the history, physical exam, or ECG.

External or implantable cardiac monitors are often helpful in finding a heart rhythm problem related to syncope.

Extensive neurological evaluations may not be necessary and should not be routine for each syncope episode, but they may be performed on a case-by-case basis.

implantable loop recorder. The patient had a fainting episode, and the device recorded a long pause (called asystole) in which the patient essentially went flatline for nearly 30 s. This patient required a permanent pacemaker.

For a summary of facts about syncope, see Table 10.2. The American Heart Association website has additional information. See www.heart.org.

Part III

Heart Muscle Problems

The structure and function of your heart will determine how it performs during stress (what I call the three E's: **E**xcitement, **E**motion, and **E**xertion). This section of the book will help you understand the types of problems that you can have with your heart, whether the problem is in the arteries, the valves, or the muscle itself. Heart muscle problems can lead to heart rhythm problems (and vice versa). So, Parts II and III of this book are interrelated.

Coronary Artery Blockages and Heart Attacks

11

Todd J. Cohen

Atherosclerosis is the process in which plaque builds up inside the arteries supplying the heart (coronary arteries) following an insult to the arterial walls. The plaque consists of fat, cholesterol, calcium, and other substances. Over time, the plaque can accumulate and cause the arterial wall to harden and narrow (referred to as "occlusion" or "stenosis" by your cardiologist). This buildup is typically the result of a combination of your genetics and your environment (lifestyle, diet, exercise, along with medications), but not always. It is a very common problem, and the coronary artery disease process is the number one cause of heart disease, mortality, and even sudden death in the United States. When people think or talk about heart disease, they're usually referring to coronary artery disease and not other problems that can happen, like the heart rhythm disorders we discussed in the previous section.

If you have a very strong family history (a first-degree relative: mother, father, sister, or brother with coronary artery disease), you too are at risk for this problem. You can modify your risk for coronary artery disease with lifestyle (diet and exercise) and medications. Common risk factors for coronary artery disease that lead to coronary artery blockages are listed in Table 11.1. They are family history of early heart disease, smoking history, high blood pressure, high cholesterol, diabetes, obesity, physical inactivity, diet, and age. Family history (your genetics) is a strong determinant of your baseline risk of heart disease. You can't change your genes, but if your genes predispose you to the other risk factors of coronary artery disease, you can modify those. Those other risks, such as high blood pressure, can be treated with diet, exercise, and medications. You need to be diligent to achieve an *acceptable blood pressure (preferably below 130/80 mmHg and optimally <120/80).* The latter may be hard to achieve, but it is an important target (see Chap. 38).

T. J. Cohen (✉)
NYIT College of Osteopathic Medicine, New York, NY, USA
e-mail: tcohen03@nyit.edu

Table 11.1 Risk factors for coronary artery disease and heart attacks

Family history
Smoking/alcohol
High cholesterol (high LDL; low HDL)
Diabetes
Poor diet
Obesity
Age
Physical inactivity

High cholesterol may be familial or diet/lifestyle related. *Specifically, a high LDL (greater than 100 mg/dL) and a low HDL (less than 40 mg/dL in a man and less than 50 in a woman) may place you at risk for heart disease (see Chap. 37).* A diet that is low in saturated fats is preferable to a high-saturated or trans-fat diet. The latter can still be found in certain baked goods, fried foods, and foods cooked with shortening. The American Heart Association recommends that trans-fat consumption be limited to no more than one percent of your daily caloric intake. In addition, adding salt to your foods can elevate your blood pressure and hinder achieving your target blood pressure.

More than moderate alcohol consumption (one modest drink per day) may also elevate your risks. If your blood pressure and cholesterol cannot be controlled via lifestyle modification (diet and exercise), medications are an important treatment option. If you have diabetes, diet, exercise, and medications are important elements of therapy. Modifiable risks also include obesity and smoking. It is important to work with your healthcare provider to come up with a plan to lose weight and stop smoking. Medications, such as varenicline (Chantix) or nicotine replacement, may help you quit smoking (see Chap. 40). Smoking is clearly linked with an increased risk of heart disease and heart attacks.

Most people think that a heart attack typically occurs in an artery that slowly clogs with fats from the diet. The coronary arteries typically accumulate plaque with age. A heart attack typically occurs in an artery that may not be severely blocked but rather undergoes an acute process of plaque rupture or erosion. This plaque quickly breaks open, causing an inflammatory process in which platelets accumulate and may block the entire artery (see Fig. 11.1). This prevents adequate oxygen and nutrients from getting to the heart muscle, which may initially impair heart function (called ischemia). The patient might experience symptoms, which are described in Table 11.2, but not always. These include mid-sternal chest pain or pressure that radiates to the neck and arms, although atypical symptoms such as abdominal discomfort and no pain might also occur.

The patient can feel short of breath, might start sweating profusely (diaphoretic), might feel lightheaded and dizzy, or might even collapse from a heart rhythm problem (ventricular tachycardia or fibrillation/sudden cardiac arrest; see Chap. 7). Women may occasionally report somewhat different symptoms than men, such as nausea, back and shoulder blade pain, and fatigue. It is important to call an ambulance (911) to get help as soon as possible to increase your chance of having a successful outcome. If you have an aspirin available, it is helpful to chew this as well. Some patients may have atypical or even no symptoms when they are having a heart

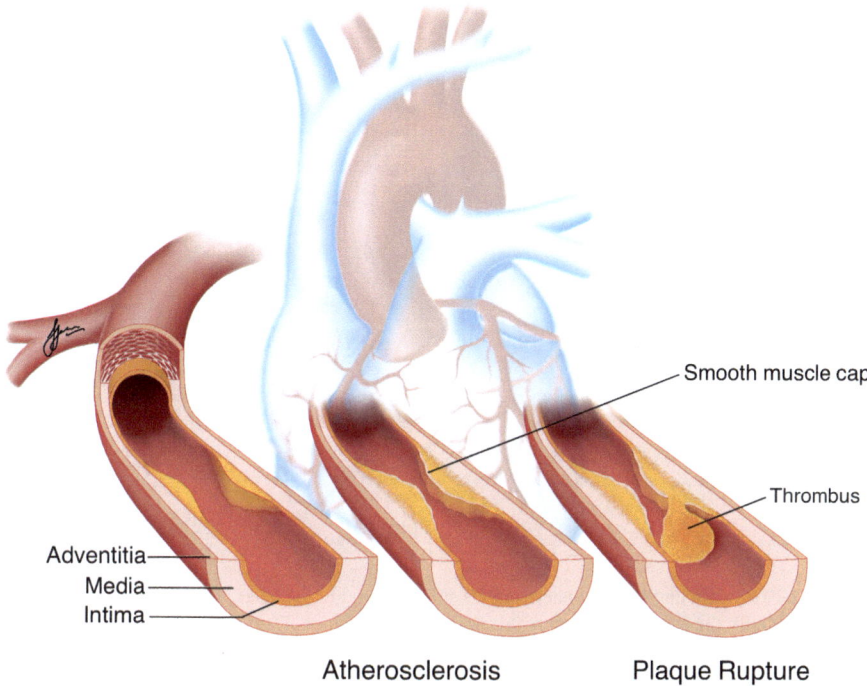

Fig. 11.1 This figure demonstrates the buildup of atherosclerosis and plaque formation that occurs with age. Risk factors and diet lead to progression of coronary artery disease. Plaque rupture and its associated inflammatory response is the trigger for a blockage in a coronary artery which causes a heart attack (also called a myocardial infarction). (Figure drawn by Jerry Jose, DO)

Table 11.2 Symptoms of a heart attack

Chest pain or discomfort; can also be in the abdomen or neck
Pain or discomfort that can radiate to the neck or arms
Pain or discomfort may be absent
Shortness of breath
Sweating
Lightheaded and dizzy; may have palpitations
Collapse/loss of consciousness
Heart attacks may sometimes have minimal or no symptoms (more common in diabetic patients and women)

attack. This is more common in both women and diabetic patients. Atypical chest pain may include abdominal pain or indigestion.

The heart is supplied oxygen and nutrients through its two coronary arteries (the right and left coronary arteries). The left coronary artery branches into the left circumflex and left anterior descending artery. When a coronary artery is blocked for a period of time, irreversible damage can occur to the heart muscle (this damage is called a heart attack or myocardial infarction [MI]). Figure 11.2 shows how a

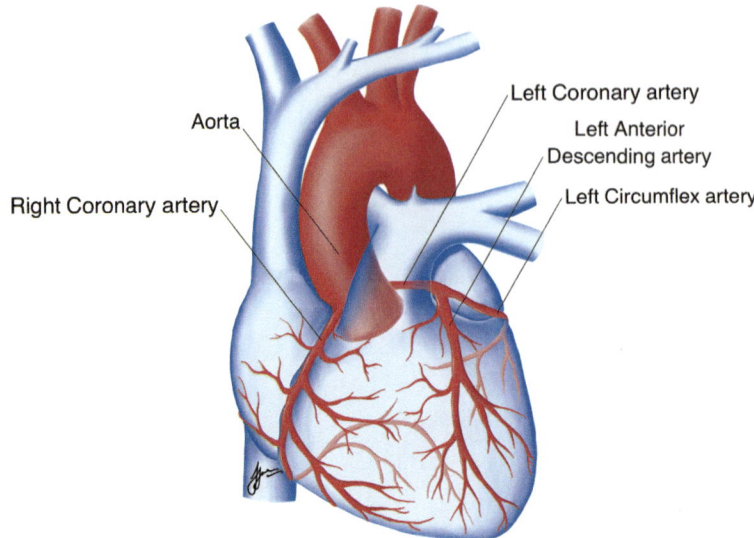

Fig. 11.2 The right and left coronary arteries supply blood to the heart. They arise from the aortic root and usually the left coronary artery is more important since it supplies the vast majority of the left ventricle (main pumping chamber of the heart). The left coronary artery begins as a left main coronary artery and branches into the left circumflex and left anterior descending coronary arteries. The latter artery typically gives off branches to the interventricular septum (called septal perforators). Severe disease in the left main coronary artery is called the widow maker, due to the large proportion of the heart that is in jeopardy, should this vessel occlude. Infarction in that area can affect the conduction of the heart and cause a heart block requiring a pacemaker. The figure demonstrates that an acute blockage in a coronary artery may result in severe damage to the heart muscle called a heart attack or myocardial infarction. (Figure drawn by Jerry Jose, DO)

coronary artery can supply a territory of heart muscle and result in a heart attack (irreversible damage to the territory of muscle downstream from the blockage). When an acute blockage occurs, time is of the essence.

The quicker you get to the hospital, the better chance that you will have for the medical team to reverse the problem either through a clot-busting medication (called thrombolytics) or through a procedure known as a PCI (percutaneous coronary intervention), in which a catheter is placed in a coronary artery and a balloon opens up the vessel and a stent is placed (see Chap. 24). Sometimes, coronary artery bypass surgery is required to effectively treat this problem (see Chap. 33).

The presence of severe coronary artery blockages (70% or more narrowing of a blood vessel's diameter, such that blood flow and oxygen delivery to the heart muscle are severely limited) and a heart attack can make you susceptible to heart rhythm problems such as atrial fibrillation, ventricular tachycardia, and ventricular fibrillation. The latter two are the common causes of sudden cardiac arrest (also called sudden death). If your heart muscle is significantly weakened after a heart attack (as indicated by testing that demonstrates an ejection fraction of 30% or less) and that persists for more than 40 days, you may qualify for an implantable defibrillator to prevent sudden death. If your heart function is better than that 3 months after a heart attack, but you are still having bouts of non-sustained ventricular tachycardia (short runs of three beats or more from the ventricle), you might require an electrophysiology study (see Chap. 21) to determine whether you are at high risk of sudden death and qualify for an implantable defibrillator. Remember to talk to (and follow up with) your cardiologist after any heart event or related procedure (such as stent placement or coronary artery bypass surgery).

Valvular Disease

12

Thomas Chengot and Matthew Tarrash

Valvular Disease

Valvular disease occurs when any valve in the heart is damaged or diseased. Valvular heart disease is a common cardiac condition, which affects about 2.5% of older adults (Table 12.1). There are four valves in the heart; this chapter will focus on the left heart valves, specifically the aortic and mitral valves (though all heart valves are important). These valves more frequently require surgical or minimally invasive therapies for repair/replacement.

Valvular heart disease falls into two basic categories: stenotic and regurgitant. A stenotic valve is unable to open easily (possibly due to calcium buildup or thickening). If the stenosis is severe enough, it's difficult for blood to flow out of the heart toward the rest of the body. A regurgitant valve is a leaky valve, because it does not close completely, so some of the blood flow is in a backward direction. Table 12.2 describes the pathology of the types of valvular diseases discussed in this chapter. Figure 12.1 offers an illustration to help differentiate between valve stenosis and regurgitation.

T. Chengot (✉)
Department of Cardiology, Amityville Heart Center, Amityville, NY, USA
e-mail: tchengot@gmail.com

M. Tarrash
Department of Anesthesiology, Hackensack University Medical Center, Hackensack, NJ, USA
e-mail: matthew.tarrash@hmhn.org

Table 12.1 Valvular disease facts

Around 2.5% of the US population has valvular heart disease and it is most common in older adults.
Aortic valvular disease in young people is most commonly caused by a birth defect where they have two cusps instead of three in the aortic valve.
The most common cause of valvular disease in the USA is valve degeneration, with rheumatic fever being more common in underdeveloped countries.
Aortic valve stenosis is the most common form of cardiovascular disease in the Western world after hypertension and coronary artery disease.

Table 12.2 Pathology of valvular disease

Diagnosis	Pathology
Aortic valve stenosis	Narrowing of the aortic valve, decreasing the amount of oxygenated blood that flows to the body
Mitral valve stenosis	Narrowing of the mitral valve, decreasing the amount of blood that fills the left ventricle
Aortic valve regurgitation	Leakage of the aortic valve, causing the backflow of blood into the left ventricle during diastole
Mitral valve regurgitation	Leakage of the mitral valve, causing the backflow of blood into the left atrium during systole

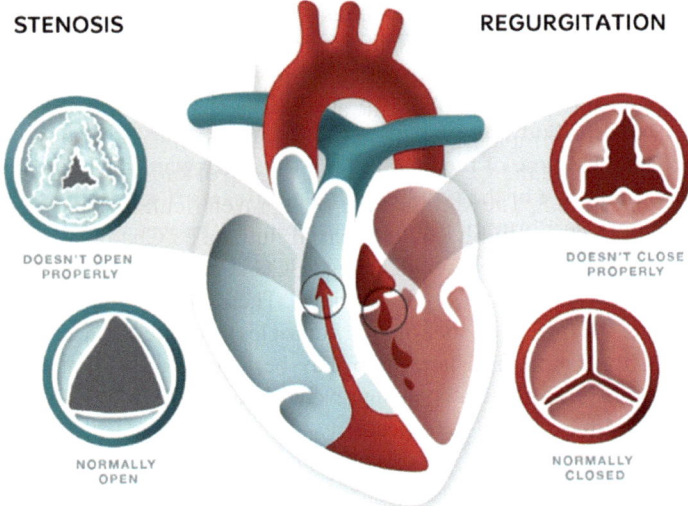

Fig. 12.1 This illustration shows an example of a three-cuspid valve (such as the aortic valve). A stenotic (or tight) valve doesn't open properly, whereas a regurgitant (or leaky) valve doesn't close properly. (This figure is reproduced with permission from The Heart Foundation, Australia)

Aortic Stenosis

Aortic stenosis ("stenosis" means narrowing) is common and more typically seen in the elderly (seventh decade or later), though it also may be congenital. The aortic valve is the gatekeeper that allows freshly oxygenated blood from the lungs to be distributed to the rest of the body. In aortic stenosis, the aortic valve has "stiffened," preventing the valve from functioning properly and preventing easy flow of blood out of the heart to the rest of the body. This stiffening can be due to thickening or fibrosis of the valve secondary to stress, rheumatic fever, or birth defects (the most common being an aortic valve with two instead of the normal three cusps, called a bicuspid aortic valve).

When the aortic valve cannot open completely, the heart works harder to pump the same amount of blood out to the body. This results in the pressure within the heart being much greater than the peripheral blood pressure. Over time, this increased pressure can lead to increased muscle thickness, known as concentric left ventricular hypertrophy (similar to what may occur from long-standing high blood pressure; see Chaps. 13 and 38).

Common symptoms of severe aortic stenosis may include chest pain (lack of blood flow into the coronary arteries), dizziness and lightheadedness, loss of consciousness (syncope), palpitations (arrhythmias such as ventricular tachycardia), and heart failure. Although rare, some patients with aortic stenosis can form an arteriovenous malformation in the intestines, which may lead to gastrointestinal bleeding.

Mitral Valve Stenosis

The mitral valve separates the left atrium (top chamber) from the left ventricle (bottom chamber). Similar to aortic valve stenosis, mitral valve stenosis occurs when the valve is stiff and does not open completely. This reduces the amount of blood that enters the left ventricle from the left atrium as the heart relaxes and increases the amount of blood remaining in the left atrium. The increase in blood volume in the left atrium leads to increased pressure. The left atrium is a relatively thin-walled structure, and, unlike the left ventricle, its response to increased pressure is dilation (expansion of the atrium) rather than thickening (hypertrophy). This expansion of the atrium can increase the risks of atrial fibrillation and atrial flutter (Chap. 9). Eventually, blood from the left atrium may back up into the lungs and cause heart failure (Chap. 14).

Aortic Valve Regurgitation

Aortic valve regurgitation occurs when the blood pumped out of the left ventricle into the aorta flows back into the left ventricle due to the incomplete closure of the valve. This means for every heartbeat, the heart must work harder to propel blood forward. This leads to an elevated pulse pressure (difference between systolic and diastolic blood pressure). Symptoms include those associated with heart failure like fatigue, shortness of breath, and an abnormal heart rhythm.

Mitral Valve Regurgitation

Mitral valve regurgitation occurs when blood leaks back into the left atrium from the left ventricle during the heart's contraction. The mitral valve is visually likened to a parachute, with the parachute-like valve being anchored to the heart via thread-like chordae tendons. When the left ventricle contracts, the parachute effect of the valve closing prevents blood flow back into the left atrium. Severe regurgitation may be acute or chronic. In the acute scenario, it may be caused by a heart attack leading to a break in the chordae tendon and resulting in a severely leaky valve (severe mitral regurgitation). In chronic situations, it may be due to the dilation (enlargement) of the left ventricle, which prevents closure of the mitral valve. Either way, the increased blood volume leads to increased pressure on the heart during contraction, which may result in fluid buildup in the lungs (heart failure). Another consequence of this increased pressure in the left atrium is an increase in the size of the left atrial chamber. Chamber dilation usually happens over time, and in the acute scenario, the atrium may not dilate. Elevated left atrial pressure and enlargement can lead to atrial fibrillation (Chap. 9).

Treatment of Valvular Diseases

Treatment of valvular disease is based on the diagnosis and the severity of associated symptoms. In many cases, valvular disease is asymptomatic and may be initially treated with medications such as ACE inhibitors. Many times, moderate valvular disease is initially detected when the physician hears a sound (murmur) when listening to the heart. Most patients develop valvular disease slowly over time; only a minority of patients develop acute symptoms. Symptoms should prompt immediate evaluation by your doctor and cardiologist and are often an indication for some form of intervention (medications, surgery, or a minimally invasive procedure; see Chap. 27).

An ECG (Chap. 18) is often the first test to confirm the presence and severity of valvular disease. It is also useful for identifying whether multiple valves may be dysfunctional and the status of the heart structures and function (such as the presence of heart muscle thickening, chamber enlargement, and the left ventricular ejection fraction).

Medications may mitigate symptoms of heart failure but typically do not cure valvular heart disease. Heart failure symptoms (shortness of breath at rest or with exertion) may be a sign that the valvular disease is severe and requires intervention. The latter can be performed by minimally invasive procedures or open heart surgery. Some of the minimally invasive approaches have been very effective for those with severe aortic stenosis and mitral regurgitation. The risk of death is typically higher for open heart surgery procedures, and the length of hospitalization and associated complications may also be higher from a surgical approach. That being said, there are situations in which a surgical approach is the best option long term. The decision to have open surgery versus a minimally invasive procedure should be discussed with your doctor, and the risks, benefits, and alternatives should be individually considered.

Heart Muscle Problems: Cardiomyopathy

13

Todd J. Cohen

The heart is composed of muscle cells. In a healthy heart, all the heart cells work together to complete their tasks, which together allow the heart to pump blood effectively throughout the body. Figure 13.1a shows a normal heart with proper-sized chambers and wall thicknesses. The healthy heart contracts and relaxes normally. When the heart is diseased, however, it cannot accomplish its tasks efficiently and so blood transport through the body is compromised.

Cardiomyopathy is a term used to describe a weak or abnormal heart muscle: *cardio* (heart), *myo* (muscle), and *pathy* (disease process) = heart muscle disease. The three main types of cardiomyopathy are *dilated*, *hypertrophic*, and *restrictive*, as shown in Fig. 13.1b–d. This chapter discusses these three types of cardiomyopathy, their causes, and possible treatments.

People with cardiomyopathies may be symptom-free or highly symptomatic or have a range of symptom severity. Symptoms differ from one person to the next. The most common are those of heart failure, including shortness of breath and leg swelling. People who have a cardiomyopathy may experience periods of dizziness or syncope (passing out). They may appear pale or experience chest pain. Many people with cardiomyopathy are at risk for abnormal heart rhythms (arrhythmias), particularly ventricular arrhythmias. Let's look at each type of cardiomyopathy.

T. J. Cohen (✉)
NYIT College of Osteopathic Medicine, New York, NY, USA
e-mail: tcohen03@nyit.edu

T. J. Cohen, R. S. Blumenthal (eds.), *Surviving and Thriving With Heart Disease*,
Contemporary Cardiology, https://doi.org/10.1007/978-3-032-00579-3_13

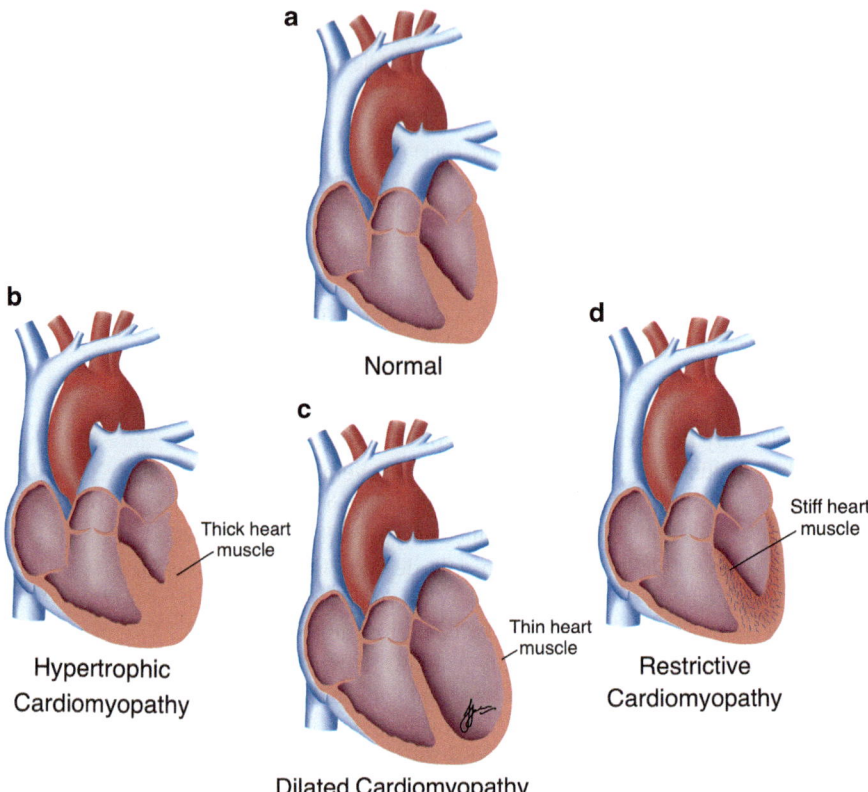

Fig. 13.1 (**a**) shows the normal heart with normal wall thickness and chamber sizes. (**b**) shows hypertrophic cardiomyopathy in which the ventricular septum and walls are markedly thickened. These patients may have obstruction to flow outside of the heart (outflow tract obstruction) and specific characteristics known as "asymmetrical septal hypertrophy (ASH) and systolic anterior motion of the mitral valve (SAM). An interventricular septum greater than or equal to 3 centimeters in thickness reports a very high risk of sudden death in these patients and is an indication for an implantable defibrillator. (**c**) shows a dilated cardiomyopathy which may be the result of long-standing hypertension, viral infection, or coronary artery disease and impaired flow to the heart muscle (ischemia) and/or damage to the heart muscle (heart attack or infarction). (**d**) shows an example of a restrictive cardiomyopathy in which substances such as iron (hemochromatosis) or an abnormal protein called amyloid (amyloidosis) can impair the stiffness of the heart and its ability to relax. In amyloidosis, the heart appears as "ground-glass" during an echocardiogram and is depicted by the crystalline structures illustrated in the drawing. (Figures drawn by Jerry Jose, DO)

Dilated Cardiomyopathy

Dilated cardiomyopathy is a common cause of heart failure. The heart muscle enlarges, and the muscle walls become thin (Fig. 13.1c). When the heart muscle enlarges and its walls get thinner, the heart has trouble contracting properly. Sometimes the heart also may have difficulty relaxing. This is because the heart muscle gets stiffer and less flexible.

There are many causes of dilated cardiomyopathy, including blood flow problems through the coronary arteries (ischemia), hypertension, heart valve problems, chemotherapy/radiation, pregnancy, genetics, and alcohol use (also known as alcohol-related dilated cardiomyopathy). Ischemia is the most common cause of dilated cardiomyopathy and is the direct result of coronary artery disease. The term *ischemia* refers to the heart being deprived of oxygen because the coronary artery circulation is impaired, which then impacts the heart's ability to contract.

Chapter 11 discusses the process of atherosclerosis (hardening of the arteries) and its link to sudden cardiac arrest. Acutely, plaque can rupture within a coronary artery, depriving a specific region of the heart of oxygen. An abrupt coronary artery blockage may cause death of heart muscle tissue (also called a heart attack or myocardial infarction [MI]). The scar from a heart attack may create other heart problems, such as ventricular tachycardia or ventricular fibrillation. Although I am discussing ischemic cardiomyopathy under the category of dilated cardiomyopathy, it is possible that the heart itself may not dilate, even though there is a focal area of scar from a prior heart attack. In many people, however, the heart muscle thins and eventually dilates.

When dilated cardiomyopathy occurs but the cause is unknown, we call that idiopathic dilated cardiomyopathy. Possible causes are an unknown genetic cause or infection. Cardiomyopathy may result from long-standing high blood pressure (hypertension). Initially, the heart muscle may thicken as a result of the high blood pressure. Years later, the heart muscle may dilate and develop into a dilated cardiomyopathy.

Disease of the heart valves (also called *valvular disease*) occurs as a result of a leaky or tight mitral or aortic valve. Both these valves are located on the left side of the heart (see Chap. 1). The mitral valve separates the left atrium (top chamber) from the left ventricle (bottom chamber), and the aortic valve is the valve that controls the outflow of oxygen-rich blood that leaves the left ventricle through the aorta and is distributed to the rest of the body. If there is backflow of blood, valvular cardiomyopathy may result. When heart valves leak, the chambers (atria and ventricles) do not empty completely, and the heart muscle may stretch and, over time, may weaken, causing those chambers to dilate. When valve disease is severe or when symptoms occur, valve repair or replacement surgery may be necessary.

Chemotherapeutic agents and radiation used in some cancer treatments may also cause dilated cardiomyopathy. Additional cardiac testing is needed in those who receive certain chemotherapeutic agents. Individuals who have an underlying cardiac disease are at greater risk for developing this type of cardiomyopathy.

Pregnant women or women who have given birth within the previous 6 months are at risk of developing what is called *peripartum dilated cardiomyopathy*. This type of heart problem is usually limited and resolves on its own. Alcohol abuse, a toxin to the heart, may cause dilated cardiomyopathy. Binge drinking can bring on heart rhythm problems (called *holiday heart*).

An inherited condition in which the right ventricle dilates as the result of fat deposited in the right ventricular muscle is called arrhythmogenic right ventricular dysplasia (see Chap. 15). The name essentially explains the condition: *arrhythmogenic*, meaning it causes heart arrhythmias, specifically ventricular; and *dysplasia*, referring to an abnormality of the right ventricular muscle. This dysplasia makes the person more likely to develop ventricular tachycardia, and an ICD may be required.

Myocarditis

Inflammatory causes and known infections can also weaken the heart muscle. This includes the coronavirus disease caused by the SARS-CoV-2 pathogen during the COVID-19 pandemic as well as a common enterovirus—coxsackieviruses. Direct inflammation of the heart muscle is called *myocarditis*. Noninfectious causes of heart inflammation include those caused by autoimmune disorders such as systemic lupus erythematosus. In addition, myocarditis may be present in patients with peripartum dilated cardiomyopathy; however, heart inflammation is most often caused by a viral infection. Specific viruses, parasites, and bacteria may attack the heart muscle and weaken it. Myocarditis may arise from the bacteria *Borrelia burgdorferi*, which is transmitted by deer ticks. *B. burgdorferi* is the cause of Lyme disease. If the bacterial infection goes untreated, the organism spreads to organs in the body, sometimes including the heart. This leads to inflammation and myocarditis.

When a microbial infection of the heart is confirmed, it can be treated with antiviral medications or antibiotics. In other cases, there are no specific targeted treatments available other than supportive measures. In some instances, the effects of the infections are short-lived and heart function improves. In others, the infection inflicts permanent damage to the heart, and medication plus device therapy should be considered. In severe cases, heart transplantation may be considered.

Treatments for Dilated Cardiomyopathy

The treatments for different types of dilated cardiomyopathy are listed in Table 13.1. If the cause of the cardiomyopathy is ischemia (due to coronary artery disease and a lack of oxygenated blood being effectively delivered to the heart), specific medications are often recommended (see Chap. 25). In addition, testing (Chaps. 16, 17, 18, 19, 20, 21, 22, and 23) and treatments such as percutaneous coronary intervention (PCI), including stent placement, and/or coronary artery bypass surgery can be helpful in ameliorating symptoms and, in some cases, prolonged survival (Chaps. 24, 25, 33, 34, and 35). In a person with a history of a heart attack and symptomatic

Table 13.1 Dilated cardiomyopathy types and treatments

Types	Treatments
Ischemic	ACE inhibitors, ARBs, beta-blockers, device therapy, revascularization
Idiopathic	ACE inhibitors, ARBs, beta-blockers, device therapy
Hypertensive	ACE inhibitors, ARBs, beta-blockers, device therapy
Valvular	ACE inhibitors, ARBs, hydralazine/nitrates, valve surgery (repair or replacement), device therapy
Chemotherapeutic/radiation induced	ACE inhibitors, ARBs, beta-blockers, device therapy
Pregnancy induced	ACE inhibitors, ARBs, beta-blockers, device therapy if the condition persists
Alcohol related	ACE inhibitors, ARBs, beta-blockers, abstinence from alcohol, device therapy
Inflammation- or infection induced	ACE inhibitors, ARBs, beta-blockers, device therapy, treatment of specific cause
Inherited (arrhythmogenic right ventricular dysplasia)	ACE inhibitors, ARBs, beta-blockers, sotalol, device therapy

ventricular tachycardia, the underlying condition (coronary artery disease) might require the opening of at least one blocked coronary artery and placement of a stent and medical treatment with acetylsalicylic acid, clopidogrel, statins, and a beta-blocker. Please see those chapters for more information and speak to your doctor regarding the risks, benefits, and alternatives to any of these interventional procedures.

For those with dilated cardiomyopathy that is not due to coronary artery disease, heart failure medications and a low-salt diet are important in treating and improving heart function. In those with a depressed ejection fraction (less than 50%) or who have heart failure, medications typically include a beta-blocker and an angiotensin-converting enzyme inhibitor (ACEI) or an angiotensin II receptor blocker (ARB). More recently, the benefits of an angiotensin receptor-neprilysin inhibitor (ARNI) have replaced the ACEI or ARB in many patients with heart failure. Please see Chap. 14 for more information on the treatment of heart failure.

The implantable cardioverter defibrillator (ICD) can be an important medical device that can improve survival in those with a history of a previous heart attack(s) and an ejection fraction of 30% or less. These patients are at risk of sudden cardiac death from ventricular tachycardia and ventricular fibrillation, so an ICD can help prevent death by terminating these dangerous rhythms should they occur in the future. Medical societies (such as the Heart Rhythm Society) use the term "primary prevention" when a defibrillator is placed in those who have never experienced ventricular tachycardia or ventricular fibrillation but remain at risk for sudden cardiac death.

The term "secondary prevention" is used to describe those who have already experienced an episode of sudden death or ventricular tachycardia/fibrillation and require an ICD to prevent another episode. In some patients with mild to moderate heart failure despite optimal medical therapy, an ICD can help prolong survival.

Additionally, specific types of devices can improve the contraction of the heart by either conduction system or biventricular pacing (called cardiac resynchronization therapy), especially if symptoms persist despite optimal medical therapy and the presence of a specific pattern on ECG (called a left bundle branch block pattern). For more information, please see Chap. 30. Cardiac transplantation is the last resort for patients with cardiomyopathies whose symptoms are not resolved using standard medical or surgical treatments.

Hypertrophic Cardiomyopathy

Hypertrophic cardiomyopathy (HCM) is a condition typically characterized by a thickened heart muscle. Hypertrophic means "enlargement." In this disease, the heart muscle's cells are enlarged, which makes the walls of the heart thicker in diameter. Think of a thin rubber band that can be easily stretched (just as the heart can easily stretch), and then think of a thicker rubber band. You can feel the increased tension when you try to stretch the thicker rubber band. Figure 13.1b illustrates hypertrophic cardiomyopathy with its thickened (hypertrophied) walls and inter-ventricular septum. These patients typically have a hypercontractile heart, rather than a weakened contraction as seen in dilated cardiomyopathy. Another term for hypercontractile is hyperdynamic, meaning the ejection fraction is greater than 70%.

More than half of HCM cases are caused by genetic mutations (a good resource for researching genetic disorders is the National Institutes of Health). Another cause for this type of cardiomyopathy is long-standing high blood pressure, which may also cause heart wall muscles to thicken. Hypertrophic cardiomyopathy may be associated with an obstruction that blocks blood from leaving the heart, called *hypertrophic obstructive cardiomyopathy.* Patients may have characteristic findings on echocardiogram, which include an abnormal thickening of the heart muscle between the two ventricles, called the septum (the medical term is "asymmetrical septal hypertrophy [ASH]"), and an abnormal movement of the mitral valve (the medical term is "systolic anterior motion [SAM] of the mitral valve").

Ventricular hypertrophy (thickened ventricular muscle) makes it more likely that a person will have ventricular tachycardia or ventricular fibrillation. HCM is the leading cause of sudden death in athletes younger than 35 years old. Patients with HCM may benefit from an ICD, especially if they have a very thick ventricular septum (3 cm or more), are symptomatic with syncope and ventricular arrhythmias, and/or have a significant family history of sudden death. Diagnostic evaluations usually include an ECG and echocardiography; the latter will give the clinician images of the heart and show the ventricular wall thickness and degree of outflow tract obstruction. Your doctor may recommend that you have a cardiac magnetic resonance imaging test (cardiac MRI; see Chap. 20). Genetic testing is available for those suspected of having a genetic component (see Chap. 15 for a discussion of hereditary conditions).

Treatment usually relates to the symptoms and includes medications such as beta-blockers and calcium channel blockers (see Chap. 25). Amiodarone may be useful for treating persistent abnormal heart rhythms such as atrial fibrillation. It may also be useful in suppressing recurrent ventricular tachycardia in patients with an ICD. Interventions may include a surgical procedure to remove part of the heart muscle (septal myotomy-myomectomy) or a catheterization procedure in which alcohol is delivered down a coronary artery to injure the middle of the heart and improve overall function (alcohol septal ablation procedure; see Chap. 36). ICDs are usually recommended for patients who are symptomatic from ventricular arrhythmias (including syncope) or who are at risk for ventricular arrhythmias and sudden death. Eventually, genetic medical therapies (which are currently investigational) may have a role in the treatment of this disorder.

Restrictive Cardiomyopathy

A restrictive cardiomyopathy, as shown in Fig. 13.1d, occurs when the ventricles are rigid and stiff (the medical term is "noncompliant") and cannot fill properly during the resting phase (diastole) of the heart cycle. The most common cause is a disease called *cardiac amyloidosis*, in which an abnormal protein builds up in the muscle. Amyloid protein buildup can occur in any organ in the body, not just the heart. Diagnosis is usually made by an echocardiogram and a heart or tissue biopsy, which helps to confirm the diagnosis.

Other causes of restrictive cardiomyopathy include cancer, radiation therapy, heart transplantation, and other disease in which substances build up in the heart muscle itself (the medical term is "infiltrative disorders"), such as iron buildup in the heart (called "hemochromatosis").

Treatment includes medications such as nitrates, beta-blockers, and calcium channel blockers. Patients are advised to avoid products containing salt (sodium) and to carefully manage their weight. Diuretics may worsen symptoms and should be used with caution. An ICD may be useful to treat patients at risk for ventricular tachycardia or ventricular fibrillation.

Heart Failure

14

Todd J. Cohen

Heart failure is a condition where the heart weakens and cannot effectively pump blood to the rest of the body. When the left side of the heart is affected, blood backs up from the heart into the lungs, leading to congestion and shortness of breath. This is called *left heart failure*. Alternatively, blood may back up on the right side of the heart, resulting in leg swelling and swelling of other tissues and organs (called edema). This is called *right heart failure*. A person may have either right or left heart failure or both. Causes of heart failure include anything that results in heart disease (Table 14.4), such as ischemia or lack of blood flow to the heart, a heart attack, a weak or thickened heart muscle, leaky or tight heart valves, inherited conditions, viral infections, and drug toxicities, including alcohol abuse.

Another classification of heart failure is related either to an impaired ability of the heart to pump blood (systolic dysfunction) or to an increased stiffness of the ventricles, which impairs blood filling (diastolic dysfunction). Figure 14.1a, b shows diastolic and systolic heart failure, respectively. The heart muscle's contraction, relaxation, or both may be affected. The primary differences between systolic heart failure and diastolic heart failure are shown in Table 14.1.

Symptoms of heart failure have been classified by the New York Heart Association (NYHA) into four classes (Table 14.2). These classes progress from asymptomatic to mild, moderate, and finally severe heart failure symptoms. Specifically, people with **class I** heart failure essentially don't have symptoms and have no limitations on their activities. Those with **class II** heart failure have mild symptoms that occur

T. J. Cohen (✉)
NYIT College of Osteopathic Medicine, New York, NY, USA
e-mail: tcohen03@nyit.edu

© The Author(s), under exclusive license to Springer Nature Switzerland AG 2025
T. J. Cohen, R. S. Blumenthal (eds.), *Surviving and Thriving With Heart Disease*,
Contemporary Cardiology, https://doi.org/10.1007/978-3-032-00579-3_14

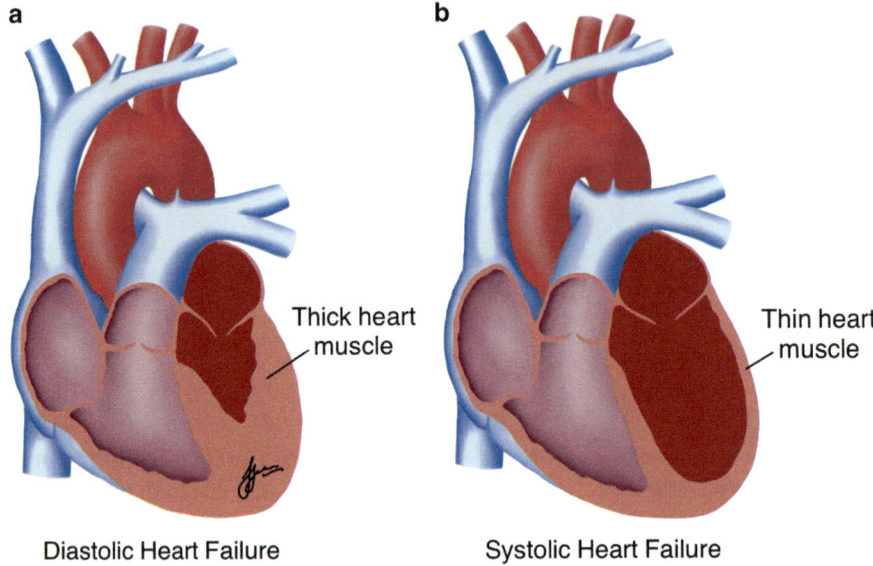

Fig. 14.1 (**a**) This figure shows diastolic heart failure in which the chambers are thickened and/or stiff and filling into the ventricles is impaired. (**b**) shows systolic heart failure in which the chambers are weak and dilated and the ability of the heart to contract is impaired. (Figure drawn by Jerry Jose, DO)

Table 14.1 Differences between systolic heart failure and diastolic heart failure

Systolic heart failure	Diastolic heart failure
More common	Less common
Muscle weak or enlarged	Muscle thick or stiff
Impaired heart contraction	Impaired heart filling

Table 14.2 The New York Heart Association classification of congestive heart failure

Class I: No limitation of activities; they suffer no symptoms from ordinary activities
Class II: Slight limitation of activity; they are comfortable at rest and with mild exertion
Class III: Marked limitation of activity; they are comfortable only at rest
Class IV: Symptomatic even at rest, and physical activity brings on discomfort

only with a great degree of exertion, such as running or other exercise. Individuals with **class III** heart failure have marked limitation of activity, and symptoms occur upon mild exertion. Those with **class IV** have symptoms at rest, which include shortness of breath, leg swelling, decreased exercise tolerance, fatigue, lightheadedness or dizziness, and confusion (Table 14.3).

Table 14.3 Symptoms of heart failure

Shortness of breath
Leg swelling
Decreased exercise tolerance
Fatigue
Light-headedness, dizziness
Confusion
Coughing or wheezing
Weight gain
Palpitations

Cardiac Remodeling

Many cardiac conditions, including heart failure, can cause remodeling. This remodeling is a process in which the heart reshapes itself due to some injury or insult, such as long-standing fluid accumulation in the heart, which causes the heart muscle to stretch until it can no longer pump efficiently. Heart failure and many other cardiac disorders can cause remodeling.

In long-standing (or chronic) heart failure, many of the heart's repair mechanisms, which were initially compensating and allowing the heart to pump effectively, turn maladaptive and worsen the condition. When your heart is not ejecting enough blood to support the rest of your body, your body feels as though it is under attack, and defense mechanisms come into play. The body has "feelers" outside the heart that determine whether these areas are getting enough blood. If these feelers realize the blood supply is low, they command blood vessels to become smaller and narrower. Think of a garden hose. When it is wide open, the water flows out smoothly. When you crimp the hose, it doesn't allow all the water to flow out at the prior quick pace. When the vessels clamp down, a strain is placed on the heart, causing fluid to be retained and preventing the heart from emptying. The result is an increase in symptoms such as shortness of breath.

Your Ejection Fraction

Chapter 4 describes an important heart function number called the ejection fraction (EF). To review, the EF is reported as a percentage and is determined by the difference in the amount of blood within the ventricle(s) during complete relaxation and complete contraction, divided by the amount of blood in complete relaxation, multiplied by 100.

Every heart patient should know their EF! This number is a measure of how well the heart contracts and, when used alone, typically represents how well the left ventricle contracts. It is determined by a variety of imaging tests including an echocardiogram (heart ultrasound; see Chap. 18), cardiac MRI, left ventricular angiogram, or nuclear study (such as a gated blood pool or positron emission tomography [PET] scan). A normal EF is between 50% and 70%. Those with systolic heart failure have a reduced EF (typically less than 50%).

The degree of left ventricular dysfunction is broken down further, in Chap. 4's Table 4.2, as mild dysfunction (EF of 40–49%), moderate dysfunction (EF of 30–39%), or severe dysfunction (EF less than 30%). Those with EFs greater than 70% are called hyperdynamic, which may be seen in hypertrophic cardiomyopathy (see Chaps. 15 and 36). It is important to remember that you can have heart failure with a normal EF. This is typically the result of diastolic dysfunction of the heart.

Diagnosing Heart Failure

If your doctor is concerned about the possibility of heart failure, they may order diagnostic tests, such as an echocardiogram, chest X-ray, a noninvasive stress test, an angiogram, cardiac MRI, CT angiogram, and/or PET scan (see Chap. 20). Lab tests may include blood chemistries, complete blood counts, electrolytes, liver enzymes, BNP (brain or B-type natriuretic peptide), and troponin levels. For those with a low EF (less than 50%) who are asymptomatic and have no heart failure symptoms (NYHA class I), taking medications such as an ACE inhibitor or ARB plus a beta-blocker is advisable (along with diet, exercise, stress reduction, and smoking cessation). For those with heart failure and mild to moderate symptoms, moderate exercise and a healthy diet (salt restriction) are important. Again, stopping smoking and reducing your stress are important. Table 14.4 lists some of the causes of heart failure.

Table 14.4 Causes of heart failure

Lack of blood flow to the heart (ischemia)
Presence of a heart attack (myocardial infarction)
Weak heart muscle (cardiomyopathy)
Thickened heart muscle (e.g., occurs with hypertrophic cardiomyopathy)
Leaky heart valves (valvular regurgitation)
Tight heart valves (stenosis)
Inherited conditions
Drug toxicity
Heart rhythm problems (arrhythmias) that weaken the heart muscle (tachycardia-induced cardiomyopathy)
Infection (e.g., caused by a virus)

Medications

In 2017, the American College of Cardiology and American Heart Association Task Force along with the Heart Failure Society of America updated their guidelines to include the use of angiotensin receptor-neprilysin inhibitors (ARNIs) and ivabradine. Your doctor should prescribe medications such as a beta-blocker, an angiotensin-converting enzyme (ACE) inhibitor or angiotensin II receptor blocker (ARB), and an aldosterone inhibitor. Suppression of the renin-angiotensin system with either or both an ACE inhibitor or an ARB has been important in improving morbidity and mortality. In 2022, heart failure guidelines replaced ACE inhibitors or ARBs with angiotensin receptor-neprilysin inhibitors (ARNIs) for the first line treatment of heart failure with a reduced ejection fraction.

Diuretics and digitalis may also help address persistent symptoms despite treatment with beta-blockers, aldosterone inhibition, and renin-angiotensin system inhibition (see Chap. 25). Heart cells also contain specialized channels in their outer membranes, which help control the flow of ions in and out of the cells. One such channel, the *If channel*, is specific to the sinus node and functions as a pacemaker control channel for the heart. An If channel inhibitor (ivabradine) may reduce hospitalizations with those on renin-angiotensin system suppression and maximal beta-blocker therapy with heart rates of 70 beats per minute or more.

Table 14.5 shows some recommended therapies for those with heart failure and structural heart disease (a reduced EF) with symptoms. In general, an ARNI is preferable to either an ACE inhibitor or an ARB in those with mild to moderate heart failure, but avoided in those with a history of angioedema (a life-threatening condition in which swelling of the skin and tissue occurs, in particular around the breathing tubes (larynx), which may make it very difficult to breathe).

Table 14.5 General CHF recommendations for structural heart disease with symptoms

Diet (salt restriction) and exercise.
Stress reduction and smoking cessation.
Renin-angiotensin system inhibition with ACE inhibitors, ARB, or ARNI along with evidence-based use of beta-blockers and aldosterone antagonists.
ARNI should replace ACE inhibitor or ARB in those with NYHA Class II or III CHF and good blood pressure, but not used in those with a history of angioedema.
Ivabradine for those with NYHA Class II/III CHF and heart rate of 70 beats per minute or more (despite optimal beta-blocker dose).
Digitalis and diuretics as needed to treat symptoms.
Defibrillator should be considered for (a) NYHA Class II or III CHF and EF less than 36 percent; (b) cardiac resynchronization therapy (biventricular defibrillator) for symptomatic CHF despite optimal medical therapy and very wide QRS complex on ECG.

Implantable Defibrillators

People who have heart failure are at risk for sudden cardiac arrest caused by ventricular tachycardia or ventricular fibrillation. Implantable defibrillators prolong life in people who have heart failure. Devices that can pace both the left and right ventricles are called *biventricular devices (also called cardiac resynchronization therapy)*; they can improve heart function beyond what can be achieved with medications.

A person may qualify for a biventricular defibrillator with an EF of less than 36% and symptomatic congestive heart failure despite optimal medical therapy with a very wide QRS complex on ECG (left bundle branch block pattern). Improvement in symptoms may be observed in about two of every three patients who have met the preceding criteria. A patient may qualify for a defibrillator, even without symptoms (NYHA class I heart failure) if they had a heart attack over 40 days ago and have an EF of 30% or less.

The MADIT-CRT study demonstrated that biventricular defibrillators improve survival with fewer heart failure interventions even in asymptomatic or mildly symptomatic heart failure patients (NYHA class I or II) with an EF of 30% or less and a wide QRS complex. If you are experiencing symptoms of heart failure or have a very weak heart (indicated by an EF of 30% or less) with a left bundle branch block on the EKG, you may want to discuss the option of a biventricular device with your doctor (see Chap. 31).

Hereditary Conditions and Congenital Heart Disease

15

Todd J. Cohen

Each cell in your body contains genes, which are the body's blueprints for development, growth, and functioning. Located within these genes are proteins called *deoxyribonucleic acid* (DNA). Genes are programmed before birth to provide our cells and to tell the organs of our body to perform specific tasks. Let's say a gene is named H-E-A-R-T, and its programmed function is to pump blood throughout the body. If that same gene is misspelled, say E-H-A-R-T, the programmed function would change, just as if you were reading the word E-H-A-R-T and did not recognize it to mean "heart." In this way, how genes are spelled (or coded) gives meaning to their function.

One major function of the heart is to support a normal heart rhythm. If the function (the spelling of the code) is altered, arrhythmias can arise. One major problem with these hereditary cardiac disorders is the risk of ventricular arrhythmias and sudden cardiac arrest. Tragically, some patients who possess genetic disorders are not identified (unless a strong family history is present) until they experience sudden cardiac death.

With many genetic disorders, it is necessary for only one parent (not both parents) to have the harmful gene to pass it on to the child. Most diseases have a genetic basis that may or may not be passed from parent to child. For the purpose of this section, the focus is on genetic diseases related to heart rhythm problems that *can* be passed this way. Your environment can affect how these genetic disorders express themselves. Genetic defects discussed in this chapter are arrhythmogenic right ventricular dysplasia, hypertrophic cardiomyopathy (see Chap. 13), long QT syndrome, and Brugada syndrome. See Table 15.1 for a list of the common gene subtypes of

T. J. Cohen (✉)
NYIT College of Osteopathic Medicine, New York, NY, USA
e-mail: tcohen03@nyit.edu

Table 15.1 Common associated gene subtypes for inherited rhythm disorders

Disorder	Gene subtypes
Arrhythmogenic right ventricular dysplasia (fat deposits in right ventricular wall)	PKP2, DSP, GSG2
Hypertrophic cardiomyopathy (thickened heart muscle)	MYH7, MYBPC3
Long QT syndrome (has a specific pattern)	ECGKCNQ1 (long QT1); KCNH2 (long QT2); SCN5A (long QT3)
Brugada syndrome (has a specific ECG pattern)	SCN5A

Source: T. J. Cohen, *Practical Electrophysiology,* Third Edition (Malvern, PA: HMP Communications, 2016), p. 215

these disorders. Later in this chapter, genetic testing is discussed as well as the treatment for people with hereditary cardiac disorders. Finally, this chapter touches on congenital heart diseases that present at birth and may require surgical intervention.

Arrhythmogenic Right Ventricular Cardiomyopathy/Dysplasia (ARVC/D)

ARVC/D (also called arrhythmogenic cardiomyopathy or ACD, arrhythmogenic right ventricular cardiomyopathy or ARVC, or arrhythmogenic right ventricular dysplasia) is a rare genetic heart disorder of the desmosome (a protein that helps hold heart cells together) typically seen in young adults. A genetic defect, called a mutation, in one or more components of this protein can affect the heart's structure by impairing how heart cells are connected. It occurs in 1 in 5000 people and is associated with ventricular tachycardia and sudden cardiac arrest. In this disorder, fat deposits in the heart muscle make these patients, especially young individuals or athletes, more likely to develop ventricular arrhythmias and possibly sudden cardiac death.

Patients with this disorder often present with symptoms of palpitations, presyncope, and/or syncope, and some present with cardiac arrest. ECG monitoring (external or implantable) can demonstrate that these symptoms are from ventricular tachycardia. ARVC/D patients may have a family history of this disorder. The ECG typically has an abnormal pattern (flipped T waves in V1 to V3 and/or an epsilon wave – a low-amplitude wave at the end of the QRS complex). A specialized signal-averaged ECG can be useful in identifying this condition (by finding an abnormality called late potentials).

The echocardiogram or cardiac MRI often shows abnormal right ventricular contractions and/or enlargement; the MRI may also show fat deposits in the right ventricular wall. A genetic abnormality, known as genetic mutation, is positive in about half the patients. Treatments include antiarrhythmic medications such as sotalol, catheter ablation, and an implantable defibrillator. Figure 15.1 shows an ECG from a patient with arrhythmogenic right ventricular dysplasia with a specific pattern called an incomplete right bundle branch block pattern. It also shows symptomatic bursts of ventricular tachycardia (short bursts of ventricular tachycardia that

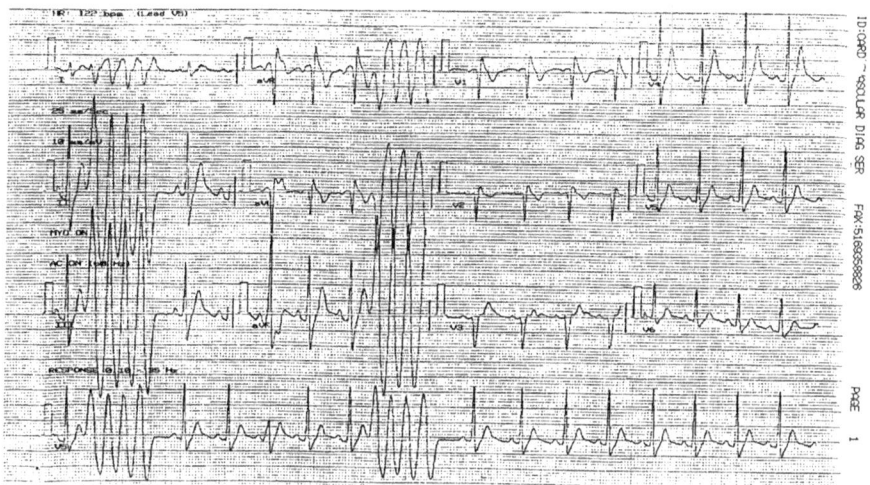

Fig. 15.1 This 12-lead ECG demonstrates areas of a near normal ECG (the more narrow complexes show an incomplete right bundle branch pattern; also localized widening at the end of the QRS in V1 through V3) and runs of rapid nonsustained ventricular tachycardia. This patient underwent a cardiac MRI which demonstrated fat deposition in the right ventricular wall and was diagnosed as having arrhythmogenic right ventricular dysplasia. He was treated with an implantable defibrillator. (Reproduced with permission from HMP Communications LLC from Practical Electrophysiology, Third Edition)

terminate spontaneously are called *nonsustained*), and the patient eventually received an implantable defibrillator.

Hypertrophic Cardiomyopathy

Numerous genes have been implicated in causing hypertrophic cardiomyopathy, which may cause thickening of the heart muscle. These genetic mutations affect the sarcomere, the basic contractile unit of heart muscle fibers. Mutations can occur in specific areas of the sarcomere (specifically the beta-myosin heavy chain, myosin binding protein C, and less commonly in troponin). These genetic abnormalities, if identified, can help with the diagnosis. The echocardiogram and cardiac MRI help define the thickness of the heart wall (hypertrophy) and the presence of features of the disease, which may include asymmetric septal thickening or hypertrophy (ASH), systolic anterior motion of the mitral valve (SAM), and left ventricular outflow tract obstruction (LVOT gradient).

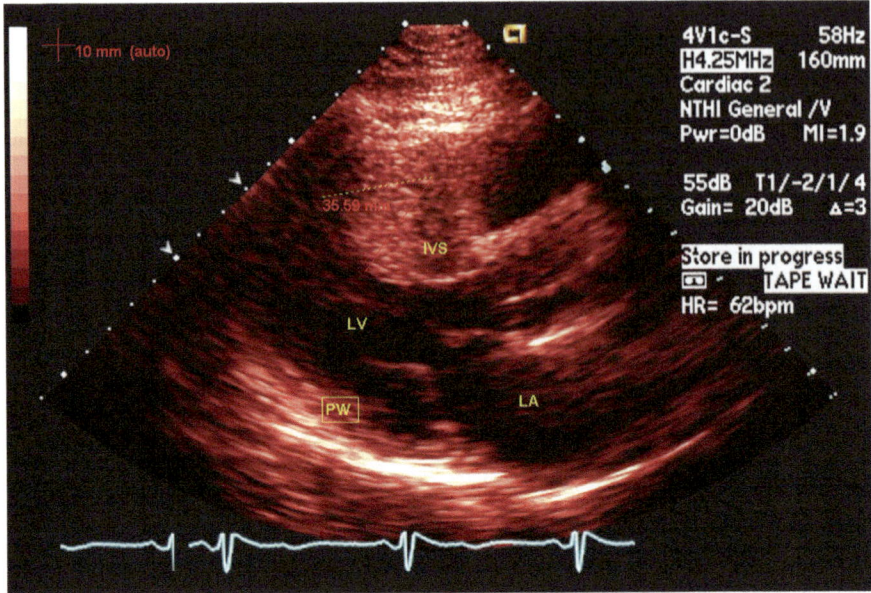

Fig. 15.2 This echocardiogram shows a very large interventricular septum (IVS of 3 cm) compared to the normal left ventricular posterior wall (PW). This patient was diagnosed as having hypertrophic cardiomyopathy and received an implantable defibrillator. (Reproduced with permission from HMP Communications LLC from Practical Electrophysiology, Third Edition)

Those with a history of loss of consciousness, ventricular tachycardia, a family history of sudden death, prior sudden cardiac arrest, or a very thick heart muscle (greater than 3 cm) may benefit from an implantable defibrillator. Figure 15.2 shows a very thick interventricular septum seen during an echocardiogram in a patient with hypertrophic cardiomyopathy. The patient received an implantable defibrillator to protect him from sudden death. For more information regarding hypertrophic cardiomyopathy, see Chaps. 13 and 36.

Long QT Syndrome

The first family identified as having long QT (LQT) syndrome was reported in 1957. This disorder was originally called Romano-Ward syndrome, though that term is outdated. Research has since demonstrated that many different genetic defects cause long QT syndrome; in fact, scientists have identified many mutations in many different genes. With this knowledge, long QT syndrome has subsequently

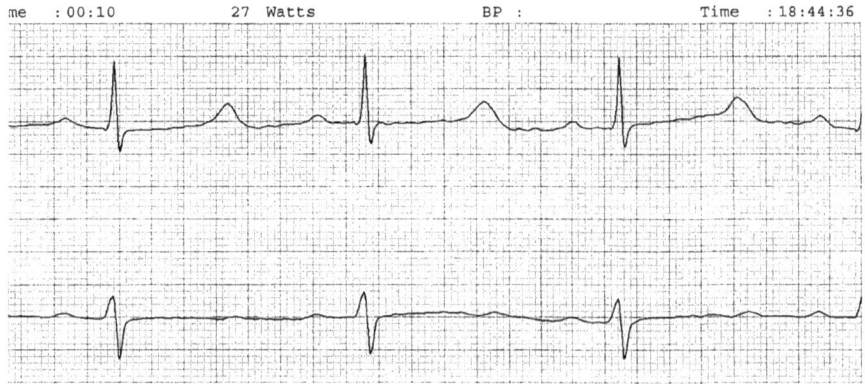

me   : 00:10   27 Watts   BP :   Time   : 18:44:36

Fig. 15.3 An ECG rhythm strip (recorded at a paper speed of 10 mm/s) from an 8-year-old girl genotyped as long QT3 (sodium channel type) and demonstrates a long corrected QT interval. The QT interval can be corrected for heart rate using the Bazeet formula and is called the QTC. (Reproduced with permission from HMP Communications LLC from Practical Electrophysiology, Third Edition)

been divided into numbered categories (LQTS1, LQTS2, LQTS3, and so on). Abnormalities in potassium ion channel genes (KCNQ1 and KCNQH2) may result in type 1 long QT and type 2 long QT. Type 3 may be caused by abnormalities in the SCN5A gene.

The most common type of LQT syndrome is type 2, which was identified in 1994. The disorder is demonstrated by a prolongation of the QT segment on the ECG. On a routine ECG, this QT change may not always be apparent. Your doctor may send you for exercise a treadmill test to elicit changes in the QT interval that would raise suspicion of this disorder. Genetic testing is very important in this disorder. Figure 15.3 shows an ECG strip with long QT in an 8-year-old girl. Treatment may include medications such as beta-blockers, environmental restrictions such as a modified exercise regimen and avoidance of noise or startling events, and possibly even an implantable defibrillator. The latter device-based treatment should be considered for people with serious symptoms that cannot be controlled by medications and lifestyle modifications.

There are many drugs you should avoid if you have LQT syndrome (Table 15.2), as they tend to lengthen the QT interval. These include diuretics (which can cause electrolyte abnormalities that can lengthen the QT interval), stimulants, and certain "anti" drugs such as antibiotics, antidepressants, antipsychotics, antihistamines, anticonvulsants, and antiarrhythmics. In 2019, Farzam and Tivakaran published a comprehensive review on QT-prolonging drugs in StatPearls, which can be found at https://www.ncbi.nlm.nih.gov/books/NBK534864/.

Table 15.2 Some drugs to avoid in long QT syndrome

"Anti" drugs (*see also* "Psychiatric medications" below)
Antiarrhythmics
Ibutilide
Procainamide
Quinidine
Disopyramide
Sotalol
Dofetilide
Propafenone
Antibiotics
Macrolides such as erythromycin
Fluoroquinolones
Anticonvulsants
Antihistamines
Antihypertensives
Diuretics (can lower electrolytes such as potassium and lengthen QT interval)
Gastrointestinal motility drugs
Migraine medications
Psychiatric medications
Stimulants such as methylphenidate
Antidepressants such as tricyclic antidepressants and SSRIs
Antipsychotics such as haloperidol
Tranquilizers

Brugada Syndrome

Brugada syndrome is an inherited condition placing the patient at risk of sudden death. It accounts for nearly half the sudden cardiac arrests in those with structurally normal hearts. In the 1980s, the Centers for Disease Control and Prevention reported a high incidence of sudden death in young Asian immigrants from Thailand. In Thailand, the disorder was known as LaiTai (death during sleep). In 1992, the Brugada brothers identified the disease now known as Brugada syndrome. Genetic investigation led researchers to identify the culprit as a defective gene affecting specialized channels within heart cells (mutation of SCN5A gene).

An ECG may show a specific pattern with an incomplete right bundle branch block and ST segment elevation in leads V1 through V3 (identifiable to your cardiologist). The details of the ECG's QRS complex and ST segment contour can help him or her define the type of Brugada pattern (type 1, 2, or 3). The most specific Brugada Pattern, type 1, may be diagnostic of the disorder if correlated with symptoms, such as syncope, ventricular tachycardia, and/or sudden cardiac arrest. Sudden death is usually caused by ventricular fibrillation. The condition is best treated with an implantable defibrillator. Figure 15.4a, b shows two ECGs from the same patient with Brugada syndrome. Note the differences in the end of the QRS complex and ST segment elevation in V1–V3, which may occur in this disorder. The patient had an electrophysiology study, which induced sustained ventricular tachycardia, and the patient received an implantable defibrillator.

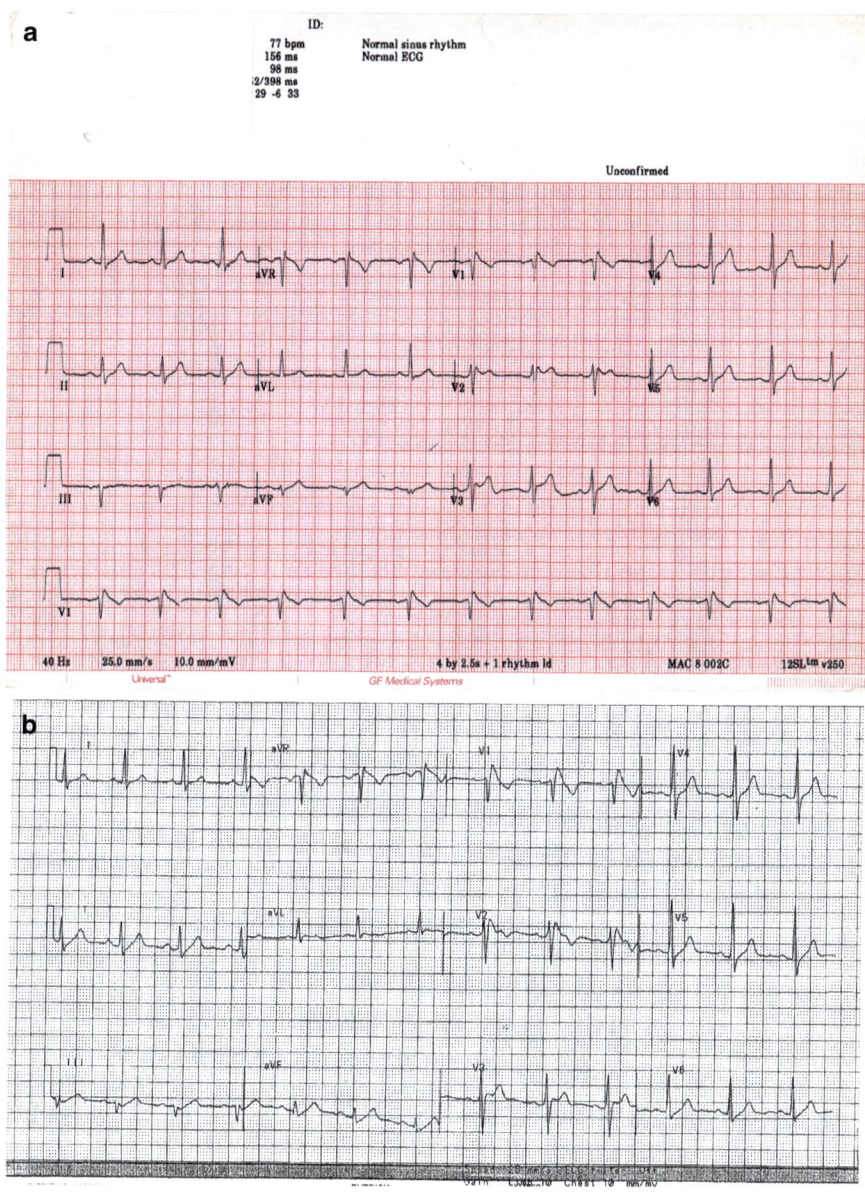

Fig. 15.4 (a, b) Two ECGs with variations in the ST segment elevation in V1 through V3. This patient had a family member with Brugada syndrome and had ventricular tachycardia induced during an electrophysiology study. Brugada syndrome is typically much more lethal than long QT syndrome, and this patient received an implantable defibrillator. (Reproduced with permission from HMP Communications LLC from Practical Electrophysiology, Third Edition)

Catecholaminergic Polymorphic Ventricular Tachycardia (CPVT)

Like Brugada syndrome, this is a genetic disorder that usually occurs in children and young adults with structurally normal hearts. Symptoms of palpitations, presyncope, and/or syncope are triggered by catecholamines (adrenaline) typically during exercise or stress and are attributable to ventricular tachycardia. The term polymorphic refers to the many shapes of the ventricular tachycardia on an ECG. CPVT is usually caused by a mutation in the ryanodine receptor gene or the cardiac calsequestrin receptor gene. The condition can be effectively treated with beta-blocker therapy and an implantable defibrillator.

Diagnostic Tests for Hereditary Disorders

A patient's history, physical examination, and 12-lead ECG are the initial steps in diagnosing a hereditary heart rhythm condition. Cardiopulmonary symptoms and signs can steer the cardiologist in the right direction of testing. The presence of a history of cyanosis (blue lips and extremities), a heart murmur, and a detailed family history are very useful. In those with heart palpitations, presyncope, and/or syncope, extended telemetry monitoring with either an external wearable device or an implantable loop recorder can help with making the diagnosis. Additional testing can include a special computerized ECG called *signal-averaged ECG*, exercise stress testing, CT angiography, coronary angiography (cardiac catheterization), and/ or a cardiac MRI to help with diagnosis.

A genetic counselor can be particularly helpful to those with a hereditary disorder. They will get a very detailed history and focus even more in-depth on family history. The genetic counselor can target a panel of genes and disorders in order to define inherited conditions. These tests have historically been expensive and have sometimes not been covered by routine health insurance. As the tests are more commonly practiced and more readily available, the costs have started to decrease, and some insurance companies and government-sponsored health plans are offering reimbursement. An important step in expanding genetic testing occurred in 2008 when the Genetic Information Nondiscrimination Act (GINA) was signed into law. This law prohibits discrimination based on information obtained through genetic testing as it relates to employment and insurance coverage.

Since its inception, genetic testing has raised ethical issues for some people. Whether patients are tested with traditional diagnostic tools or with genetic testing, they need to be aware of the implications to other family members when one person is identified as having a genetic disorder. Some patients do not want others to know about their condition, and some individuals do not want to deal with the psychological effects of knowing they have a life-threatening condition. Generally, however, identifying the risk factors through diagnostic or genetic testing is important to patients and other family members so that they can be properly treated with drugs or other medical therapies.

Unfortunately, many families only learn about genetic testing after the tragedy of sudden cardiac death strikes a parent or child. Now that the privacy of genetic testing is protected and discrimination is prohibited through federal law, there are fewer obstacles for patients to fully discuss the option of genetic testing with their physician if there is a family history or suspected history of these hereditary conditions.

Make your physician aware if you have a family history of passing out (syncope), with or without sudden death. If a close family member has died suddenly, even if it was a parent or grandparent and it occurred 20 years ago, share that information with your physician. If a family is identified as being at risk for sudden cardiac death, your doctor can increase surveillance of all family members, which will make appropriate and timely treatment options more likely.

Treatment Options for People with Hereditary Cardiac Disorders

The goal for individuals who are identified with hereditary disorders is the prevention of sudden cardiac death. Treatment may include lifestyle modifications (avoiding strenuous exercise, avoiding caffeine and cigarettes, limiting alcohol intake), medications (beta-blockers help treat long QT syndrome), ablation therapies, and possibly an implantable defibrillator. Treatment in the future may include genetic therapies, such as the delivery of engineered genes into a patient's cells to treat the specific genetic defect.

Case 4: My Hereditary Heart Disorder

My family consisted of myself, my mother, father, and two siblings. In the early 1970s, my mother experienced an unexplained syncopal event. Some 6 or 7 years later, my brother, then 15 years old, had a similar fainting spell and was in a semi-comatose state for about 24 h. During his subsequent hospitalization, various tests were conducted, and doctors concluded that he might have had a drug overdose or drug reaction. To this day, my family does not understand why doctors would have made such a diagnosis since they never identified a drug in his system that may have caused the event.

Several years later, while on vacation, my brother collapsed again. Friends administered CPR, and he was taken to a local hospital. When he was well enough to return home, my parents took him to a local cardiologist, who referred him to a well-known university hospital several hours away. Physicians and researchers there were doing extensive work on arrhythmias and had identified the patterns and traits of long QT syndrome, which can result in arrhythmias, syncope, and even sudden death. An extensive cardiology exam identified my brother as having long QT. At their recommendation, my family was given ECGs, and my mother's ECG also showed the patterns of the condition (essentially an elongated pause at the end of the heartbeat). Both my mother and my brother were put on beta-blocker therapy. No other family members were identified as having the condition.

During this time, my family agreed to participate in a clinical research project, which eventually led to the first identification of genetic markers for long QT as well as the first commercial genetic tests for patients. Some 12 years later, I was married and had children. While my ECG had shown no trait of long QT, I routinely took my young children for an ECG, given the family history. At the age of 5, my eldest daughter's ECG showed the traits. While genetic tests for long QT were not widely available and were not covered by insurance, my children and I were genetically tested. All three of us were identified as carriers of one of the genetic abnormalities associated with long QT.

We are all on beta-blocker therapy and have shown no symptoms, but every year, we consult with an electrophysiologist, who monitors our heart health. The kids are now teenagers, and as a precaution, they do not play competitive sports, but they dance, play tennis, and are otherwise normal and active. My family has donated and advocated for the placement of automatic external defibrillators (AEDs) in our children's schools. My younger brother, who was the source of the original diagnosis, has had an implantable cardioverter defibrillator for more than 15 years because of chronic issues related to his condition.

While not happy with the diagnosis, I am certainly thankful that my wife and I took the family history seriously and consulted with medical experts to get the appropriate care. My wife and I also make sure that the physicians we see for other health issues understand the condition and do not prescribe drugs that can trigger arrhythmias. Finally, we work very hard to make sure that our children learn to take responsibility for their condition. Just like people with diabetes must watch what they eat and take insulin, our kids understand the importance of watching their diet, sticking to a regular exercise routine, and taking their medicine on time.

Congenital Heart Disease

Congenital heart disease (or CHD) is a category of heart conditions in which the normal anatomy of the heart fails to develop properly and leads to a defect(s) in the heart that may present in infancy or childhood. One simple variety is a hole in the heart (or septal defect). This can occur in the upper chambers (atrial septal defect or ASD) or lower chambers (ventricular septal defect or VSD). Occasionally, patients may have a smaller interatrial connection covered by a flap, which may be discovered during an echocardiogram and bubble study. This bubble study is performed by injecting agitated saline into a vein while the patient bears down. If this maneuver forces bubbles from the right side to the left side of the heart, a patent foramen ovale (PFO) or septal defect is present. This type of connection is an important cause of a stroke of unknown origin.

If a septal defect or PFO is the only finding in a patient who has experienced an embolic stroke (a stroke from a clot that has broken off) and occurs even after treatment with blood thinners (anticoagulants), the hole (or flap) will need to be closed either percutaneously (via a catheterization procedure) or surgically. The larger the size of the hole in the heart, the more likely the defect will lead to heart wall thickening, blueness of the skin and lips from blood not flowing to the lungs and being properly oxygenated (cyanosis), weakness, shortness of breath, exercise intolerance, and heart failure.

Johns Hopkins University made headlines in the treatment of congenital heart disease in 1944 by pioneering the treatment of a rare congenital heart disease called tetralogy of Fallot. The condition consists of pulmonary atresia (preventing deoxygenated blood that has returned to the heart from going to the lungs and getting oxygen); a VSD (that permits the pumping of deoxygenated blood to go directly to the body), thereby causing cyanosis; an overriding aorta; and right ventricular thickening from the hard work performed by the heart. This condition requires surgical repair, which was pioneered by two Johns Hopkins physicians.

In 1944, Drs. Helen Taussig and Alfred Blalock and research lab manager Vivien Thomas developed a shunting operation called the Blalock-Taussig shunt (or Blue Baby Operation) in which a surgical conduit is created to bring blood from the right subclavian artery to the right pulmonary artery. The procedure was first performed on Nov. 29, 1944, at Johns Hopkins Hospital on a patient by the name of Eileen Saxon. The procedure was only minimally successful, and the patient required a second operation and died shortly thereafter.

The work of Drs. Taussig and Blalock began an entire field of cardiac shunts and surgical repairs that are currently used to treat those with congenital heart defects such as individuals born with a single ventricle, those with transposition of the great arteries, and coarctation of the aorta to name a few. Only specialized heart hospitals and centers such as Mount Sinai Hospital, Stanford University Hospital, and Johns Hopkins Hospital perform this type of pediatric heart surgery. For more information on congenital heart conditions and the pediatric population, see Chap. 44.

Your Vital Signs and Common Blood Tests

In this part of the book, we will look at all of the common cardiac tests, both noninvasive and invasive ones. This includes the electrocardiogram, echocardiogram, stress testing, other heart imaging tests, heart rhythm monitoring, tilt table testing, electrophysiology testing, and the cardiac catheterization test. Tests are an important way to determine whether you and your heart are healthy. Before any tests begin, your doctor will obtain your medical history. Following this, they will perform a physical exam, which includes your vital signs. Vital signs include your heart rate and your blood pressure. A healthy resting heart rate in an awake adult is typically between 50 and 100 beats per minute (though it may be as low as 40 beats per minute) and a healthy blood pressure is 120/80 mm Hg or less. It also will include your temperature (may be elevated with infection or an inflammatory process), your respiratory rate (normally 12–20 breaths per minute; if abnormal, it may be a sign of heart failure or distress), and oxygen saturation (SpO_2; normally 95% or more). It also includes your weight and a calculation of your body mass index (or BMI; normal is 18.5–24.9, 25–29.9 is overweight, and 30 or more is obese; see Chap. 39). Since so many Americans have high blood pressure, blood pressure is commonly above the normal 120/80 mm Hg value and may need attention.

After your examination, an electrocardiogram is typically performed (see Chap. 16). Your doctor may order some blood tests, which can show the status of your electrolytes (which can make you prone to arrhythmias if outside of the normal range), BUN and creatinine (shows the status of your kidneys), and your cholesterol (total cholesterol, LDL, HDL, and triglycerides; see Chap. 37 on high cholesterol). As a cardiologist, I focus on the LDL, HDL, and triglyceride numbers (all numbers you should know), rather than your total cholesterol.

They can also order liver function tests (sometimes affected by alcohol, liver disease, or medications). Your doctor may order tests to show levels of injury to the heart muscle. These tests measure the amount of troponin (a heart muscle protein) that is released during a heart attack. Troponin-i and/or troponin-t can be measured.

Additionally, brain natriuretic peptide (BNP) may be tested to see if you have heart failure (normally less than 125 pg/ml if under 74 years old, or under 450 pg/ml if over 75 years old).

Blood tests can identify markers of inflammation, such as high-sensitivity C-reactive protein, often abbreviated as hsCRP (less than 1 is low risk, 1–3 mg is intermediate risk, and greater than 3 mg signifies a higher risk for heart disease). A high hsCRP is strongly associated with abdominal obesity. Elevated and circulating high levels of troponin-t, CRP, and BNP are all associated with heart disease. It is also helpful to know your fasting blood sugar to see if you are pre-diabetic or diabetic, along with your hemoglobin A1C (A1C). A normal fasting blood sugar is 100 mg/dl, 100–125 mg/dl is prediabetic, and 126 mg/dl or more is diabetic. An A1C below 5.7% is normal; above 5.7–6.4 is prediabetic; and above 6.4 is diabetic.

A common theme throughout this book is to know your numbers. *At a minimum, know your blood pressure, your cholesterol values (LDL, HDL, and triglycerides), and your weight (perhaps more importantly, your BMI).* It is also helpful for you to know your fasting blood sugar, A1C, ejection fraction, and the other numbers listed above. *In other words, it can be tailored to you and your personal situation!*

Electrocardiogram (ECG or EKG)

16

Todd J. Cohen

An ECG is a simple, painless, noninvasive test that can be performed in virtually any clinic, doctor's office, or medical facility. Small electrodes are attached to the chest, arms, and legs and connected to a machine that can record the electrical activity of the heart over time. The ECG is a map of electrical activity generated by the heart as it contracts and relaxes. The ECG is printed on paper that runs through the recording device. The ECG can show changes that suggest a blocked coronary artery or a heart rhythm abnormality (fast rhythms such as atrial fibrillation that may require blood thinners and slow rhythms such as complete heart block that may require a pacemaker). It can show the effects of electrolyte abnormalities, evidence of heart chamber enlargement, and abnormalities such as QT prolongation that can make a patient more likely to have ventricular tachycardia, ventricular fibrillation, and sudden cardiac arrest. For a summary of ECG facts, see Table 16.1.

T. J. Cohen (✉)
NYIT College of Osteopathic Medicine, New York, NY, USA
e-mail: tcohen03@nyit.edu

Table 16.1 ECG facts

An ECG is a simple, noninvasive test.

Ask your physician for a copy of the paper tracing from your ECG and place it in your personal records. It is useful to have a copy available in case of an emergency or if you change or add physicians.

Your ECG can show changes that could suggest a blocked coronary artery or a heart rhythm abnormality.

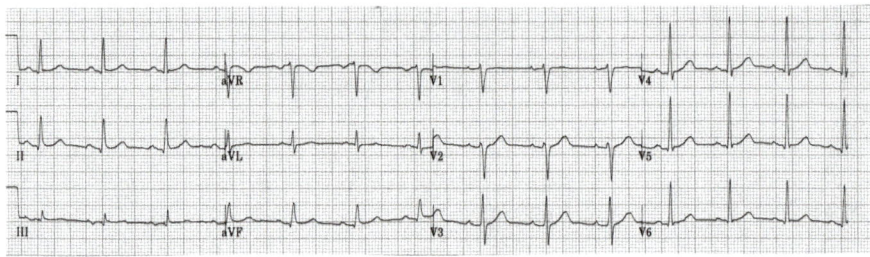

Fig. 16.1 Standard 12-lead electrocardiogram (ECG or EKG) showing a reading from a normal heart. A 12-lead ECG is a baseline assessment of your heart. From this, your doctor can determine heart rhythm abnormalities. Your doctor may compare a previous 12-lead ECG with your current ECG to see if there have been any significant changes. (Adapted from T.J. Cohen, *A Patient's Guide to Heart Rhythm Problems* (Baltimore, MD: The Johns Hopkins University Press, 2010), p. 60)

Basics of the ECG

A typical 12-lead ECG for a heart in which the upper and lower chambers beat in a normal sequence is shown in Fig. 16.1. This normal rhythm is called *normal sinus rhythm* (since it originates in the sinus node), and a normal heart rate is between 60 and 100 beats per minute.

From an ECG, it is possible to determine whether your rhythm is normal or abnormal. Abnormal rhythms include slow rhythms (bradycardias), fast rhythms (tachycardias), and heart block (in which impulses from the atria fail to conduct to the ventricles). In addition, the ECG can show the effects of electrolytes (normal or abnormal blood chemistry) and medications on the heart.

A single ECG signal is depicted in Fig. 16.2. This figure shows the normal sequence of electrical activity of the heart recorded from the surface ECG. The electrical signal may be broken into different waves. The medical terms P, QRS, T, and U are used to describe waves when referring to the ECG. The P wave represents atrial electrical activity, the QRS complex represents ventricular electrical activity, and the QT interval (from the beginning of the Q wave to the end of the T wave)

Fig. 16.2 A single ECG recording of a heartbeat. This figure shows the normal electrical sequence of the heart. The electrical signal may be broken into different waves. The P wave represents atrial electrical activity; the QRS complex represents ventricular electrical activity; and the QT interval (from the beginning of the Q wave to the end of the T wave) represents the ventricles returning to a resting state. (Adapted from T.J. Cohen, *A Patient's Guide to Heart Rhythm Problems* (Baltimore, MD: The Johns Hopkins University Press, 2010), p. 60)

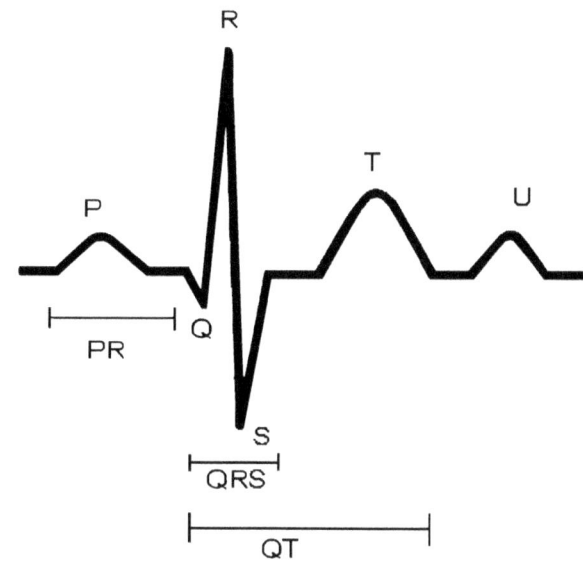

represents the ventricles returning to a resting state or repolarization, while the U wave represents the relaxation of the Purkinje fibers of the conduction system.

Abnormal ECGs

A slower-than-normal rhythm (*sinus bradycardia*), in which the heart rate is below 60 beats per minute, is demonstrated in Fig. 16.3. If the rhythm remains the same, but the heart rate *exceeds* 100 beats per minute, this would be called sinus tachycardia. In atrial fibrillation (Fig. 16.4), there are no discrete P waves present, but chaotic atrial activity can be seen between the QRS complexes. The atria quiver and fail to efficiently pump the blood into the ventricles. An example of atrial flutter on an ECG, which can be identified by sawtooth P waves, is shown in Chap. 9 (see Fig. 9.3).

Wolff-Parkinson-White (WPW) syndrome is a condition in which there is an extra connection between the atrium and ventricle (accessory pathway). People with WPW have supraventricular tachycardia plus a characteristic baseline ECG in which a delta wave is present (fusion of the P wave and the QRS complex; Fig. 16.5).

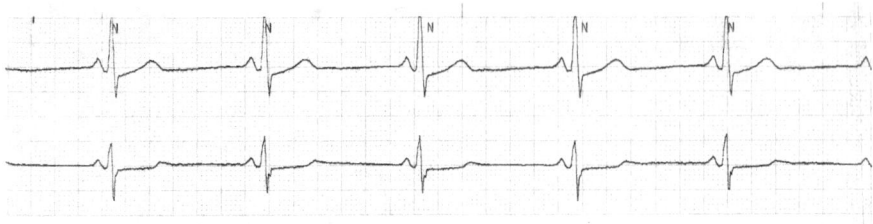

Fig. 16.3 An ECG tracing demonstrating sinus bradycardia (slow heart rhythm) in which the heart is beating at approximately 46 beats per minute (normal is 60–100 beats per minute). (Adapted from T.J. Cohen, *A Patient's Guide to Heart Rhythm Problems* (Baltimore, MD: The Johns Hopkins University Press, 2010), p. 63)

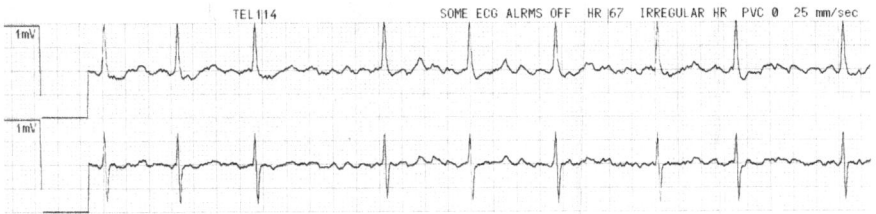

Fig. 16.4 An ECG tracing demonstrating atrial fibrillation, a rapid atrial rhythm in which the P waves are irregular and chaotic. (Adapted from T.J. Cohen, *A Patient's Guide to Heart Rhythm Problems* (Baltimore, MD: The Johns Hopkins University Press, 2010), p. 64)

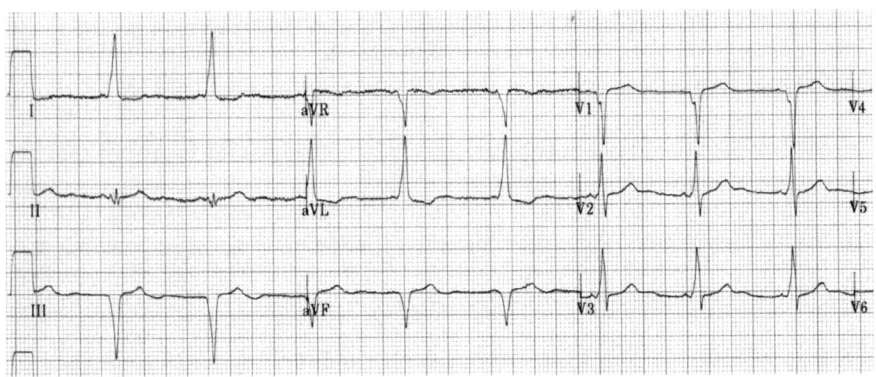

Fig. 16.5 Part of a 12-lead ECG of a patient with Wolff-Parkinson-White (WPW) syndrome. Note fusion from the end of the P wave to the QRS complex. This is called a delta wave. Patients with WPW syndrome may be at risk for sudden cardiac arrest and may benefit from catheter ablation. (Adapted from T.J. Cohen, *A Patient's Guide to Heart Rhythm Problems* (Baltimore, MD: The Johns Hopkins University Press, 2010), p. 62)

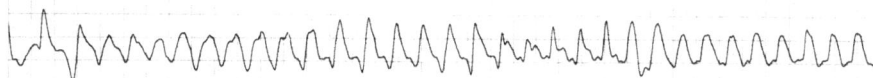

Fig. 16.6 An ECG tracing of ventricular tachycardia. This is considered a life-threatening arrhythmia and requires prompt medical attention. If the condition is not due to a reversible cause, an ICD should be considered. (Adapted from T.J. Cohen, *A Patient's Guide to Heart Rhythm Problems* (Baltimore, MD: The Johns Hopkins University Press, 2010), p. 62)

An example of *ventricular tachycardia* is shown in Fig. 16.6. These impulses are originating in the ventricles and are firing at a rapid rate. The QRS complexes of ventricular tachycardia are typically wider than the normal baseline QRS complexes. If it does not resolve spontaneously, ventricular tachycardia usually requires defibrillation.

Stress Testing and Preparation for Cardiac Procedures

17

Todd J. Cohen

Cardiologists use the diagnostic and imaging tests and procedures described in Chaps. 16, 17, 18, 19, 20, 21, 22, and 23 to assess the heart's structure and function. Not every test is appropriate for every patient. To identify whether your heart is performing normally, your doctor may order a stress test. It is considered a functional test because it determines how well your heart functions under stress. While you exercise, your heart must pump more blood to your body, because it requires more oxygen. A doctor recommends a stress test to patients when they are diagnosing or ruling out obstructive coronary artery disease, evaluating worsening stamina, or checking the effectiveness of a previously performed PCI procedure (such as angioplasty or stenting). This test is also useful in predicting a person's risk of a heart attack. For people with a normal ECG who have been sedentary prior to beginning an exercise program, the stress test can evaluate their fitness for exercise. In addition, this test may be useful in determining patient fitness before having major surgery.

In a stress test, you exercise on a treadmill while the ECG is monitored. Your walking or running speed is progressively increased along with the grade (or slope) as the doctor continuously analyzes your blood pressure as well as the ECG. Changes in the EC G recording and the development of arrhythmias during exercise-induced stress may indicate the presence of coronary artery disease. A standard exercise test typically uses a "Bruce protocol," increasing the speed and grade while exercising on a treadmill every 3 minutes. Each 3 minute segment is called a stage. The workload of each stage is calculated in metabolic equivalents (or METs). During a Bruce protocol, a patient exercises until a target heart rate is reached, which is 85% of the

T. J. Cohen (✉)
NYIT College of Osteopathic Medicine, New York, NY, USA
e-mail: tcohen03@nyit.edu

maximal predicted heart rate, or until symptoms develop and the test is terminated. If the test is terminated for symptoms, it is called a symptom-limited exercise stress test.

Maximal predicted heart rate can be calculated by subtracting one's age from 220. For example, a maximal predicted heart rate in a 70-year-old is 150 beats per minute. The target heart rate is 85% of the maximal predicted heart rate or 128 beats per minute. If the target heart rate is not reached during the test, the results may be inconclusive. The inability to increase heart rate with exertion may be called chronotropic incompetence and may be related to sinus node disease or medications being taken.

During the test, the doctor monitors the patient's blood pressure and ECG looking for abnormal ST segment changes (ST segment depression or elevation may indicate a lack of blood flow and oxygen to a region of heart muscle, also called ischemia), an abnormal heart rate and blood pressure response, the presence of arrhythmias or heart block, as well as more general symptoms of shortness of breath, chest pressure or discomfort, and fatigue. The higher the stage the patient achieves during exercise, the greater their functional capacity.

The stress testing protocol can be modified, called a modified Bruce protocol, to accommodate more frail individuals (i.e., those with weaker hearts and the elderly). To accomplish this, the stress testing protocol is modified with two lighter stages (or warm-up periods) before reaching the same speed and grade as the Bruce protocol. Similar endpoints are used with a modified stress test; however, the target heart rate may be reduced in those who had a recent heart attack or coronary intervention procedure.

Your doctor may also perform a nuclear stress test. Here, a radioisotope is injected into your vein, and images of your heart are taken during the stress test to identify whether all areas of the heart muscle are receiving enough blood. This study can thus help determine if blockages are present. This test might be more useful in people with an abnormal ECG, with a prior heart condition or heart-related risk factors, or having a body that is unusual or large.

In addition to a regular nuclear stress test, certain drugs such as dipyridamole (Persantine), adenosine, or dobutamine may be administered to help facilitate the test if the patient cannot walk or run for a sufficient length of time. These medications allow the test to be performed without the patient exercising. Specifically, the patient can remain supine during the test, and the medication administered produces a pharmacologic stress test.

Alternatively, a stress test may be followed by an echocardiogram to help demonstrate whether the heart muscle itself functions appropriately under stress. This technique is called a stress echocardiogram and provides very similar information as is obtained during a nuclear stress test. The CT angiogram, cardiac MRI, and/or PET scan (see Chap. 20) may also be useful in evaluating possible obstructive coronary artery disease.

The most definitive test for coronary artery disease (although invasive) is a cardiac catheterization, also known as a coronary angiogram (see Chap. 23). During this procedure, a tube (catheter) is inserted into the radial artery in the wrist or the

Table 17.1 Stress test facts

Stress tests are useful for diagnosing blockages and predicting heart attacks.
They can reveal rhythm problems by bringing on symptoms.
They are not as definitive as a CT angiogram or cardiac catheterization, which both show pictures of the coronary arteries (the vessels that supply the heart with oxygenated blood).
Stress tests are useful for sedentary patients before they begin an exercise regimen, to evaluate whether exercise is safe for them.
Stress tests are useful as part of the preoperative work-up for elderly patients and those with heart risks before they undergo major surgery.

Table 17.2 Indications for stress testing

Determination of physical fitness before exercise regimen or stressor
Evaluation of chest pain/discomfort or shortness of breath
Evaluation of heart failure
Assessing for functional capacity and exercise-induced arrhythmias
Preoperative clearance for surgery
Following heart attack, coronary artery bypass surgery, or PCI to assess status and effectiveness of therapy and to prescribe activities

Note: Stress test is contraindicated in those with a very recent heart attack, unstable angina, severe heart failure at rest, and suspected severe aortic stenosis or aortic dissection

femoral artery in the groin, and a catheter is inserted into the arteries that lead to the heart. Contrast dye is injected, and imaging may be performed through cinefluoroscopy (a type of radiation) to help diagnose a blockage. Discrete blockages can often be effectively treated with a stent, and more extensive disease can be treated by coronary artery bypass surgery.

A review of some stress test facts is presented in Table 17.1. Table 17.2 shows some common indications for stress tests. Stress tests are very useful for evaluation of chest pain or shortness of breath of unknown etiology, for assessing arrhythmias or heart block related to exertion, before beginning a new exercise regimen or stressor, for clearance before surgery, for evaluating heart failure, for evaluating the effects of medications, for determining the need for bypass surgery or PCI, and for risk assessment following a heart attack. Note that stress testing may be contraindicated in those with a recent heart attack, unstable angina (chest pain at rest), severe heart failure, severe aortic stenosis, or suspected aortic dissection.

Preparation for Cardiac Procedures

Before any of these procedures, patients typically need instructions from their healthcare provider in order to get the most out of a test. For noninvasive tests, this may include information regarding medications as well as information regarding the location, time, and attire for the test (running shoes, etc.). For invasive procedures, patients may need presurgical testing, which may be provided by an outside laboratory (organized by the operating physician) or provided by the hospital or medical center (organized by the facility).

Table 17.3 Preparation for cardiac procedures

"Nothing by mouth," also known as "nil per os" (NPO)
For many cardiac procedures, you may be directed by your physician not to eat or drink after midnight before the scheduled procedure, including coffee and orange juice. Only a sip of water with routine medications is allowed, and only if permitted by your doctor. Ask your doctor if you can take all your medications, or if you should take only some of them—or even none of them.

Blood thinners and antiplatelet medications
Ask your doctor if you should continue taking blood thinners and antiplatelet medications before surgery. Some invasive procedures may require that you stop taking these medications a few days before the procedure. **Always check with your physician before stopping blood thinners or antiplatelet medications**. In most circumstances, antiplatelet medications should not be discontinued. Sometimes, the physician will choose to stop the oral blood thinner and instead prescribe an injectable form or admit you to the hospital for intravenous blood thinners. This is done to bridge your anticoagulation therapy and decrease your risk of stroke.

Testing before an invasive procedure may include analysis of your electrolytes, blood count, urinalysis, coagulation status, an ECG, type and screen, and a chest X-ray. A type and screen of your blood can help identify your blood type, in case a transfusion is required. Information for patients preparing for cardiac procedures is detailed in Table 17.3. For all stress tests and all invasive procedures, the patient must have nothing by mouth (also called NPO) for at least 8 hours before the procedure. Other noninvasive tests, such as an echocardiogram, may not be affected by eating before the procedure.

In the early period following the COVID-19 pandemic, all patients required testing for the viral antigen within 48 hours of their in-hospital procedure. In addition, the doctor may ask the patient to stop taking blood thinners (or continue them) and antiplatelet medications, such as acetylsalicylic acid (aspirin) and clopidogrel (Plavix), before a procedure. If you have any questions about how to prepare for a diagnostic test or a surgical procedure, ask your doctor well before the test is scheduled.

Echocardiogram

18

Todd J. Cohen

An echocardiogram, also called an echo or a cardiac ultrasound, is an ultrasound technique that uses sound waves to create images of the heart. It is one of the most useful cardiac tests performed by the doctor and is a noninvasive and safe test. It specifically provides information about your heart's structure and function. This test can reveal your heart's ejection fraction (EF), the presence of leaky or tight (stenotic) valves, weak heart muscles (cardiomyopathies), thick heart muscles (hypertrophy), blood clots or masses in your heart, or fluid in the sac around the heart (the pericardium).

The EF, when specified alone, refers to how well your left ventricle contracts. The doctor would specify "right ventricular EF" if that chamber's function is being referenced. The EF is a number that all heart disease patients should know and can be recorded in Appendix I: Know Your Numbers at the end of this book. A normal EF is between 50% and 70% (see heart failure, Chap. 14). The echocardiogram is also useful in showing the presence and location of a heart attack. Figure 18.1 shows a standard echocardiogram machine. Figure 18.2 shows an echocardiographic image obtained during this test, which is very similar to that which may be seen during a regular echocardiogram. Note the color in the image, which shows the flow of blood through the mitral valve (called color Doppler). Typically, the heart structure is shown in black and white, and valve function and flow can be seen using the color Doppler ultrasound function.

T. J. Cohen (✉)
NYIT College of Osteopathic Medicine, New York, NY, USA
e-mail: tcohen03@nyit.edu

© The Author(s), under exclusive license to Springer Nature Switzerland AG 2025
T. J. Cohen, R. S. Blumenthal (eds.), *Surviving and Thriving With Heart Disease*,
Contemporary Cardiology, https://doi.org/10.1007/978-3-032-00579-3_18

Fig. 18.1 This figure shows an echocardiogram machine that uses ultrasound and Doppler technology to evaluate the structure and function of the heart

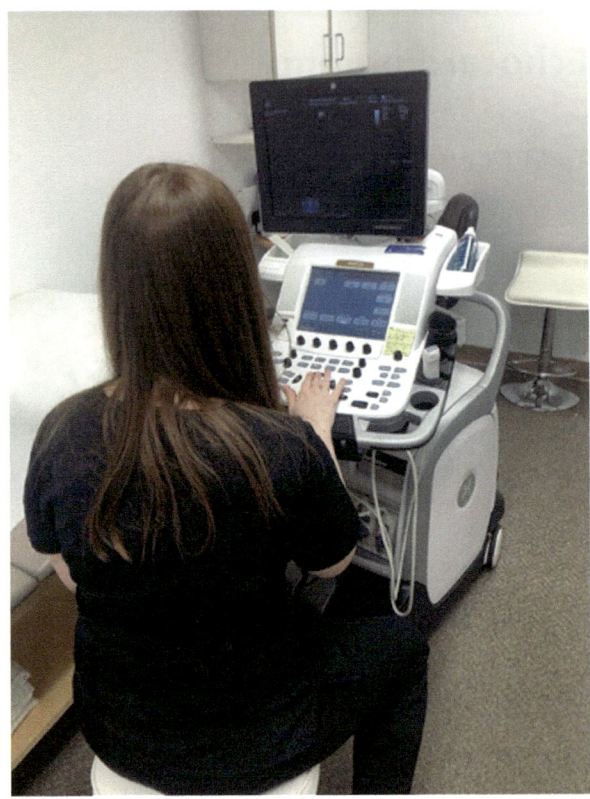

Sometimes this test is performed through the esophagus (called a *transesopha-geal echocardiogram*), where it is particularly useful in looking for the presence of blood clots in the left atrium. The patient is typically sedated by an anesthesiologist, and a transesophageal probe is inserted down the esophagus to image the heart and valvular structures, as well as the aorta. Blood clots may form in the left atrial appendage (a site that is not well visualized by standard echocardiogram but can be visualized by the transesophageal procedure). This test is used frequently in patients who have a history of atrial fibrillation and have not been taking adequate blood thinners, or taking blood thinners long enough. If no clot is seen on the transesopha-geal echocardiogram, it may be safe to proceed with electrical cardioversion (shock) to convert atrial fibrillation safely (see Chap. 26). The transesophageal echocardio-gram is also important to perform before the Watchman-type procedure (see Chap. 32), in which a device is placed in the left atrium in order to prevent an embolic stroke. If a left atrial appendage clot is identified, it would be unsafe to proceed with this test, since device placement might dislodge the clot and cause a stroke.

Fig. 18.2 This figure shows an echocardiographic image of the heart. Doppler is particularly helpful at demonstrating valvular function (stenosis and regurgitation) as well as shunts in the heart wall. It is indicated by the white, red, and blue colors that traverse the valve. Color Doppler can help identify stagnant flow in the atrial appendage which may put a patient at risk for clot formation and a possible stroke

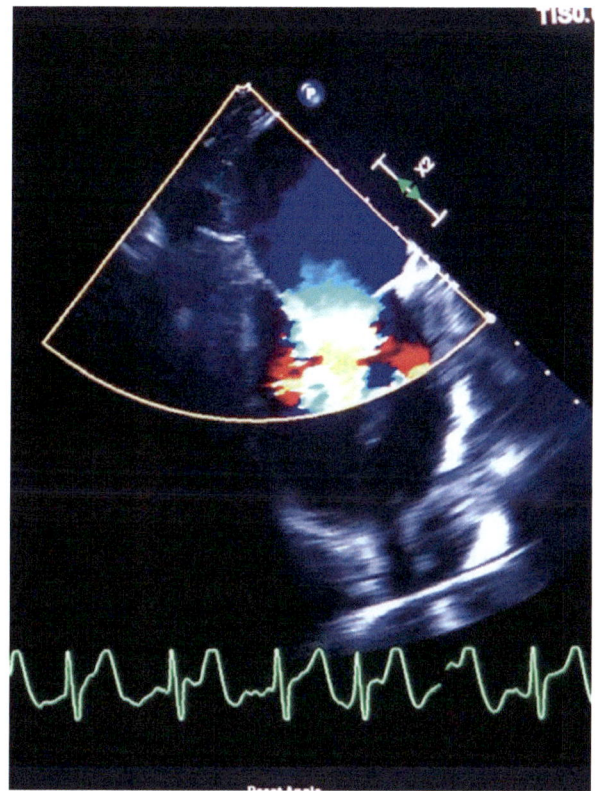

An echocardiogram can be performed together with a stress test (a stress echocardiogram procedure) to identify the presence of a significantly blocked coronary artery. As described in the stress testing chapter (Chap. 17), this test can provide similar information as that obtained during a nuclear stress test. Imaging may be difficult in obese individuals, and a nuclear study may be preferable. Additionally, agitated saline could be administered during a standard echocardiogram while the patient bears down (Valsalva maneuver). This could reveal a hole in the heart (septal defect in the atrium or ventricle), or the presence of a functional flap between the right and left atrium (called a patent foramen ovale). Such a hole may be important in individuals who have symptoms of heart failure or who have experienced a stroke. If the hole is large enough, it may be seen by color Doppler.

Table 18.1 Echocardiogram facts

An echocardiogram (also called an echo) is safe: it uses only sound waves.
An echo can provide useful images of the heart, its valves, its function, and the presence of fluid around the heart or masses in the heart.
It can help determine the ejection fraction (EF).
It can be used with a stress test and provide similar information as obtained during a nuclear stress test.
A bubble study can identify septal defects (holes in the heart's septum) and a patent foramen ovale (flap between the right and left atrium).
Intracardiac echocardiography (ICE) can help guide a transseptal puncture for left-sided heart procedures (such as an atrial fibrillation ablation) and can identify pericardial effusion as a complication during the procedure.

Ultrasound has been incorporated into a catheter and used for procedures such as catheter ablation. This intracardiac echo (ICE) catheter can help visualize internal structures, as well as catheter contact and lesion formation, guide the transseptal procedure, and monitor for pericardial effusion formation (a sign of a perforation) during the procedure. For a summary of key facts about this useful and safe test, see Table 18.1.

Monitoring Devices (Wearable and Implantable)

19

Todd J. Cohen

Your doctor may try to uncover the precise nature of your symptoms and your potential heart disease problem. Monitoring devices come in all shapes and sizes. Specifically, there are wearable or pocketable devices (such as a smartphone) that can record your activity, distance, steps, as well as your heart rhythm. Kardia (or KardiaMobile) is a commercial application (available through AliveCor; www.alivecor.com) that combines with your smartphone and allows the recording of your ECG, which can then be shared with your healthcare provider. Figure 19.1 shows an ECG strip used with Kardia, showing a sinus rhythm. Some smartphones can pair with a wearable watch that itself can record health-related information, including your ECG.

Throughout the book, useful information is provided to educate patients and their families on a wide variety of wearable and implantable heart monitoring devices. Table 19.1 reviews some of the devices that can help monitor patients with heart disease. Please see the individual chapters throughout the book to learn more about these devices.

T. J. Cohen (✉)
NYIT College of Osteopathic Medicine, New York, NY, USA
e-mail: tcohen03@nyit.edu

© The Author(s), under exclusive license to Springer Nature Switzerland AG 2025
T. J. Cohen, R. S. Blumenthal (eds.), *Surviving and Thriving With Heart Disease*,
Contemporary Cardiology, https://doi.org/10.1007/978-3-032-00579-3_19

EKG Summary

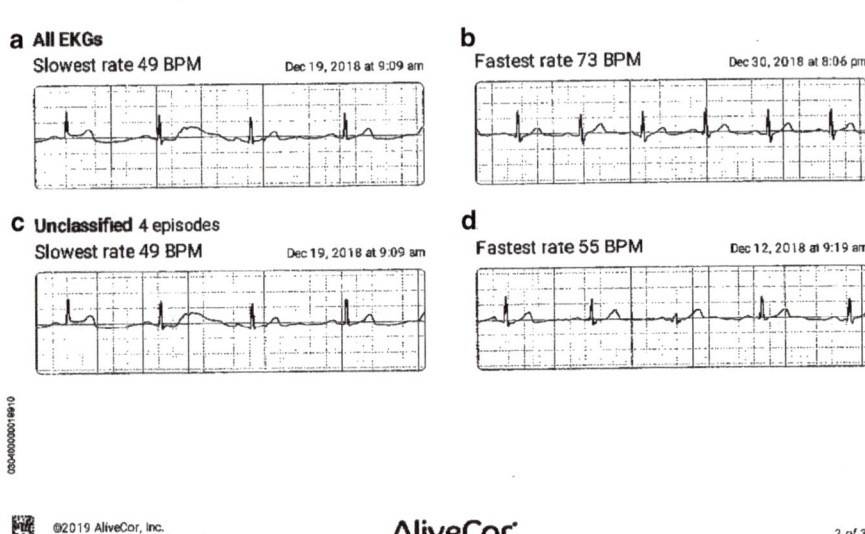

Fig. 19.1 This figure shows a tracing obtained using a smartphone and the KardiaMobile (or Kardia) application (App). The figure shows a sinus rhythm, though at other times this detected atrial fibrillation. The system is available through AliveCor (www.alivecor.com)

Table 19.1 Some wearable and implantable devices useful to those with heart disease

Holter monitor, loop recorder, and event recorder
Smartphones and accessories such as Kardia
Smartwatches such as those made by Apple, Fitbit, and Google
Implantable loop recorder, pacemaker, and implantable defibrillator
Wearable blood pressure monitor (arm and wrist)
Vagus nerve stimulator and insulin pump
Ventricular assist device and artificial heart

Wearables

The Apple Heart Study demonstrated that the Apple Watch is capable of identifying atrial fibrillation in a large population. The nice thing about the Apple Watch and other smartwatches (such as those manufactured by Google) is that they do not have to be prescribed by a physician. Family members and relatives of those with heart disease may use these devices as an adjunct to monitor their health, since those individuals may be at higher risk of also getting heart disease.

Other wearable devices exist in the form of skin patches that contain ECG electrodes and recording circuitry (such as the CAM Patch, manufactured by Bardy Diagnostics Inc., Bellevue, WA, and the Zio Patch, manufactured by iRhythm Technologies, San Francisco, CA), which can record heart rhythm telemetry and

Fig. 19.2 This figure shows a small compact white medical device (DMS 300, DM Software, Stateline, Nevada) that is battery-powered and hooks up to disposable electrodes. The device was extremely helpful during the COVID-19 pandemic, as point-of-service care was provided to patients even during sheltering in place orders, allowing them to receive Holter monitoring and real-time telemetry monitoring without coming into the office

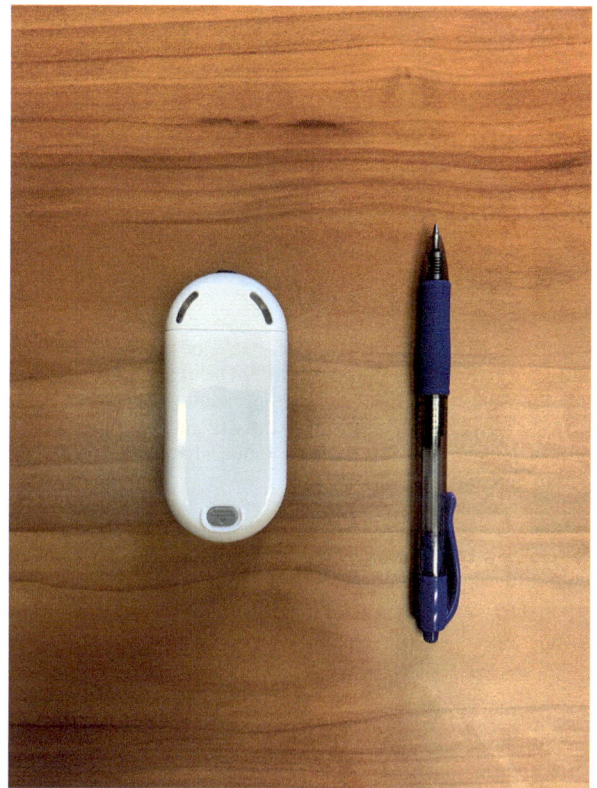

events for 24 hours (called a Holter monitor) or longer (extended telemetry up to 14 days). A similar device can be used for real-time telemetry recordings over a longer period of time, such as 1 week.

Figure 19.2 shows one example of a real-time telemetry recorder called the DMS 300 (DM Software, Stateline, Nevada), which clips to electrodes and is placed on the chest. Wearable short- and long-term blood pressure monitors (wrist and around arm) also have high utility to patients and their physicians. Wearable devices are only useful when "worn." These devices may occasionally create artifacts through the electrode or sensor skin interface and may not always be reliable. Chapter 49 tells you more information about some useful applications that may help improve your quality of life.

Implantables

An alternative to wearable devices is implantable devices, which can continuously monitor heart rhythms (ECGs) as well as other physiologic events. Implantable devices, although placed through an invasive procedure, have a "set it, forget it" utility. These devices do not require recharging, and one can shower and swim

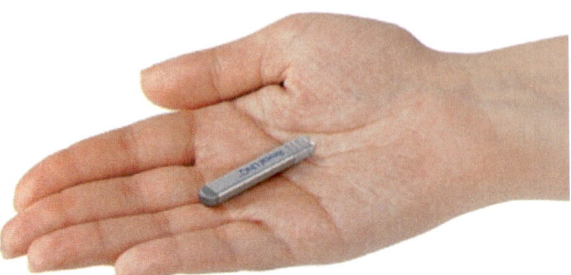

Fig. 19.3 This figure shows an injectable loop recorder (called the Revel LinQ, manufactured by Medtronics Inc.). This device can record heart rhythms remotely for up to 3 years and is useful for detecting and correlating heart rhythms with symptoms, as well as identifying atrial fibrillation in patients with a history of embolic stroke of unknown etiology. (Reproduced with permission from HMP Communications LLC from Practical Electrophysiology, Third Edition; Reproduced with permission of Medtronic, Inc.)

without having to remove the device. One example of an implantable device is the implantable loop recorder (Fig. 19.3). This is a tiny, paperclip-sized device that can be injected under the skin (typically to the left of the chest bone). This device pairs either with a phone or an external communicator to send regular reports and programmed detected alerts to the monitoring healthcare provider. Implantable loop recorders can last over 4 years and allow the clinician the ability to identify infrequent heart rhythm problems, correlate symptoms, and assess the efficacy of treatments.

Other heart rhythm-controlling devices (such as pacemakers, defibrillators, and cardiac resynchronization devices) can record similar and even more complicated events. Certain pacemakers and most implantable defibrillators can also record fluid accumulation (typically the result of congestive heart failure) and may help treat this chronic disease. Additionally, a small implant can be placed in the pulmonary artery, which can permit the remote monitoring of heart failure and its response to treatment.

Other Devices

Other wearable and implantable devices exist to control diabetes (glucose sensors and pumps), as well as seizure disorders (EEG sensors and vagus nerve stimulators). Other drug delivery pumps can be worn or implanted to routinely deliver critical medical therapy. Patients with heart failure can benefit from cardiac resynchronization devices to improve their performance. Finally, ventricular assist devices exist in both a temporary or more permanent form that enhance the severely diseased patient who is refractory to medications and other more routine implantable devices.

Many of these patients will improve, but younger patients without terminal diseases that don't improve may require a heart transplant. If a heart is not readily available, patients may temporarily be given a total artificial heart.

Computerized Axial Tomography (CT) Angiogram, Cardiac Magnetic Resonance Imaging (MRI), and PET Scan

20

Todd J. Cohen

A variety of imaging techniques exist that can help reveal the heart and its function and structures. Table 20.1 reviews some similarities and differences between a CT angiogram, cardiac MRI, and PET scan. Cardiologists and radiologists skilled in using these imaging modalities may help the electrophysiologist gain a better understanding of your heart and help guide the electrophysiologist's interventions.

Table 20.1 CT angiogram, cardiac MRI, and PET scan

CT angiogram, cardiac MRI, and PET scan are all noninvasive heart imaging procedures.
CT angiogram is associated with a heavy dye load.
CT angiogram can image the coronary arteries and detect blockages.
Cardiac MRI does not utilize dye or a nuclear tracer injection.
Cardiac MRI can diagnose arrhythmogenic right ventricular cardiomyopathy/dysplasia (ARVC/D).
PET scan uses a nuclear tracer (similar to a nuclear stress test).
PET scan can detect heart metabolism and lack of blood flow to the heart muscle.

T. J. Cohen (✉)
NYIT College of Osteopathic Medicine, New York, NY, USA
e-mail: tcohen03@nyit.edu

© The Author(s), under exclusive license to Springer Nature Switzerland AG 2025
T. J. Cohen, R. S. Blumenthal (eds.), *Surviving and Thriving With Heart Disease*,
Contemporary Cardiology, https://doi.org/10.1007/978-3-032-00579-3_20

127

CT Angiogram

A test called a CT angiogram may be useful in demonstrating heart function and visualizing the arteries to the heart. CT angiogram helps diagnose coronary artery disease by looking directly at the coronary arteries. Direct visualization of the heart is difficult since it is constantly moving, and techniques continue to be developed to obtain adequate images.

During this procedure, you are given contrast dye intravenously and exposed to an amount of radiation comparable to having a cardiac angiogram. Notify your doctor if you have any known allergies to contrast dye, so he or she can take measures to avoid you having an allergic reaction during the procedure.

Cardiac Magnetic Resonance Imaging (MRI)

Similar to a CT angiogram, the cardiac MRI also takes images of the heart to diagnose coronary artery disease, assess damage caused by a previous heart attack, and diagnose heart failure as well as valve problems. This form of MRI is a useful test that usually poses no serious threat to the patient, except for some with a metallic implantable device (such as an implantable defibrillator).

The cardiac MRI provides limited visualization of arteries but is particularly useful for looking for an inherited condition called *arrhythmogenic right ventricular cardiomyopathy/dysplasia* (in which fat deposits are seen within the wall of the right ventricle). The cardiac MRI can determine whether certain criteria exist that can help confirm this diagnosis. Patients with this disorder may be at high risk for sudden cardiac arrest and ventricular tachycardia and should be considered candidates for an implantable cardioverter defibrillator (ICD). In addition, CT angiography and cardiac MRI may both be useful for visualizing the pulmonary veins and the left atrium (which is useful during an atrial fibrillation ablation).

PET Scan

A positron emission transmission (or PET) scan can be very useful for seeing how well the heart muscle itself is working. A nuclear tracer is injected through a vein (similar to what happens during a nuclear stress test) to identify differences in heart metabolism. Although it might not always be available, it can provide additional information above and beyond the normal nuclear stress test. Please talk to your cardiologist to see if you might benefit from this test, especially if a nuclear stress test is inconclusive.

Electrophysiology Study (EP Study)

21

Todd J. Cohen

Introduction

The electrophysiology study (EP study) is a crucial procedure for identifying heart rhythm problems. This invasive test is typically administered to patients who are thought to have some type of arrhythmia and can reveal if you need a pacemaker or defibrillator. In addition, this test can help to identify the precise type of rapid heart rhythm (tachycardia) that you have. An EP study is useful for diagnosing unexplained rhythm problems, syncope, unexplained palpitations, or lightheadedness. It is also effective for performing a curative procedure such as catheter ablation or determining whether there is a need for an implantable device therapy (see Table 21.1). Appendix A presents a more in-depth list of the indications for an EP study obtained from a consensus statement from the American College of Cardiology, American Heart Association, and Heart Rhythm Society guidelines.

Table 21.1 When do you need an EP study?

To diagnose unexplained rhythm problems
To determine the cause of fainting or blacking out (syncope)
To diagnose unexplained palpitations, light-headedness, or dizziness (presyncope)
To cure a rhythm problem with a catheter ablation procedure
To determine if you need a pacemaker or defibrillator

T. J. Cohen (✉)
NYIT College of Osteopathic Medicine, New York, NY, USA
e-mail: tcohen03@nyit.edu

Procedure

An EP study is performed in a specially equipped room called the EP lab, using specialized stimulating equipment and recording technology to assess the heart's electrical system (Fig. 21.1). The electrophysiologist (heart rhythm specialist) may choose to use mapping equipment to locate the area where the abnormal heart rhythm is originating. For this procedure, you must have specialized pads placed on your chest and upper back (which can be used to shock you if necessary), and an

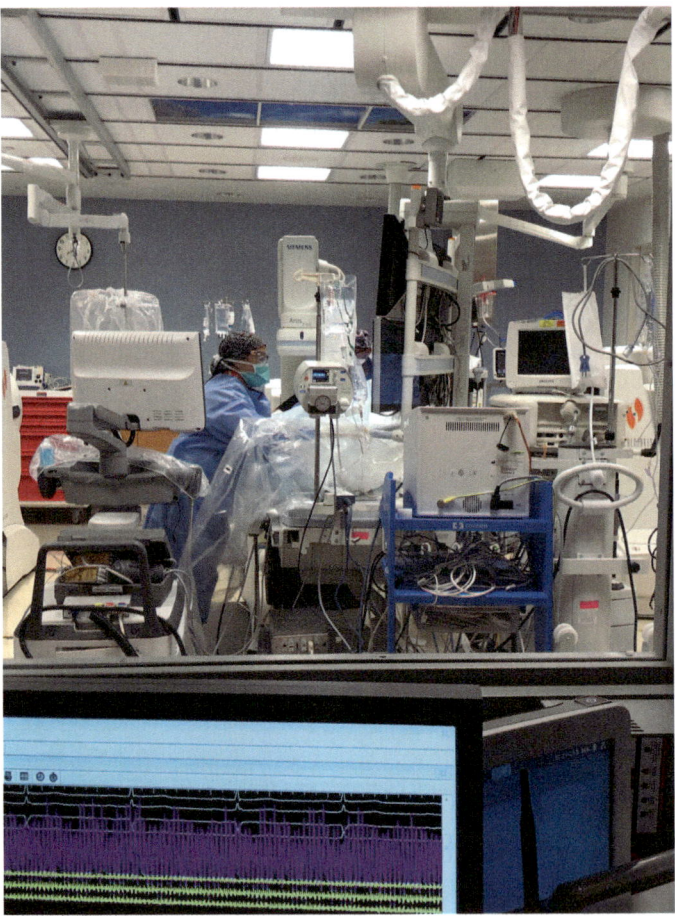

Fig. 21.1 An electrophysiology laboratory. A typical lab consists of a procedural table; X-ray imaging equipment; computerized equipment for monitoring, recording, analyzing, and imaging; mapping/ablation equipment; electrical stimulating equipment; and a defibrillator. Shown here is a state-of-the-art laboratory from Mount Sinai Morningside Hospital, one of the author's preferred hospitals. This laboratory includes a Stereotaxis system which can be used for remote magnetic navigation. The laboratory is also often used to implant heart rhythm-controlling devices such as pacemakers and defibrillators. The Watchman procedure may also be performed in this laboratory

intravenous line must be inserted. Continuous monitoring of the ECG and blood pressure is essential throughout this procedure.

During the EP study, catheters are guided through blood vessels into the heart using an X-ray technique called *fluoroscopy imaging*. The catheters are placed through the veins, arteries, or both up into the chambers of the heart. Electrical signals are recorded directly from the heart. From this electrophysiology (EP) catheter, the doctor is capable of pacing (stimulating) your heart at a faster rate than normal and recording the signals.

Concurrent Procedures

Sometimes during this test, the doctor decides to utilize another procedure at the same time called catheter ablation, in which the rhythm is mapped and treated with energy, such as radio waves, to cure the abnormality. While undergoing such a procedure, you may be given a shock by the doctor, if necessary, to terminate a significant arrhythmia such as ventricular tachycardia or fibrillation. When a shock is unsynchronized, it is called *defibrillation*; when it is synchronized, it is called *cardioversion*. An external defibrillator, which can be used to shock a patient out of tachycardia, is pictured in Fig. 21.2. As with any test, it is important to communicate

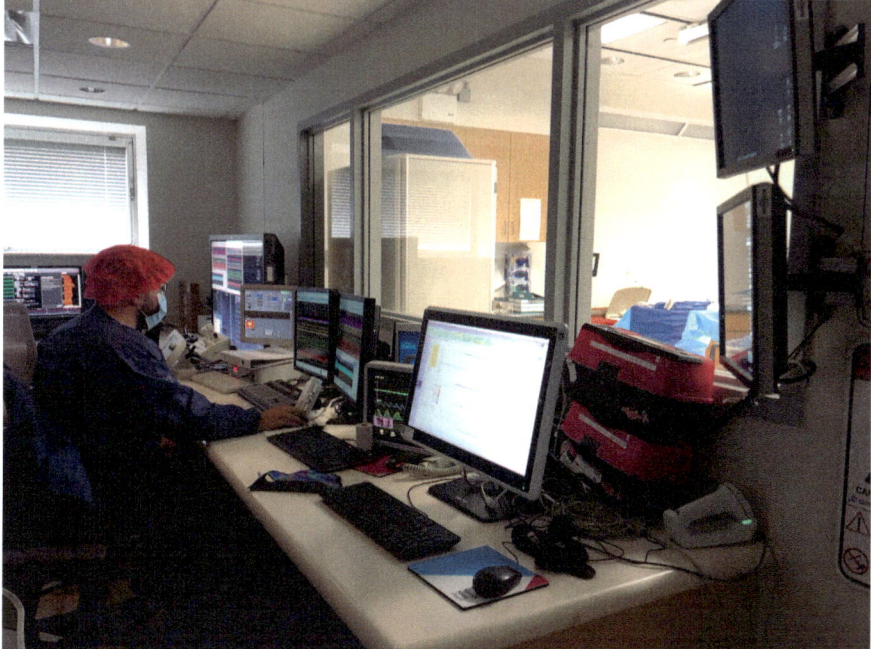

Fig. 21.2 The control room where the operator and staff can remotely stimulate and treat heart rhythm problems without wearing lead. Stereotaxis permits the remote manipulation of mapping and ablation catheters using a magnetic field in the lab, all controlled from this control room

Fig. 21.3 The book's co-author (Dr. Todd Cohen) wearing an SR headband for radiation protection, as well as the EZ Holder TM, both his inventions. The former helps minimize radiation to the operator, and the latter helps hold the catheters in position, and minimizes radiation to both patient and operator, by avoiding unnecessary catheter repositioning under fluoroscopy

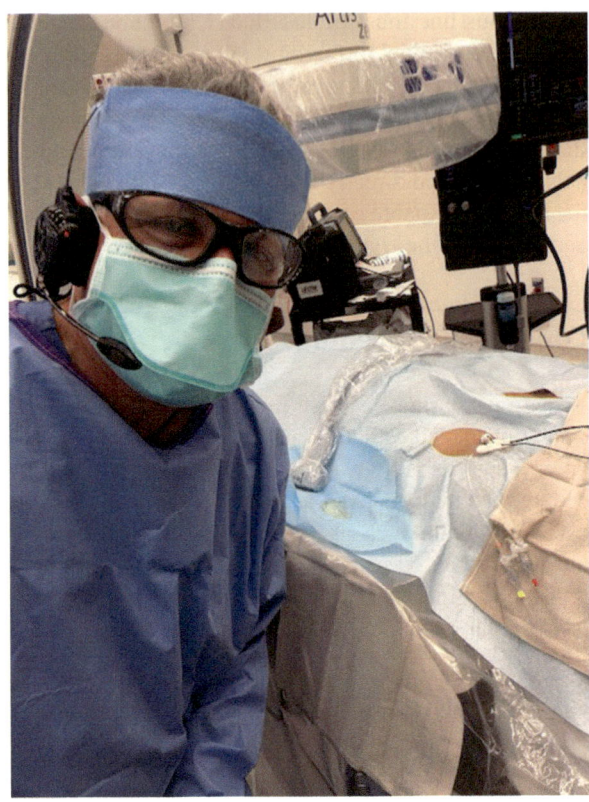

with the facility's staff and let them know if you are experiencing symptoms such as palpitations, chest pain, or any discomfort.

Figure 21.3 shows coauthor, Dr. Todd Cohen, in the electrophysiology laboratory with two of his inventions. First, he is wearing the SR Headband manufactured by TZ Medical in Oswego, Oregon, which helps prevent radiation exposure to the operator's brain. Second, the EZ Holder TM is a simple inexpensive adhesive device (also manufactured by TZ Medical) that helps hold electrophysiology and ablation catheters in place, avoiding unnecessary patient and operator exposure to radiation, which can occur when these catheters lose their position and require fluoroscopic repositioning.

Risks and Benefits

Patients need to understand the risks, benefits, and alternatives to this invasive procedure. The risks include bleeding, clot formation, perforation, heart attack, cardiac arrest, stroke, and death. Major complications are uncommon. Your doctor may provide some sedation during the procedure to make you more comfortable. You may feel the sensation of a fast heart rate, which may be similar to your symptoms of palpitations or flutters in the chest. This procedure is performed in a carefully controlled setting in the presence of the doctor and qualified and trained support staff.

Tilt Table Test

22

Todd J. Cohen

A tilt table test is a simple, noninvasive test used to investigate lightheadedness, dizziness, and loss of consciousness (syncope). The purpose of this test is to try to replicate your symptoms and potentially provoke a syncopal episode. A positive test result may show a drop in blood pressure with or without a significant change in heart rate.

During this procedure, you lie down on a specialized table that can be tilted nearly upright at an angle prescribed by the doctor (usually 60–80°) for up to 45 minutes (Fig. 22.1). Electrodes are placed on your chest, and an intravenous line is put in a vein. The test may be performed passively, that is, without any medication infused. Alternatively, a medicine may be infused into the intravenous line to provoke the response and possibly elicit a positive test result—an abnormal heart rate or rhythm and possible blood vessel response in which your blood pressure may drop and your heart rate slows down. This reaction is called neurocardiogenic, or vasovagal, syncope.

If this reaction occurs, the table will be adjusted downward, you will be placed flat, and your symptoms will normally subside within seconds. If your heart rate drops significantly and symptoms such as unresponsiveness or persistent slow heart rate (bradycardia) occur, you will be treated immediately with medications or the doctor may choose to pace (stimulate) your heart through specialized pacing pads.

T. J. Cohen (✉)
NYIT College of Osteopathic Medicine, New York, NY, USA
e-mail: tcohen03@nyit.edu

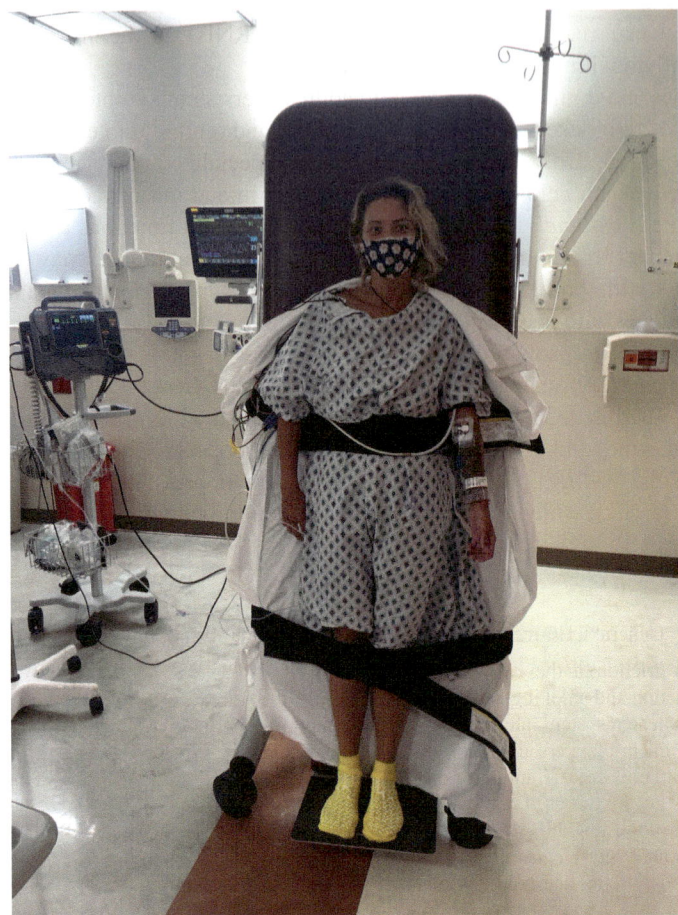

Fig. 22.1 An upright tilt table, which is used to elicit syncope in susceptible patients. The patient is fastened to the table, and it is brought nearly upright in order to evaluate the patient's heart rate and blood pressure response to an upright position. An intravenous medication may be administered to facilitate the test

Vasovagal Syncope

Figure 22.2 shows the mechanism behind neurocardiogenic (or vasovagal) syncope. Blood pools in the lower extremities while standing that triggers a release of adrenaline and vigorous heart contraction. This stretches specialized heart receptors that trigger a vagal response, causing a drop in blood pressure (hypotension) and slowing of the heart rate (bradycardia). Neurocardiogenic (or vasovagal) syncope is an exaggerated response to a normal reflex and can be treated with conservative measures including increasing hydration with electrolyte solutions, compression stockings, education about moving your lower extremities, not standing still for a long

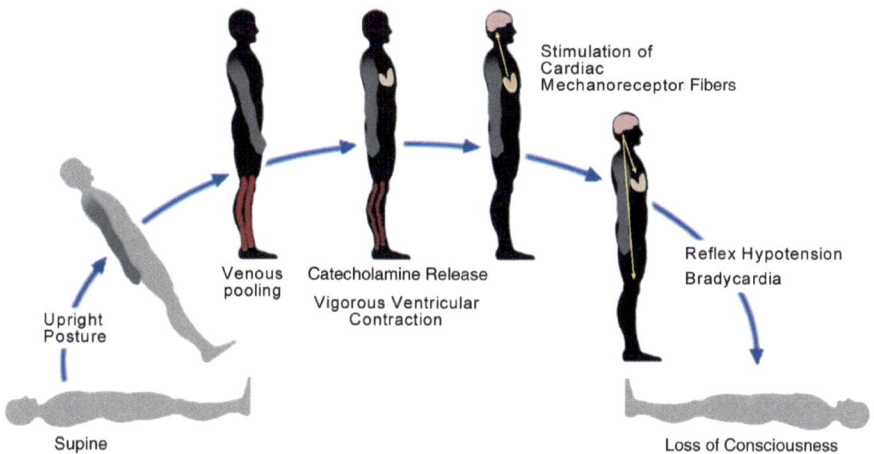

Fig. 22.2 This figure demonstrates the reflex that triggers a vasovagal response (neurocardiogenic syncope). Patients may be standing upright and blood pools in the legs. The lack of blood returning to the heart triggers a release of adrenaline that causes the heart to contract, which stimulates specialized fibers that cause the blood pressure to drop and heart rate to slow. (Courtesy of HMP Communications LLC from Practical Electrophysiology, Third Edition)

period of time, and increased salt intake. Occasionally, medications such as beta-blockers, midodrine (Proamatine), and fludrocortisone (Florinef) may help (see Chap. 10).

Postural Orthostatic Tachycardia Syndrome (POTS)

Many patients have a condition in which their heart rate races when they stand up. Sometimes this is associated with a drop in blood pressure and can make the patient lightheaded and even pass out. When the heart rate increases by 30 beats per minute or more within 10 minutes of standing, or exceeds 120 beats per minute, the patient may have a condition called postural orthostatic tachycardia syndrome (POTS). People with this condition have an abnormal autonomic nervous system, also called dysautonomia. POTS is more common in women and can be associated with autoimmune disorders like systemic lupus erythematosus, Sjogren's syndrome, mast cell disorders, Chiari malformation, diabetes, deconditioning, mononucleosis, Lyme disease, and paraneoplastic diseases. POTS is also common in connective tissue disorders such as Ehlers-Danlos syndrome, hypermobility spectrum disorder, and Marfan's syndrome (see Chap. 45).

POTS is usually treated initially with conservative measures, which include increased hydration with electrolyte solutions, increased salt intake, and compression stockings. If this condition persists or is more severe, medications (such as beta-blockers, midodrine, and fludrocortisone) may be warranted. Rarely, more aggressive measures including stronger medications and/or a port for regular intravenous saline infusions may be needed. Please talk to a specialist if you are diagnosed with this condition.

Risks and Benefits

Many patients have a misconception that the tilt table test is one in which the patient's head is tilted back. Some patients come in for the test thinking it is going to be much like a ride at an amusement park (the Tilt-a-Whirl). This test is more like standing straight upright for a prolonged period in the same spot, as though you were waiting in a long line. The tilt table test is relatively safe and is unlikely to result in any serious complications. Frequent and clear communication between the patient and the staff is essential. Also, like other heart tests, this test is not perfect and can miss the diagnosis in some patients. Table 22.1 lists some important facts on tilt table testing.

Table 22.1 Tilt table facts

Simple noninvasive test
You are not placed upside down but rather stood up for a period of time
Useful at diagnosing vasovagal, orthostatic hypotension including POTS, dysautonomia
Can be performed without any medication infusion (passively); or with an infusion (actively)
Can take an hour including hook-up, monitoring, etc.
May miss the diagnosis in some people

Cardiac Catheterization: Coronary Angiogram, Left Ventriculogram, and Aortogram

23

Todd J. Cohen

Based on your history and medical condition, your doctor may recommend an invasive procedure called a *cardiac catheterization*. This procedure is performed in a specialized laboratory (called a catheterization laboratory or cath lab) under X-ray visualization (called cinefluoroscopy) by placing catheters (tubes) through sheaths into the blood vessels (artery and/or vein) and threading the catheters into the heart. This procedure is typically performed from a blood vessel (artery) from the groin or the wrist. Patients are given sedation before or during the procedure so they feel more comfortable. Contrast dye is administered to visualize structures, and pressures are recorded to determine heart and valve function. *Please tell your doctor if you have a contrast dye allergy or a shellfish allergy before the procedure. In addition, you should notify your doctor if you are allergic to latex.*

A cardiac catheterization may have several components. The following are just some of the types of cardiac catheterization procedures that may be performed. Table 23.1 shows some important facts related to cardiac catheterization, left ventriculogram, and aortogram.

T. J. Cohen (✉)
NYIT College of Osteopathic Medicine, New York, NY, USA
e-mail: tcohen03@nyit.edu

© The Author(s), under exclusive license to Springer Nature Switzerland AG 2025
T. J. Cohen, R. S. Blumenthal (eds.), *Surviving and Thriving With Heart Disease*,
Contemporary Cardiology, https://doi.org/10.1007/978-3-032-00579-3_23

Table 23.1 Cath/LV angiogram/aortogram facts

Cardiac catheterization or angiogram is an invasive test.

Performed from groin or wrist.

Requires dye typically containing iodine (please tell your doctor if you have an iodine, dye, or shellfish allergy).

LV angiogram can define your ejection fraction (or EF); your EF is an important number to know if you have heart disease, and typically should be greater than 50%.

Aortogram can visualize the aortic root, identify aneurysms and dissection, or aortic valve disease.

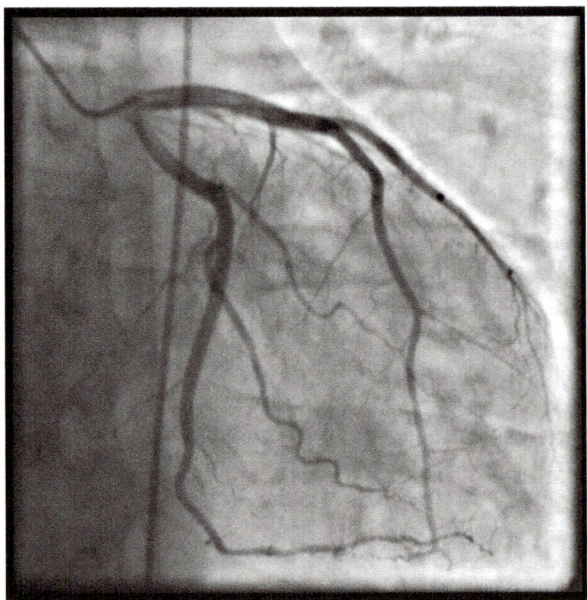

Fig. 23.1 Visualization of the left coronary artery during a coronary angiogram. A catheter was inserted into the femoral artery in the groin and manipulated around the aorta into the opening of the left coronary artery. Contrast dye was then injected and cinefluoroscopic images were recorded. Additional images and views were recorded to completely image the coronary artery anatomy. (Adapted from T.J. Cohen, *A Patient's Guide to Heart Rhythm Problems* (Baltimore, MD: The Johns Hopkins University Press, 2010), p. 74)

Coronary Angiogram

The coronary arteries and any blockages can be visualized by injecting contrast dye. The type of image obtained from a coronary angiogram is shown in Fig. 23.1.

Left Ventriculogram

A pigtail catheter (one in which the end curls around like the tail of a pig in order to provide a safe blunt end) is advanced around the aorta and across the aortic valve, and contrast dye is injected into the left ventricle to visualize its function and calculate the ejection fraction (EF). Your EF is an indicator of the heart's function and is normally above 50%. If you have heart disease, know your EF. During a left ventriculogram, a leaky mitral valve may be seen when the dye is injected back into the left atrium (called mitral regurgitation). The degree of mitral regurgitation can be quantified by this test.

Aortogram

This is typically performed with a pigtail catheter placed in the root of the aorta, and dye is injected to visualize the aortic root, coronary artery origins, and other blood vessels such as the left common carotid artery, left subclavian artery, and brachiocephalic artery. It can show enlargement of the aorta and leakiness of the aortic valve (aortic regurgitation). Sometimes the doctor may choose to cross the aortic valve into the ventricle and measure pressures to determine whether the aortic valve has a small or tight opening (called aortic stenosis). This test is useful in determining the degree of aortic stenosis.

Part V

Treatments (Surviving)

To survive and thrive with heart disease, you may need to undergo certain procedures. These could include percutaneous coronary intervention (PCI), cardiac catheter ablation, transcatheter aortic valve replacement (TAVR), coronary artery bypass surgery, stenting, a pacemaker or defibrillator implant, or even a heart transplant. Whatever it may be, read about it in this book, research it, and ask questions before you undergo any procedures. It is fine to get a second opinion, especially if you are uncomfortable about going through with the recommended treatment.

Percutaneous Coronary Intervention (PCI)/Stenting

24

Todd J. Cohen

Percutaneous Coronary Intervention

Procedure

Percutaneous coronary intervention (PCI) is an invasive procedure used to treat blockages within the coronary arteries. This procedure may include percutaneous transluminal coronary angioplasty (PTCA), in which a balloon catheter is placed across a coronary artery blockage to open up the occlusion, and stenting, in which metal mesh (called a *stent*) is deployed at the site to keep the blood vessel open after PTCA. Figure 24.1 shows the process in which a guidewire is placed across the blockage, and then a catheter is inserted over the guidewire, which contains the stent and balloon to open the blockage and deploy the stent (left-sided figure).

The central figure shows the balloon inflation of the catheter, which compresses the blockage and opens the stent. Once the stent is opened, the balloon can be deflated and the catheter removed (right-sided figure). The balloon itself provides angioplasty, a procedure in which the vessel is open, while the stent helps keep the vessel open. A stent may be made of bare metal, or it may be drug-coated (the latter may help prevent the artery from blocking again, in stent stenosis). Antiplatelet medications also help keep the artery open (see below). Talk to your doctor about the type of stent he or she may use prior to the procedure and understand his or her rationale.

T. J. Cohen (✉)
NYIT College of Osteopathic Medicine, New York, NY, USA
e-mail: tcohen03@nyit.edu

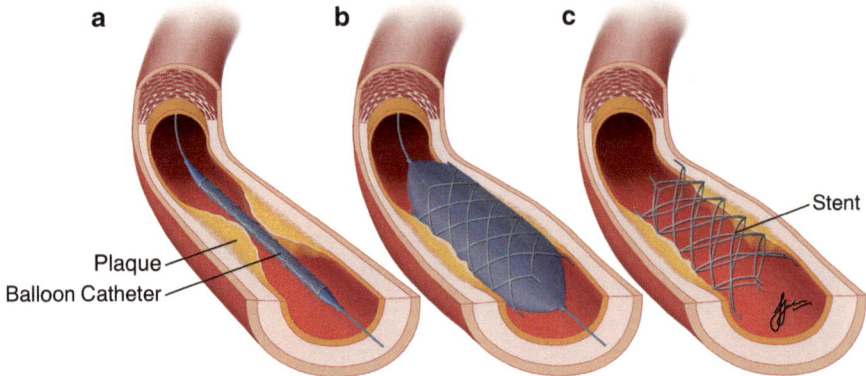

Fig. 24.1 The process in which a guidewire is placed across the blockage and then a catheter is inserted over the guidewire which contains the stent and balloon in order to open the blockage and deploy the stent. (**a**) shows a guidewire containing a balloon and the stent is placed across a blockage. (**b**) shows the balloon inflation of the catheter which compresses the blockage and opens the stent. Once the stent is open, the balloon can be deflated and the catheter removed. (**c**) shows a stent helps keep the vessel open. A stent may be made of bare metal or may be drug-coated. The latter may help prevent the artery from blocking again, in stent stenosis. Antiplatelet medications also help keep the artery open. (Figure drawn by Jerry Jose, DO)

Risks and Benefits

The risks of these procedures are less for the diagnostic studies (coronary angiogram and LV angiogram) and slightly more for the PCI procedures. These risks include bleeding, clot formation, damage to the blood vessels or heart (including perforation), contrast dye reaction (including possible injury to the kidneys), dissection of a blood vessel, coronary artery occlusion, heart attack, heart rhythm abnormality, stroke, cardiac arrest, and death. Understand that if your doctor decides to deploy a stent, there is a small risk that you might require emergent open-heart surgery.

Recovery

After any of these procedures, patients go to a recovery room for monitoring. In the recovery room, the sheaths are removed, and pressure is applied to the access sites for 15–30 minutes. To prevent bleeding, patients must lie flat for 6 hours or more after these procedures. Occasionally, special tools and devices may be used to help close the blood vessels. Your doctor will explain the test results to you and your family. Additionally, there are certain medications that your doctor will prescribe following any PCI or stent placement. These typically include aspirin and other antiplatelet agents, such as clopidogrel (Plavix), and almost always cholesterol-lowering medications such as statins. See Chap. 25 for more information on these

Table 24.1   PCI/stenting facts

Less invasive than open heart surgery.
Percutaneous coronary intervention (PCI) or stenting can treat coronary artery blockages
without cracking the chest.
Afterward, you will need to be on medications like aspirin, a cholesterol-lowering drug like a
statin, and an antiplatelet drug like clopidogrel (Plavix).
Get your stent card and have it with you at all times.

and other coronary artery disease-related medications. After stenting, you will be given a card with the manufacturer and serial number of any stents that are implanted. The card should be kept in your wallet or smartphone and always be available. Ask your doctor what you can and cannot do following a stent before your discharge from the hospital. Table 24.1 shows some PCI/stenting facts.

Case 5: A Two-Stenter

I had never given much thought to undergoing an angiogram before I had one. I had heard that angiograms were the gold standard for diagnosing cardiovascular disease, but I also knew that they were not routinely performed on patients without a medical reason. I did not have a single symptom to justify an angiogram: no chest pain, no shortness of breath, and a normal stress test the previous year.

After I suddenly collapsed, I was still having trouble comprehending what had happened to me and why I was being told that I was lucky to be alive. In the hospital, when I heard the doctor mention the need for an angiogram that evening, I began to appreciate the significance of what had happened to me. My first thoughts were of my wife's mother, who had died from cardiac disease 30 years ago. I can still remember her describing to me the pain associated with cardiac catheterizations at that time and how she feared having to undergo several such procedures. I was as much concerned about the pain involved in the procedure as I was about what my doctor would find.

My doctor reassured me that it would be a painless procedure and that he would be looking for an explanation of what had happened to me. He thought that it was sudden cardiac arrest, based on my lack of symptoms, and he was hoping that he could place stents in my arteries if he found treatable blockages. If he could not treat me with stents, I would have to be transferred to another hospital for coronary artery bypass grafts. I began to root real hard for the stents.

The next morning was a blur. I recall being wheeled out from my room with wishes of good luck from the wonderful nursing staff and then arriving in an intimidating white room. I was placed on a table and spoke with some very caring people in the room. The doctor came in and once again explained that I could watch the procedure on the monitors next to me, but I politely declined the invitation. I was told that I would feel a warm sensation, and that's the last thing I remember until I woke up to the good news from my doctor that he had found two significant blockages that he was able to treat with stents. The procedure was quick, uneventful, and painless. Even the wound in my groin healed quickly and with minimal discomfort.

Dealing with the stents has been less cumbersome than I would have expected. They are truly a medical miracle. I have no surgical marks on my chest. I sometimes try to feel if they are there, but of course, I don't feel a thing. I have met a surprising number of people who have had stents inserted. One client sent me a get-well message addressed to a "two-stenter" from a "three-stenter." I found out that a friend of mine, who happens to be a doctor, is a "six-stenter," as he calls himself with great pride.

With the ability to exercise now and to raise my heart rate, I feel much more confident that the stents are doing their job and that I can live a normal life. My doctors have done their job well. Now it is my job to eat properly, to exercise, to take my medications, and to try to manage stress better. I'm still working on the last one.

Heart Medications

25

Slava Gitelman and Todd J. Cohen

Prescription medications are an important treatment option for patients with heart disease. They are useful in treating risk factors such as high blood pressure and high cholesterol. Early treatment with medication can lower a person's risk of developing a heart attack and/or subsequent sudden cardiac arrest. This chapter discusses many of the drugs taken by people with heart disease or by people who are at risk for heart disease.

The following five general principles about medications are applicable to most people with heart disease or risk factors for heart disease:

1. Certain medications, such as beta-blockers, are useful in treating many different conditions such as high blood pressure (hypertension), coronary artery disease, and heart failure. Your doctor may prescribe a medication for one or more of these conditions.
2. You should pay close attention to instructions on how to take your medications. Instructions include the timing (when and how often) and dosage of the medication, as well as whether you should take the medication with meals. If you miss one pill, take the next regularly scheduled pill. In addition, some medications are less active if a person has eaten grapefruit or grapefruit juice or has taken non-steroidal anti-inflammatory drugs (also called NSAIDs) such as ibuprofen. You may be instructed not to consume grapefruit products or not to take NSAIDs while you are on these medications. *Follow the instructions for any prescribed*

S. Gitelman (✉)
Department of Osteopathic Manipulative Medicine, St. Barnabas Hospital, Bronx, NY, USA

T. J. Cohen
NYIT College of Osteopathic Medicine, New York, NY, USA
e-mail: tcohen03@nyit.edu

© The Author(s), under exclusive license to Springer Nature Switzerland AG 2025
T. J. Cohen, R. S. Blumenthal (eds.), *Surviving and Thriving With Heart Disease*,
Contemporary Cardiology, https://doi.org/10.1007/978-3-032-00579-3_25

medication. Following medical instructions (called medical compliance) is essential to achieve the drug's desired effects.
3. Potential side effects and potential drug interactions should be covered in a discussion between you and your doctor or pharmacist before you start taking the drug. Bring any significant side effects to your doctor's attention. The more medications used, the more likely the side effects.
4. Notify your doctor before stopping *any* medication.
5. Report any suspected drug allergies to your doctor. Keep a list of your current medications and drug allergies in your wallet at all times and show the list to any healthcare provider you consult.

Heart Rhythm Drugs (Antiarrhythmics)

A number of medications are prescribed to treat heart rhythm problems and minimize complications associated with arrhythmias. The American College of Cardiology, the American Heart Association, and the Heart Rhythm Society review ongoing research and collaborate in making recommendations for the safe and effective management of patients with arrhythmias.

An arrhythmia means the heart may beat too fast, too slow, or with an irregular rhythm. There are two ways to control heart arrhythmias: physicians can attempt to control the heart rate (called rate control) or suppress the rhythm abnormality (called rhythm control). *Drugs that control either heart rate or heart rhythm are grouped into a class known as antiarrhythmic drugs, even though the mechanism by which they terminate arrhythmias is different.* Table 25.1 shows common heart rhythm medications and their effects.

Drugs That Control Heart Rate

Two drugs that attempt to control heart rate are *beta-blockers* and *calcium channel blockers*. Beta-blockers are very useful in treating patients with coronary artery disease, congestive heart failure, and high blood pressure. Beta-blockers are used to block the effects of adrenaline (by blocking beta receptors in the heart muscle), therefore decreasing the workload of the heart; they are also useful in preventing ischemia (lack of blood flow to the heart muscle) in people with coronary artery disease. Caution needs to be taken in patients with slower heart rates and lower blood pressures and those with certain circulatory and lung problems such as chronic obstructive pulmonary disease (COPD) or asthma. Beta-blockers may also hide some of the reactions that people can get to low blood sugar (hypoglycemia).

Drugs to lower blood sugar should be used with caution in patients on beta-blockers. Another category of drugs that help control the rate are the calcium channel blockers, verapamil and diltiazem. These medications work like beta-blockers, and slow conduction in the SA and AV nodes, but should be used cautiously, if at all, in those with congestive heart failure. Dietary calcium intake or calcium supplements usually do not interfere with calcium channel blockers. For more information on beta-blockers and calcium channel blockers, see the chapter on high blood pressure (hypertension; Chap. 38).

Table 25.1 Common heart rhythm (antiarrhythmic) medications and their effects

Medicine	Effects	Comments
Beta-blocker	Slows pulse (treats SVT[a]), lowers blood pressure, helps treat heart failure and coronary artery disease	Caution in patients with asthma, COPD; may cause impotence and depression; may mask hypoglycemia
Calcium channel blocker	Slows pulse (treats SVT), lowers blood pressure	Not as good as a beta-blocker if you have coronary artery disease
Amiodarone	Best drug treatment for ventricular tachycardia and atrial fibrillation or flutter	Many potential side effects: can affect thyroid, liver, and lungs; requires follow-up every three months; ventricular tachycardia (proarrhythmia) is a rare complication
Sotalol	Less effective than amiodarone for ventricular tachycardia and atrial fibrillation or flutter	Can bring on or worsen ventricular tachycardia (proarrhythmia)
Dofetilide	Can treat atrial fibrillation or flutter	Can bring on or worsen ventricular tachycardia (proarrhythmia)
Dronedarone	Can treat atrial fibrillation or flutter	Amiodarone-like drug with fewer side effects
Mexiletine	Even less effective than sotalol for ventricular tachycardia	Does not worsen ventricular tachycardia; can cause confusion, dizziness, numbness, and tingling
Flecainide	Can treat SVT and atrial fibrillation	Can bring on ventricular tachycardia (proarrhythmia)
Propafenone	Can treat SVT and atrial fibrillation	Can bring on ventricular tachycardia (proarrhythmia)

[a]*SVT* supraventricular tachycardia

Drugs That Suppress Heart Rhythm Abnormalities

There are also drugs that are used to suppress abnormal heart rhythms. These medications are targeted toward maintaining regular, continuous, and orderly contraction of the heart cells and keeping the heart in a normal sinus rhythm. These heart rhythm suppression drugs are more potent than the heart rate-controlling drugs (and typically have more side effects). They include amiodarone, dofetilide, dronedarone, sotalol, propafenone, mexiletine, and flecainide. Ibutilide, a drug used to treat atrial fibrillation and atrial flutter, is not listed in Table 25.1 because it is available only in an intravenous form; it has no orally ingested version.

Drugs That Prevent Clotting (Antiplatelet and Anticoagulant Drugs)

When there is a bleed, platelets are recruited to the site by special signals. The bleed is controlled by two steps. First, platelets stick to the blood vessels to stop the bleeding and then stick to each other by a molecule known as fibrinogen. *Antiplatelet drugs* interfere with this initial step. The next step is the conversion of fibrinogen,

Table 25.2 Common medications to treat and prevent blood clots

Medicine	Effects	Comments
Acetylsalicylic acid (aspirin)	Antiplatelet medication used to help prevent heart attack.	Helpful for patients who are having a heart attack to chew an aspirin.
Clopidogrel (Plavix)	Antiplatelet medication used with aspirin.	Used after placement of a stent to prevent the stent and coronary artery from occluding.
Warfarin (Coumadin)	Anticoagulant medication that works by blocking vitamin K; given to people who have blood clots anywhere in the body or have atrial fibrillation and subsequent increased risk of stroke.	It is useful for people with mechanical heart valves; has many interactions so it is important to discuss all foods, drugs, and supplements with your physician. The main risk is bleeding which is increased with clopidogrel and aspirin. The effects are monitored by an INR blood test which looks at the blood thinner's effect on clotting (coagulation). Green leafy foods and other substances that contain vitamin K may lower your INR (blood thinner) level and reduce effectiveness.
Novel oral anticoagulants (NOAC)	These drugs include apixaban (Eliquis), dabigatran (Pradaxa), and rivaroxaban (Xarelto). They are considered superior alternatives to warfarin for treating atrial fibrillation since there is no need for routine blood testing. Foods high in vitamin K are not a problem.	Used in people with nonvalvular atrial fibrillation. They are not indicated in people with mechanical heart valves, mitral valve stenosis, or prior mitral valve repair. Compared to warfarin, uncontrolled bleeding may be more difficult to reverse and NOAC reversal agents are in different stages of development.

which holds the platelets together, to fibrin, which strengthens the interaction between platelets. Drugs that interfere with the conversion from fibrinogen to fibrin are known as blood thinners (also called *anticoagulants*). Both types of medications function to prevent blood from clotting and blocking blood flow; therefore, both medications carry a risk of bleeding. *You should always be in touch with your doctor regarding any side effects of medications.* Table 25.2 shows common medications used to treat and prevent blood clots.

Antiplatelet Drugs

Acetylsalicylic acid (aspirin) is an antiplatelet agent useful in preventing the buildup of platelets around any atherosclerotic plaques. This minimizes the inflammatory process, thereby preventing acute coronary artery occlusion (which can occur if the plaque ruptures). Aspirin inhibits inflammation and stabilizes the plaque. In people who have a stent to treat coronary artery blockage, antiplatelet agents including aspirin and clopidogrel (Plavix) are useful in preventing the blood vessel from occluding again. In general, aspirin is a mainstay in anyone with coronary artery disease. A low-dose aspirin (81 mg) once daily may be sufficient to prevent the inflammatory reaction responsible for coronary artery occlusion. If you have chest pain, which is typically caused by acute plaque rupture within a coronary artery, chewing a full aspirin (325 mg) is a first-line therapy, after calling 911 to go to the hospital.

Clopidogrel (Plavix) is typically given in conjunction with aspirin to patients following the placement of a stent. Certain proton pump inhibitors such as omeprazole may weaken the antiplatelet effects of this medication. Ticagrelor (Brilinta) is another antiplatelet drug that is useful in those who experience side effects or are not responding to clopidogrel. Studies have shown no increase in major bleeding rate, heart attack, and stroke with this medication when compared to Plavix, though it may increase shortness of breath in some people.

Anticoagulants

Warfarin (Coumadin) is an anticoagulant drug that works against vitamin K. Vitamin K is critical in creating fibrin in the second step of forming a blood clot. By interfering with vitamin K, blood clots cannot continue to form. Specifically, this medication helps to prevent additional blood clots and facilitates blood flow, whether it be to the leg, heart, or lungs. Warfarin is given to people who have a blood clot anywhere in the body or if they have atrial fibrillation or flutter, which places them at a higher risk of a stroke. It is important to note that the risk of stroke in those with atrial fibrillation is increased fivefold and that atrial fibrillation accounts for 15% of all strokes. For more information on why this occurs, please see the section entitled "Drugs Used to Treat Atrial Fibrillation and Flutter" (below). Therefore, people with atrial fibrillation and one or more stroke factors (heart failure, high blood pressure, diabetes, 65 years of age and over, history of stroke, vascular disease, are female) can benefit from anticoagulants. These medications are also useful in preventing clot formation in those with mechanical heart valves. Many drugs, foods, and supplements interact with warfarin, and it is imperative to have a clear dialogue with your physician about this medication.

Novel oral anticoagulants (NOACs) include apixaban (Eliquis), dabigatran (Pradaxa), and rivaroxaban (Xarelto). In general, these medications are superior alternatives to warfarin (since there is no need for routine blood testing and eating foods rich in vitamin K is not an issue) for preventing stroke in those with nonvalvular atrial fibrillation. Warfarin is as effective as the NOACs, but the latter medications do not require constant blood monitoring and have many fewer drug interactions and a rapid onset and rapid offset, which all can increase patient medication compliance. NOACs are not recommended in people with mechanical heart valves, mitral stenosis, or prior mitral valve repair. In these cases, the use of warfarin for the prevention of thromboembolism is the only established option.

Bleeding from warfarin can be reversed by stopping the medication, giving vitamin K, and, if necessary, giving special blood products such as fresh frozen plasma or prothrombin complex concentrate. Uncontrolled bleeding while on a NOAC requires supportive measures including discontinuation of the medication and the use of reversal agents such as *andexanet (Andexxa)* for rivaroxaban (Xarelto) and apixaban (Eliquis) and *idarucizumab (Praxbind)* for dabigatran (Pradaxa).

To determine whether you are a candidate for NOACs for atrial fibrillation, your doctor will likely use either the CHADS2 or CHA2DS2-VASc stroke risk scoring system (discussed in more detail in Chap. 9). The latter score is preferred by the American Heart Association, the American College of Cardiology, and the Heart Rhythm Society. A CHA2DS2-VASc score of 1 or more for men, and 2 or more for women, may qualify you for anticoagulants. Your doctor will review your particular history, including any bleeding history, and determine whether you are a candidate for anticoagulants. Please talk to your doctor about the risks and benefits of these therapies, as well as possible alternatives, before choosing an anticoagulant. If you have had bleeding while on these medications, and still have a significant risk of a stroke, a Watchman™ type device should be considered as an alternative stroke prevention treatment. To learn more about this procedure, please see Chap. 32.

Drugs Used to Treat Atrial Fibrillation and Atrial Flutter

People who have atrial fibrillation and atrial flutter are at a higher risk for stroke. This is because the left atrium contracts very erratically and is unable to propel the blood efficiently forward. Therefore, due to the blood stasis and the turbulent flow, clots develop in the sac off of the left atrium (called the left atrial appendage), which may break off and travel to the brain and cause a stroke. Blood thinners such as warfarin (Coumadin) and the novel oral anticoagulants [*apixaban (Eliquis), dabigatran (Pradaxa), and rivaroxaban (Xarelto)*] all lower the risk of stroke in those with significant risk factors (see section above entitled "Anticoagulants" and Chap. 9). In patients with atrial fibrillation, structurally normal hearts, and no major risk factors for stroke, acetylsalicylic acid (aspirin) may be useful for stroke prevention. Adding antiplatelet medications such as acetylsalicylic acid (aspirin) and clopidogrel (Plavix) to the drug regimen for patients on the anticoagulants may increase the risks of bleeding and bruising.

Heart rate control can be achieved with a beta-blocker or calcium channel blocker. The drugs that regulate heart rhythm are dronedarone, amiodarone, sotalol, dofetilide, propafenone, and flecainide, and are also useful in treating atrial fibrillation.

Drugs Used to Treat Ventricular Tachycardia and Ventricular Fibrillation

The principal way to treat nonreversible or recurrent ventricular tachycardia or ventricular fibrillation (the causes of sudden cardiac arrest) is with a device (an implantable defibrillator or ICD). However, frequent and recurrent episodes, even in patients with an ICD, require treatment with drug therapy to suppress the arrhythmia and prevent frequent shocks from the device. Drugs that control heart rhythm, such as mexiletine, sotalol, and amiodarone, may all be useful in preventing ventricular tachycardia and ventricular fibrillation (see Table 25.1). Sotalol and dofetilide have a higher chance of causing arrhythmia than the other medications. Amiodarone is more effective than the rest but has the greatest toxicity. Mexiletine is less effective, but it has a low incidence of proarrhythmia and is usually well tolerated. It is also very helpful in addition to sotalol or amiodarone therapy.

Proarrhythmia and the QT Interval

The most consequential side effect of heart rhythm medications is proarrhythmia, which is a more serious rhythm disturbance than the original problem. One form of proarrhythmia caused by some antiarrhythmic medications is the occurrence of a rapid rhythm from the lower chambers of the heart called ventricular tachycardia (see Chap. 7), which on an ECG appears to twist about a point. This twisting rhythm is called *torsades de pointes*. Proarrhythmia may also occur in the form of an exacerbation of more typical ventricular tachycardia or fibrillation and/or the exacerbation of atrial fibrillation or rapid atrial flutter. A measurement on your electrocardiogram, called the QT interval (measured in milliseconds), can be important in determining if you are at risk for ventricular tachycardia and proarrhythmia. The QT interval is corrected according to your heart rate (QTc interval). A normal QTc is less than 470 milliseconds in women and less than 450 milliseconds in men.

Other problems can add to or independently cause lengthening of the QT interval and subsequent ventricular tachycardia. These include electrolyte abnormalities (such as low potassium, low calcium, and/or low magnesium), long QT syndrome (a genetic condition), and certain medications (besides antiarrhythmic medications), which are also proarrhythmic. These medications include antipsychotics, antiemetics, antifungals, antimicrobials, antidepressants, antihistamines, and diuretics. Proarrhythmia must be immediately addressed, and the first step in management is to determine the cause and remove any exacerbating agents while supporting the patient and treating/terminating the arrhythmia. Intravenous medications, such as magnesium, calcium, and isoproterenol, and electrical procedures, such as pacing faster than the baseline rhythm (called overdrive pacing) and/or defibrillation, may be required.

Common heart rhythm medications that may be prescribed by your doctor are listed in Table 25.1. Each of these medications has a version that may be taken by mouth; an intravenous version of the drug may also exist. Your doctor may monitor you more closely while starting one of these antiarrhythmic medications. Your doctor may want you monitored in real time via a wearable or implantable device or in the hospital on a telemetry floor. If your doctor has prescribed any of these medications for you, you may be asked to see your doctor more frequently for follow-up visits to avoid complications.

Other Heart Disease Drugs

Risk factors for heart disease include high cholesterol (Chap. 37), high blood pressure (Chap. 38), obesity (Chap. 39), smoking (Chap. 40), and diabetes (Chap. 41). Each of these chapters addresses an important heart disease risk factor, and each discusses common medications used to treat these problems. It is important to control these and other risk factors (including smoking and excessive alcohol consumption) in order to prevent and manage heart disease. Here, we focus on medications for treating and controlling coronary artery disease and heart failure.

Drugs Used to Treat Coronary Artery Disease

Sudden cardiac arrest is often the result of severe ventricular tachycardia or ventricular fibrillation that arises from injured areas of the heart. These injuries may be a result of scarring from a prior heart attack or may occur during sudden cardiac arrest if the person is having a heart attack at the same time. The buildup of fatty deposits, such as cholesterol, in the coronary arteries (a condition called atherosclerosis) followed by plaque rupture is one common cause of heart attacks.

Table 25.3 shows some common medications used to treat coronary artery disease. The treatment of high cholesterol is an important aspect of treating coronary artery disease, and common medications used for that purpose are listed in Table 25.4. Patients who have plaque buildup in their coronary arteries (atherosclerosis) may experience chest pain during activity or rest, if the degree of blockage in their arteries is significant (typically greater than 70%). The lack of blood flow (and oxygen) to the heart muscle from a narrowing or blockage of a coronary artery is

Table 25.3 Common medications used to treat coronary artery disease

Medicine	Effects	Comments
Nitroglycerin	Used to treat chest pain from ischemia (called angina) due to coronary artery disease. Can lower blood pressure; works by expanding blood vessels.	Should not be taken by patients using sildenafil (Viagra) or tadalafil (Cialis) because it may lead to a sudden drop in blood pressure and loss of consciousness.
Beta-blockers	A medication that blocks the beta-adrenergic receptors in the heart. As a result, this medication blocks the effects of adrenaline.	Used to limit the workload of the heart. May also slow down the heart rate and help lower blood pressure.

Table 25.4 Common medications to treat high cholesterol

Medicine	Effects	Comments
HMG-CoA reductase inhibitors (statins)	Used to prevent cholesterol buildup in the coronary arteries. Can also prevent the inflammatory response that could cause atheromatous plaques to rupture in the heart and precipitate a heart attack.	Side effects include muscle and liver injury. Side effects on muscle tissue increase when drugs are used concomitantly with a fibrate (i.e., clofibrate).
Niacin (nicotinic acid) cholestyramine gemfibrozil clofibrate	Used to treat high cholesterol and high triglycerides.	Have multiple different mechanisms of action. Typically not as effective as a statin, but may serve as an alternative if a statin does not work as well as planned.

called ischemia. Nitroglycerin can be used sublingually (under the tongue) or topically (in paste or patch form) and can help expand the coronary arteries and improve blood flow to the heart muscle. Nitroglycerin may be useful in treating chest pain from ischemia, a condition called *angina* or *angina pectoris*.

Statins (HMG-CoA reductase inhibitors) are a class of drugs that block not only the buildup of cholesterol but also the inflammatory process that can lead to plaque rupture and subsequent coronary artery occlusion. An example of a statin is Lipitor (atorvastatin). Other drugs, such as cholestyramine, niacin (nicotinic acid), and fenofibrate, are used to treat high cholesterol and high triglyceride levels, but these drugs are typically less effective than the statins, especially in patients with known coronary artery disease. For more information on cholesterol and cholesterol-lowering drugs, see Chap. 37.

Drugs Used to Treat Heart Failure (And Also High Blood Pressure)

Table 25.5 shows some common medications used to treat heart failure. According to the American Heart Association's *Get with the Guidelines* heart failure program, heart failure should be treated with a beta-blocker plus an angiotensin-converting enzyme (ACE) inhibitor or angiotensin II receptor blocker (ARB) unless the patient cannot tolerate those medications. Both ACE inhibitors and ARBs are contraindicated in pregnancy because they pose a risk to a developing fetus. They may also cause life-threatening swelling of the face, throat, and/or airways (called angioedema). ACE inhibitors and ARBs work by lowering the amount of fluid in the body and expanding blood vessels, thus lowering blood pressure.

Beta-blockers work by blocking beta receptors in the heart, allowing the heart to beat slower while also lowering blood pressure and facilitating heart remodeling. This enhances heart function, thereby conserving vital cardiac energy. Beta-blockers help to decrease the amount of work that the heart needs to perform to pump blood. If those drugs are unacceptable, alternative drugs exist. These include other vasodilators, such as hydralazine and isosorbide dinitrate.

Diuretics are useful in removing excess fluid that builds up in the body as a result of the ineffective pumping of blood by a weakened or diseased heart. These drugs may alter the body's electrolytes (such as potassium) and on occasion may cause arrhythmias. If a problem is suspected, your blood should be tested for an electrolyte abnormality.

Digitalis may help to increase the heart muscle's ability to contract, especially if ACE inhibitors or ARBs fail to improve heart failure symptoms. If the blood level of digitalis is too high, ventricular and atrial arrhythmias may occur as well as heart block. Renal failure, low potassium levels, verapamil, amiodarone, and quinidine may all contribute to toxicity. Other side effects include gastrointestinal upset, blurry yellow vision, and elevated potassium levels. A digitalis blood level test is useful in identifying toxicity.

Entresto, a combination of an ARB (valsartan) and a drug called sacubitril (the two drugs together are called an ARNI; see Chap. 14), helps rid the body of excess

Table 25.5 Common medications to treat heart failure

Medicine	Effects	Comments
Angiotensin-converting enzyme (ACE) inhibitors	Used to help improve heart function. May vasodilate the blood vessels and lower blood pressure, making it easier for the failing heart to pump blood.	It may adversely affect the kidneys and cause a cough in some people. Swelling of the face and airways is a dangerous side effect that warrants an immediate 911 call.
Angiotensin II receptor blockers (ARBs)	Similar to ACE inhibitors (see above).	Similar to ACE inhibitors, but may have less incidence of coughing as a side effect (see above).
Beta-blockers	Can improve heart function in patients with heart failure. See "Coronary artery disease medications," above. Note: some medications act by blocking both alpha and beta receptors. See "Antihypertensive medications," below.	Carvedilol is very helpful in treating heart failure and blocks the alpha-1 receptor as well as beta receptors.
Diuretics	Used to eliminate excess fluid in patients with heart failure.	May affect kidney function, lead to dehydration, and cause electrolyte abnormalities.
Digitalis	May make a weak heart pump stronger. May be useful if heart failure does not improve with ACE inhibitors or ARBs.	Side effects include worsening heart rhythm problems and yellow vision. Dosage should be reduced in people with kidney failure.
Entresto (Valsartan + Sacubitril)	Approved for people who have chronic heart failure (NYHA Class II to IV) with a reduced ejection fraction.	People treated with this drug have been shown to have a lower mortality from cardiovascular complications.

Note: ACE inhibitors or ARBs plus a beta-blocker fulfill the AHA's *Get with the Guidelines* heart failure program for treating congestive heart failure

fluid and helps alleviate symptoms of heart failure. This drug also helps lower blood pressure. This combination medication is approved for people with chronic moderate to severe heart failure (NYHA classes II–IV) and with a reduced ejection fraction. The most common adverse reactions are low blood pressure, electrolyte abnormalities (specifically high potassium), cough, dizziness, and kidney failure. The use of this medication is contraindicated in patients with any hypersensitivity to the drug components and people with a history of angioedema, with concomitant use of ACE inhibitors, and with concomitant use of a drug called aliskiren in patients with diabetes. Drug interactions are possible with potassium-sparing diuretics, NSAIDS, and lithium. People treated with this drug combination are less likely to die from cardiovascular complications. Examples of the drugs that may be used to treat heart failure while also lowering blood pressure are listed in Table 25.6. This table is not comprehensive with respect to blood pressure management. Specifically, a thiazide diuretic is typically first line for blood pressure management in the context of heart failure. For more details on blood pressure management, please see Chap. 38.

Table 25.6 Common medications to treat high blood pressure (hypertension). These medications may have an additive effect on lowering blood pressure

Medicine	Effects	Comments
Beta-blockers	Lower blood pressure by blocking beta-adrenergic receptors in the heart.	See "heart failure medications," "coronary artery disease medications," and "heart rhythm medications," above.
Alpha blockers	Block alpha-adrenergic receptors (therefore blocking noradrenaline).	There are two types of alpha receptors (alpha 1 and alpha 2). These medications may be used to treat prostate enlargement (benign prostatic hypertrophy), Raynaud's disease, and high blood pressure.
Combined alpha and beta-blockers	May block both alpha and beta receptors.	May be useful in treating high blood pressure as well as heart failure.
Calcium channel blockers	Block calcium channel receptors.	May lower blood pressure and may slow down the heart rate. Important to stay well hydrated and eat fruits and vegetables to avoid constipation as a side effect.
ACE inhibitors and ARBs	Causes vasodilation and stops the reabsorption of water in the kidneys, facilitating the lowering of blood pressure.	See "heart failure medications," above.

Summary

If you have begun taking medications for a heart problem or a risk factor for heart problems, or if you are discussing medications with your doctor, there are several things for you to be mindful of. For all your medications, you should know the name, indication (reason for taking), and dosing instructions, and you should understand what are the common and uncommon side effects and what the symptoms of these side effects might be. If you feel you are experiencing a side effect, notify your doctor. In fact, if you have any questions related to your medicines, including how and how often to take them, ask your doctor. Although your cardiologist may be taking care of your heart, you are probably seeing other physicians who are also involved in your care. *Bring a list of your medications when visiting any of your physicians.*

Cardioversion and Defibrillation

26

Todd J. Cohen

Cardioversion and defibrillation are procedures used to convert abnormal rapid heart rhythms (tachycardias including atrial fibrillation, atrial flutter, ventricular tachycardia, and/or ventricular fibrillation) back to a more normal heart rhythm (such as sinus rhythm; see Table 26.1). Cardioversion can be performed either electrically or chemically. To perform an external electrical cardioversion or defibrillation, a medical device is used to deliver a high-voltage shock to the patient's chest. Electrical cardioversion and defibrillation are similar procedures, except cardioversion is synchronized to a part of the ECG (the peak of the QRS complex; see Chap. 16), while defibrillation is unsynchronized. Synchronization takes more time than unsynchronized shock delivery. When the heart rhythm is too rapid and/or chaotic (as occurs during ventricular tachycardia and ventricular fibrillation) and the patient is unconscious (without significant blood pressure or palpable pulse), time is of the essence, and rapid defibrillation is necessary to restore a normal rhythm and circulation.

Table 26.1 Electrical cardioversion and defibrillation

Electrical cardioversion and defibrillation are useful for breaking fast rhythms
They are used to terminate (convert) atrial fibrillation, atrial flutter, ventricular fibrillation, ventricular flutter, and any rapid rhythm that does not respond to standard drugs and is not stable, such as when the patient is semiconscious or unconscious or has a low blood pressure. Pressure applied with paddles or over patches with an insulated material can help facilitate cardioversion and defibrillation.
Internal cardioversion and internal defibrillation can be lifesaving when standard means fail.

T. J. Cohen (✉)
NYIT College of Osteopathic Medicine, New York, NY, USA
e-mail: tcohen03@nyit.edu

© The Author(s), under exclusive license to Springer Nature Switzerland AG 2025
T. J. Cohen, R. S. Blumenthal (eds.), *Surviving and Thriving With Heart Disease*,
Contemporary Cardiology, https://doi.org/10.1007/978-3-032-00579-3_26

External Cardioversion and Defibrillation

In order to perform a cardioversion or defibrillation, electrical energy must be applied to the chest, using either insulated paddles or patches. Figure 26.1 shows an example of defibrillator patches connected to an external defibrillator. An external defibrillator is used to shock the patient out of rapid heart rhythms in the upper chamber of the heart (atrial fibrillation and atrial flutter) as well as to treat very serious rhythms from the lower chambers (ventricular tachycardia and ventricular fibrillation). For cardioversion of atrial fibrillation or atrial flutter, the patches are placed closer to the middle of the chest (anterior patch) and between the scapulae (posterior patch). These patches provide hands-off cardioversion and defibrillation.

Figure 26.2 shows alternative patch configurations for the treatment of ventricular arrhythmias. In one configuration, there is a posterior patch between the scapulae and an anterior one on the left side of the chest below the breast tissue or muscle (lateral). Patches and/or paddles can also be used entirely on the anterior chest. For cardioversion or defibrillation of ventricular tachycardia, the left patch or paddle should be more lateral for the shock vector to engulf more of the left ventricle muscle during the procedure.

When cardioversion or defibrillation fails after multiple attempts, pressure can be applied using an insulated material (such as an unconnected defibrillator paddle or the paddle itself). Figure 26.3 shows a specially designed medical device, called PrestoPush™, developed by Dr. Todd Cohen's Johns Hopkins University undergraduate biomedical engineering design team, which was designed for this purpose.

Fig. 26.1 A patient connected with anterior and posterior patches connected to an external defibrillator for hands-free cardioversion. (Reproduced with permission from HMP Communications LLC from Practical Electrophysiology, Third Edition)

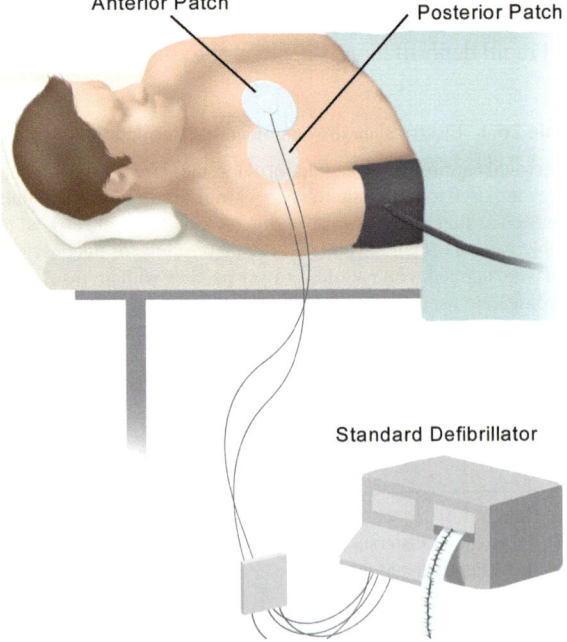

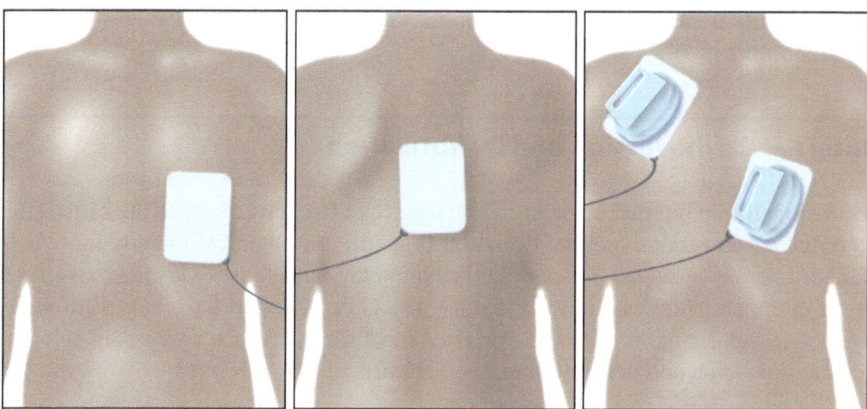

Fig. 26.2 A placement of patches for the treatment of ventricular tachycardia. Note: The first figure shows an anterior patch used in conjunction with the second figure which shows a posterior patch. The third figure shows an alternative configuration in which either patches or paddles are used anteriorly. One is placed slightly to the right of the midsternum, and another to the left of the midaxillary line of the patient (left of the nipple line) and below the point of maximum impulse of the heart (typically to the left and below breast tissue). (Reproduced with permission from HMP Communications LLC from Practical Electrophysiology, Third Edition)

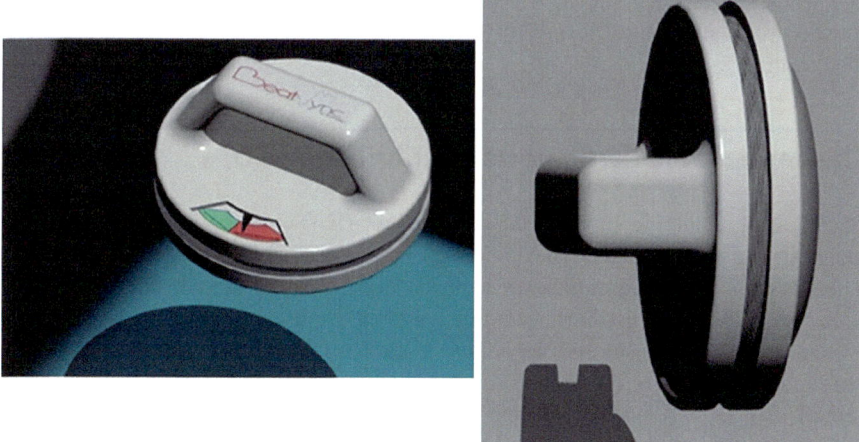

Fig. 26.3 An innovative way to improve the success of an unsuccessful cardioversion or defibrillation. Dr. Cohen previously described an active compression cardioversion method in which 20–40 pounds of pressure is applied (using an insulated material) over the patch (such as paddles or a PrestoPush™ type device) and can improve the success of the procedure. The latter device was developed by Dr. Todd Cohen's Johns Hopkins University undergraduate biomedical engineering design team, which won the National Collegiate Inventor's Competition with this invention in 2013. (Reproduced with permission from HMP Communications LLC from Practical Electrophysiology, Third Edition)

This invention helped the team win the 2013 National Collegiate Inventor's Competition.

Internal Cardioversion and Defibrillation

Occasionally, an internal catheter can be used to deliver electricity to the heart, after external cardioversion and defibrillation in addition to medical therapy have both failed. Internal cardioversion and defibrillation are failsafe methods that have been used in the electrophysiology laboratory (see Chap. 21) and have helped to break refractory ventricular fibrillation. For a review of some key factors regarding electrical cardioversion and defibrillation, see Table 26.1.

The Automatic External Defibrillator (AED)

The AED is a small lunch box-sized device that can be life-saving during a cardiac arrest (when a patient collapses from a lethal arrhythmia such as ventricular tachycardia or ventricular fibrillation). AEDs are widely available (in churches, schools, stadiums, and airports) and are simple enough to be used by non-medical personnel. The devices guide the user (often via voice command) on how to apply the patches and when to deliver a shock. AEDs can be purchased by friends and families of those with heart disease, especially if their loved one is at risk for sudden cardiac death.

The Implantable Cardioverter-Defibrillator (ICD)

Lastly, an implantable cardioverter-defibrillator (ICD) has incorporated the above technology in a pacemaker-type device and has been available for over four decades. This device is indicated in those at high risk for sudden cardiac death. Specifically, those with cardiomyopathies (ischemic, dilated, or hypertrophic) and those with certain hereditary conditions may benefit from these devices. If you have had a heart attack, a history of cardiomyopathy, a family history of sudden death, or heart failure, please talk to your cardiologist to see whether you qualify for this life-saving device. See Chap. 30 for more on pacemakers and ICDs.

Chemical Cardioversion

To perform chemical cardioversion, the doctor may use antiarrhythmic medications to help convert certain arrhythmias (such as atrial fibrillation and atrial flutter) into normal rhythms without the use of electrical energy. Some of these medications can be given orally (called *pill in a pocket*) and include propafenone and flecainide. Intravenous medications, such as ibutilide and procainamide, can also be used to facilitate conversion. Patients should be monitored during intravenous chemical cardioversion since antiarrhythmic medications can lengthen the QT interval on ECG and cause proarrhythmia (polymorphic ventricular tachycardia called torsades de pointes). In general, electrical cardioversion and defibrillation are preferred over drugs in those who are less stable.

.

Repair and Replacement of Malfunctioning Valves: Surgery, TAVR, and MitraClip

27

Thomas Chengot and Jillian Nostro

Valvular heart disease occurs when there is damage to one of the four heart valves (see Chap. 1). The appropriate opening and closing of these valves is important to the efficient functioning of the heart. To review, blood flows into the right atrium and crosses the tricuspid valve into the right ventricle and out the pulmonary artery to the lungs. Oxygenated blood then leaves the lungs into the left atrium and crosses the mitral valve into the left ventricle where it is pumped through the aorta to the rest of the body. In this chapter, we will focus on mitral valve regurgitation (MR) and aortic valve stenosis (AS) as these are the two most commonly corrected disease processes.

Treatment Options: An Overview

Patients with severe valvular disease may present with symptoms of heart failure, shortness of breath, decreased exercise capacity, or even a new weak heart muscle (cardiomyopathy, often associated with decreased left ventricular function or a low ejection fraction). These symptoms, together with severe valvular disease, often indicate the need for valve replacement and/or repair. This type of intervention is

T. Chengot (✉)
Department of Cardiology, Amityville Heart Center, Amityville, NY, USA
e-mail: tchengot@gmail.com

J. Nostro
Department of Family Medicine, Plainview Hospital, Plainview, NY, USA
e-mail: jnostro@northwell.edu

performed to improve or eliminate symptoms and reduce mortality. In the past, open heart surgery was the only option. However, with the recent development of minimally invasive procedures, many valve disorders can be corrected in a minimally invasive way, often through the skin (percutaneously) or smaller incisions in the chest, rather than cracking the chest open (sternotomy or thoracotomy) and undergoing open heart surgery. The latter is associated with increased risks, complications, and a longer hospitalization and recovery period.

There has been increasing clinical experience and progressive improvement in two specific percutaneous procedures: transcatheter aortic valve replacement (TAVR) and transcatheter mitral valve repair (TMVr). The development of these percutaneous procedures has shown comparable results to open heart replacement/repair. They may particularly be preferred in patients who are at very high risk for open heart replacement/repair. Percutaneous procedures also have the benefit of faster overall postoperative recovery and shorter postoperative hospitalization.

In the evaluation and treatment of these valvular diseases, the formation of the "Heart Team" approach has been a vital way to combine the knowledge and resources of interventional cardiologists and cardiothoracic surgeons to find the best way to treat patients. The Heart Team approach was originally formed during the initial trials for TAVR. During the early trials for TAVR, patients were considered "non-operative candidates," and the versions of the current devices were very bulky compared to the current sleeker generations used today. Now, the Heart Team approach is an integral part of structural heart disease management and has expanded its scope to include evaluation and treatment with the MitraClip™, another minimally invasive treatment for structural heart disease. Percutaneous, minimally invasive therapies in their current form are excellent options and are comparable to open chest surgical replacement/repair. If you have severe AS or severe MR, it is important to discuss your valvular disease with your cardiologist, so that you can be properly evaluated for these therapies.

Repairing Aortic Valve Stenosis

Patients with severe AS classically present in the seventh or eighth decade of life with symptoms of heart failure, chest pain (angina), or arrhythmia (ventricular tachycardia). Initial evaluation includes a series of tests including an echocardiogram, cardiac catheterization, and a CT scan of the chest and abdomen/pelvis. The latter is to look at the blood vessels as a potential conduit to the heart. The Heart Team will then gather all the information, and the interventional cardiologist and/or cardiothoracic surgeon will decide on the type of valve that will be used and where access for the procedure will be performed.

Valve Replacement

The most common access site is through one of the femoral arteries, close to the hip joint. If femoral access is not possible, other access sites are considered such as the subclavian artery, direct aortic approach, carotid artery, or trans-caval access. There are two devices that currently have the largest global market share: the Edwards SAPIEN valve and the Medtronic CoreValve. The Edwards SAPIEN valve is a relatively small artificial valve that can be delivered via a catheter (medical device) and expanded via a balloon. It is made from the pericardium (tissue outside of the heart) of a cow (bovine).

The Medtronic CoreValve is another option that is self-expanding and can be placed above the valve annulus (where the patient's native valve is located). It is made from pig (porcine) pericardium. In full evaluation of patient risk, anatomy, and presence of coronary or peripheral vascular disease, the Heart Team will decide on the best device and approach for a patient.

This procedure is usually performed in a hybrid cardiac catheterization lab (one large enough to allow for surgical equipment, i.e., heart-lung machine, ventilator, etc.) or in a modified operating room (one that has been built for the bulky fluoroscopy machine to fit in). An anesthesiologist will sedate the patient for the duration of the procedure and maintain close hemodynamic monitoring. Patients are not usually intubated during these procedures but may be if they are considered high risk. As a precaution, patients are also prepared for emergent open heart surgery.

When everything is ready, the interventional cardiologist and cardiothoracic surgeon perform the procedure together. Access is first obtained, and the delivery system with the device is moved through an artery and crossed through the aortic valve. After the device is placed in position at the site of the calcified AS, the heart rate is increased with a temporary pacing wire to decrease cardiac output to minimize valve movement when the valve is being deployed. Once deployed, the valve is evaluated with an aortogram and an immediate transthoracic echocardiography.

Fig. 27.1 An artist illustration of a TAVR procedure performed by a retrograde aortic approach. This device is deployed much like a cardiac stent. A balloon and a TAVR device are inserted across the diseased and stenotic aortic valve and then expanded and deployed through that valve. The guidewire catheter and balloon are then removed. This procedure may have less morbidity than an open-heart valve replacement. (Figure drawn by Jerry Jose, DO)

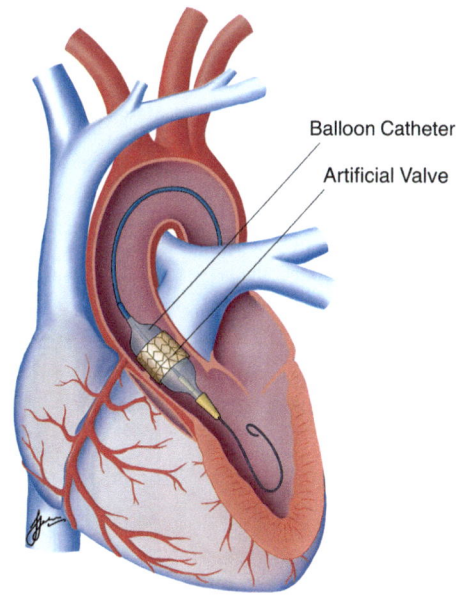

Balloon Catheter

Artificial Valve

Transcatheter
Aortic Valve Replacement

If the valve isn't well-placed, the deployed valve is re-crossed, and an appropriately sized balloon is used to fully expand the valve, decreasing any apparent paravalvular regurgitation. When results are acceptable, as illustrated in Fig. 27.1, the delivery system is removed from the body, and access sites are closed. Patients are monitored in the hospital for 1–2 days after the procedure. The most common complications post-TAVR are access site complications needing vascular repair or an abnormally low heart rate requiring a pacemaker.

Repairing Mitral Valve Regurgitation

Severe MR, discussed in Chap. 12, is the most common valvular heart disease and occurs when the mitral valve leaflets fail to close completely. This failure to close may be classified as either primary – a deformity of the mitral valve apparatus due to excess tissue, loose tissue, or chordal (attachments of the mitral valve to the left ventricle) disruption – or secondary, which results from dilation of the left ventricle stretching the mitral valve apparatus to the point that the valve cannot close appropriately. Differentiating between the etiologies of MR is dependent on the patient's history, symptoms, physical examination, echocardiography, and other advanced imaging techniques. The percutaneous, minimally invasive option for correction of MR is with the MitraClip™.

The MitraClip

The MitraClip™, shown in Fig. 27.2, is currently the only FDA-approved device used in TMVr. It reduces mortality and repeat hospitalizations and improves heart failure symptoms. In patients with severe MR, valve correction is considered if

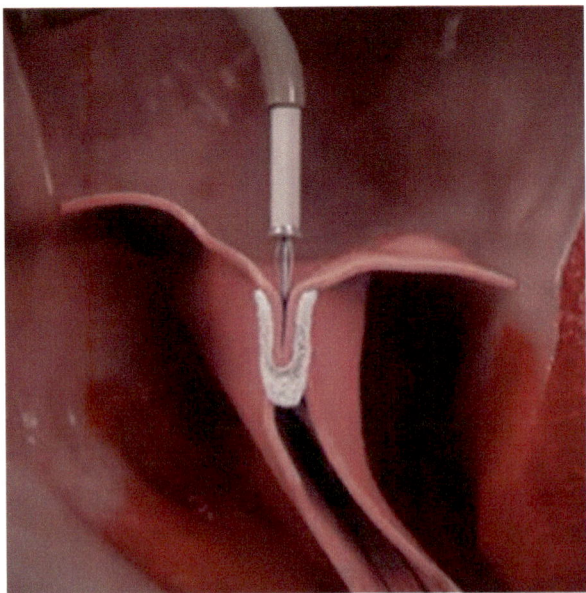

Fig. 27.2 The portion of the MitraClip (MitraClip™ NTR/XTR Clip Delivery System) procedure in which the clip is completely retracted within the left mitral valve. When properly positioned, the MitraClip closes the mitral valve leaflets and creates a double orifice within the mitral valve. (Figure obtained from Abbott Laboratories)

Table 27.1   Repair and replacement of malfunctioning valves

Surgical valve replacement
   Patients with symptomatic valvular heart disease.
   Patients with significant valve disease and decreased left ventricular ejection fraction (LVEF less than 50%).
   Asymptomatic patients with severe valve disease and progressive LV dilation.
   Patients undergoing other cardiac surgery (CABG/aortic root replacement/other valve replacement).
Mitral valve repair (MitraClip™)
   Patients with primary or secondary mitral regurgitations (MR) who are symptomatic despite optimal medical therapy and/or considered at high surgical risk.
TAVR
   Patients with symptomatic aortic stenosis (AS); initially only high surgical risk patients were considered for TAVR; FDA has more recently approved this procedure for low surgical risk patients as well.
   Asymptomatic patients with severe AS and decreased LVEF or dilated LV.
   Patients with severe AS who present with syncope, palpitations, chest pain.

repair is possible. The valve is surgically replaced in patients when repairs will most likely fail. Predisposing characteristics of valve repair failure are listed in Table 27.1. In patients who qualify for repair, MitraClip™ may be a treatment option. With the MitraClip™, the Heart Team can perform a percutaneous, minimally invasive approach, as opposed to an open surgical correction using edge-to-edge repair (also called the Alfieri stitch technique). This effectively creates a double orifice to the mitral valve, reducing the amount of regurgitation to minimal or none.

The MitraClip™ procedures are often executed in the same rooms used for TAVR implantation. Patients are prepared for the procedure with sedation provided by an anesthesiologist, and then staff will prepare the patient with anticipation of needing to perform an open chest procedure in the rare event that complications occur. The MitraClip™ device is accessed only from the femoral vein. Then, catheters are brought to the level of the heart, and using transesophageal echocardiography or intravascular ultrasound to image the intra-atrial septum (the separation between the top chambers of the heart), a procedure called a transseptal puncture is performed. During a transseptal puncture, a small needle is used to cross the intra-atrial septum into the left atrium, with imaging used concurrently to limit risk and possible complications, such as cardiac tamponade or bleeding around the heart.

Once across the intra-atrial septum, a wire is placed into the left atrium, and then over that, the MitraClip™ device and delivery system are placed. Using imaging, the clip is traversed into the left ventricle, and then the arms of the device are opened. The device is then placed in a position so that when in systole (the part of the heart cycle in which the mitral valve is closed), the arms of the MitraClip™ are closed. Imaging technology (such as a transesophageal echocardiogram) is then used to see how much the mitral regurgitation has improved.

Once the correct positioning is determined, the clip is released from the delivery system. Sometimes a second clip may be necessary given the amount or severity of the mitral regurgitation. The procedure takes 3 hours, and the patient may be monitored in the hospital for up to 3 days postoperatively. Post-procedure treatment includes anticoagulation or antiplatelet therapy, as well as possible changes to a heart failure medication regimen.

MitraClip Risks and Benefits

The benefits of the MitraClip™ and its durability have been well documented. The success of this procedure is typically greater than 90%, with an average hospital stay of 2 days and a low complication rate. The most common complication that occurs is access site bleeding. Less frequently, there is partial clip detachment, device embolization, or narrowing of the mitral valve size (called mitral stenosis). Most patients show dramatic improvement in their mitral regurgitation that persists with improvement in ventricular size and their heart failure status. References related to TAVR and TMVr including the MitraClip™ can be found in the bibliography by searching those terms.

Osteopathic Manipulative Medicine for the Cardiac Patient

28

Sheldon Yao and Todd J. Cohen

Osteopathic manipulative medicine (OMM) is a hands-on complementary medicine treatment provided by osteopathic physicians. It is a safe and easily tolerated option that corrects, or "manipulates," dysfunctional sections of the musculoskeletal system. When utilizing OMM, doctors evaluate and treat a patient's musculoskeletal system in order to improve their functionality. Some applications of OMM might impact the cardiovascular system. Table 28.1 shows some facts related to OMM and how it can benefit heart patients.

Osteopathy was founded by Dr. Andrew Taylor Still, MD, in the late 1800s. A pioneer physician, Dr. Still discovered that he could treat his patients by restoring normal healthy motion to areas of musculoskeletal restriction in their bodies. In his autobiography, Dr. Still describes how he suffered from back pain and an irregular heartbeat after being thrown from a horse. Both symptoms resolved after his spine

Table 28.1 OMM facts

OMM is a hands-on manipulative medical treatment.
OMM was founded by Dr. Andrew Taylor Still in the late 1800s.
Dr. Still applied pressure to the back, which relieved back pain and an irregular heart rhythm.
OMM is a holistic therapy connecting the mind, body, and spirit.
OMM may lower blood pressure and may have an effect on your heart rhythm.
Improves mobility, thereby facilitating ability to exercise in order to maintain cardiac fitness.

S. Yao (✉)
Department of Osteopathic Manipulative Medicine, New York Institute of Technology College of Osteopathic Medicine, Old Westbury, NY, USA
e-mail: sheldon.yao@nyit.edu

T. J. Cohen
NYIT College of Osteopathic Medicine, New York, NY, USA
e-mail: tcohen03@nyit.edu

© The Author(s), under exclusive license to Springer Nature Switzerland AG 2025
T. J. Cohen, R. S. Blumenthal (eds.), *Surviving and Thriving With Heart Disease*,
Contemporary Cardiology, https://doi.org/10.1007/978-3-032-00579-3_28

was adjusted while lying back on a clay ball. This experience led him to believe that nerves exiting the spine can influence the internal organs, including the heart. He continued to develop manual treatment to target restrictions of the musculoskeletal system in order to resolve nerve compressions and promote lymphatic and circulatory flow. Based on this principle, diseases affecting cardiovascular health may have a direct connection to the musculoskeletal system.

One of the osteopathic tenets is the connection of mind, body, and spirit. OMM aims to reduce the general level of stress and work that the body experiences, also called allostatic load. By reducing this load, OMM may improve the balance of the nervous system and facilitate the treatment of cardiac conditions. With respect to heart failure and peripheral vascular disease, some data exist that suggest that OMM may improve circulation and promote lymphatic drainage. Additionally, OMM can improve mobility, thereby facilitating the ability to exercise in order to maintain cardiac fitness.

Dr. Todd Cohen and his team at the New York Institute of Technology College of Medicine, together with the Department of Osteopathic Manipulative Medicine, performed a preliminary randomized trial of OMM versus placebo in patients with cardiac implantable electronic devices (pacemakers, defibrillators, and implantable loop recorders). Their study demonstrated improvement in activities of daily living and pain in those with cardiac devices. This study demonstrated that OMM can be safely applied to cardiac patients with no significant adverse events noted in the trial.

It is important for patients to let their cardiologist know if they are going to receive or are receiving OMM therapy. OMM typically should not interfere with the effects of cardiac treatment, except perhaps immediately after open heart surgery or immediately after receiving a pacemaker or defibrillator. Complete healing from those procedures would be recommended before receiving treatment.

Catheter Ablation

29

Todd J. Cohen

The term *ablation,* used medically, is a procedure that is performed to treat, ameliorate, and potentially cure a medical problem. Surgical ablation is used to excise and/or deliver therapy to an area of the body in order to treat and/or destroy an abnormality, such as cancer. When applied to the heart, this treatment is called cardiac ablation. Cardiac ablation is typically used to treat cardiac arrhythmias. It is most frequently used to treat atrial fibrillation, atrial flutter, supraventricular tachycardia, symptomatic premature ventricular contractions, and stable ventricular tachycardia, though it can also treat atrial tachycardia, ventricular fibrillation (via substrate ablation), unstable ventricular tachycardia, and inappropriate sinus tachycardia.

The risks of catheter ablation include heart perforation, damage to its conduction system (potentially requiring a pacemaker implant (although rare)), and collateral damage (to nearby structures such as the phrenic nerve and esophagus). Other complications include bleeding, stroke, and even death (the latter two are rare).

Procedure

Typically, cardiac ablation uses a specialized medical device to generate an electrical therapy (radiofrequency energy or pulsed field ablation) that is delivered to the heart via a catheter. In that instance, it is called cardiac catheter ablation. Cardiac ablation can also be performed with a freezing balloon (cryoablation) or via the injection of alcohol into the heart muscle in order to destroy the heart tissue that may be responsible for the arrhythmia. Radiation therapy, though not yet approved,

T. J. Cohen (✉)
NYIT College of Osteopathic Medicine, New York, NY, USA
e-mail: tcohen03@nyit.edu

© The Author(s), under exclusive license to Springer Nature Switzerland AG 2025   175
T. J. Cohen, R. S. Blumenthal (eds.), *Surviving and Thriving With Heart Disease*,
Contemporary Cardiology, https://doi.org/10.1007/978-3-032-00579-3_29

has also been used as a noninvasive form of ablation in those with difficult to treat ventricular tachycardias.

Cardiac catheter ablation may be performed as a stand-alone procedure or as an extension of an electrophysiology (EP) study to diagnose, map, and treat arrhythmias. Once the mechanism of the arrhythmia is defined, mapping and cardiac ablation can be performed. Typically, a long thin medical device called an ablation catheter is inserted through a blood vessel in the groin and guided into the heart using X-ray or mapping equipment. Occasionally, the ablation catheter can be remotely controlled using more complex robotic equipment. Heart conditions that can be treated with ablation procedures are summarized in Table 29.1.

Figure 29.1 shows a Mount Sinai electrophysiologist with a specialized contact sensing ablation catheter in hand. He will insert the catheter into the black steerable sheath's handle resting on the patient. Nonfluoroscopic (no radiation needed) mapping

Table 29.1 Heart conditions treated by ablation procedures

Easier to treat	More difficult to treat
Typical atrial flutter	Ventricular tachycardia
AV node reentry	Atrial fibrillation
AV node ablation	Atrial tachycardia
	Wolff-Parkinson-White syndrome

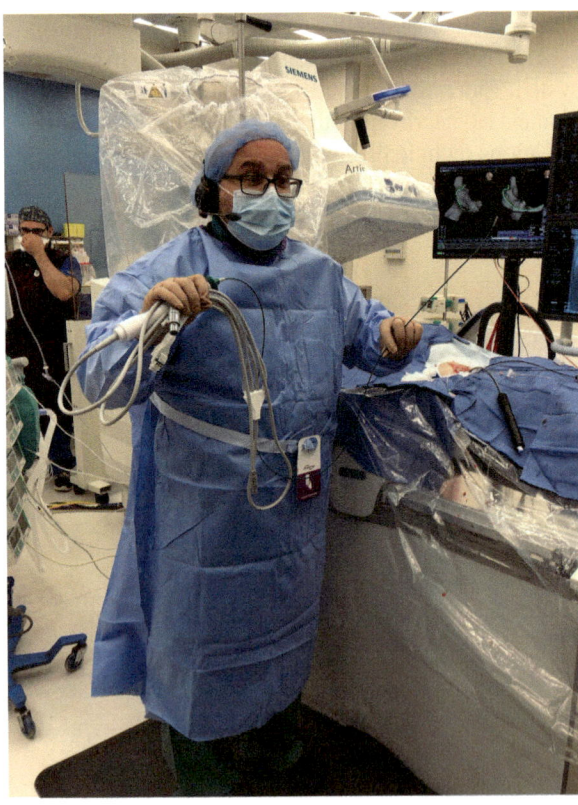

Fig. 29.1 A Mount Sinai electrophysiologist, Dr. Seth Keller, assisting in a complex ablation procedure with the author. He is holding a contact sensing catheter, to enhance the safety of the ablation, and is about to insert the ablation catheter (in his hands) into a steerable sheath, in order to control the delivery of radiofrequency energy during the ablation procedure

helps guide the ablation, and contact sensing assures that not too much force is applied to the catheter tip (an important safety feature that can minimize perforation).

Cardiac Mapping

More difficult ablation procedures are often left-sided and may require additional equipment such as intracardiac echocardiography (ICE) and a 3-D mapping system. The 3-D mapping equipment is used to identify the type of arrhythmia and assist in finding where the arrhythmia originates. It can also track the location of each ablation that is applied to the heart. Figure 29.2 shows a high-density map obtained from the Rhythmia™ mapping system manufactured by Boston Scientific.

Mapping may look like a video game to the untrained observer; however, it is a computer-intensive system that can gather many electrical points and recordings in

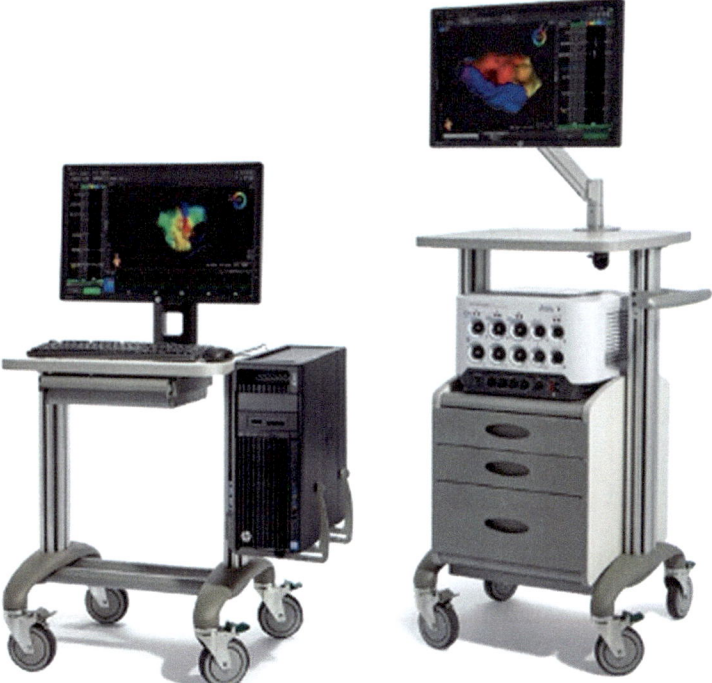

Fig. 29.2 A high-density map obtained from the Rhythmia™ mapping system manufactured by Boston Scientific. The figure shows a high-density voltage map of the left ventricle that could be useful in identifying viable tissue that could support ventricular tachycardia. The image shows a narrow corridor of low-voltage tissue within a region of dense scar. Elimination of this corridor may help eliminate the ventricular tachycardia. (Reproduced with permission from HMP Communications LLC from Practical Electrophysiology, Third Edition. Image provided with courtesy of Boston Scientific. ©2020 Boston Scientific Corporation or its affiliates. All rights reserved)

space in order to define the heart's inner structures while recording its electrical activity. In this image, a voltage map is obtained from the left ventricle. A small corridor of low-voltage tissue was detected within a dense scar. For arrhythmias that originate at a focal spot within the heart, the earliest spot may be mapped and color-coded to indicate the area where the rhythm is coming from. The tip of an ablation catheter can then be manipulated to that point in order to localize and ablate the source of the heart rhythm abnormality. These nonfluoroscopic mapping systems can facilitate ablation procedures and minimize radiation exposure to both the patient and the operator.

Some complex ablation procedures may also require more complicated mapping and ablation catheters, as well as the use of blood thinners, temporary use of an artificial airway, and general anesthesia. Atrial fibrillation ablation also typically requires a transseptal procedure in which a needle is carefully placed from the right atrium into the left atrium, along with a sheath, in order to access the left atrium for pulmonary vein isolation and other ablative maneuvers (see Chap. 9).

The transseptal procedure has the additional risk of perforation, inadvertent puncture of the aorta, and/or risk of stroke from bubble or clot formation. Figure 29.3 shows this book's coauthor, Dr. Todd Cohen, performing a catheter ablation procedure. Please note that your doctor should discuss his or her recommendations if you

Fig. 29.3 The book's coauthor, Dr. Todd Cohen, performing a catheter ablation in the state of New York, during the COVID-19 pandemic, when the hospitals permitted elective procedures

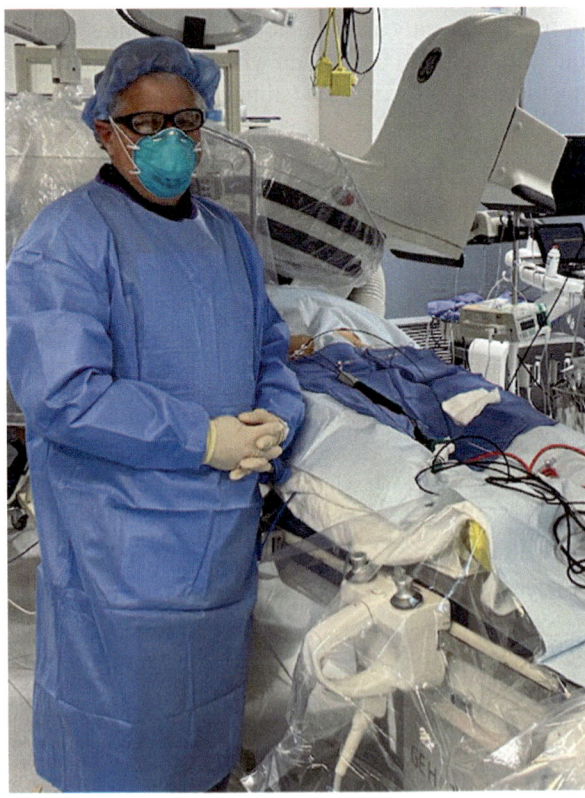

are diagnosed with an arrhythmia that might benefit from a catheter ablation procedure.

Cardiac Ablation Outcomes

The anticipated success rates for specific types of ablation procedures are presented in Table 29.2. Success rates differ based on physician experience, in this case the number of procedures the physician has performed and how long he or she has practiced electrophysiology. In general, the greater the physician's experience, the greater the success rate. Ablation of ventricular tachycardia is typically more complicated than ablation of supraventricular tachycardia. Exceptions to this rule are common. In general, success rates for ablation of supraventricular tachycardia are typically greater than 90% if treated properly.

Success rates for atrial fibrillation ablation depend on the duration and type of heart disease; rates of cure range from 50% to 85% (depending on whether the atrial fibrillation comes and goes (called paroxysmal) or is more permanent and longstanding (called persistent or chronic)). The latter type of atrial fibrillation is more difficult to cure and therefore has a lower success rate. More than one procedure may be required to achieve success from atrial fibrillation ablation.

Ventricular tachycardia that is due to coronary artery disease or a heart attack is ablated with a success rate of between 50% and 75%. Certain types of ventricular tachycardias that begin from a specific site in a more normal heart have a very high cure rate of more than 90% if treated properly. More complex and unstable forms of ventricular tachycardia, and even ventricular fibrillation, can be effectively treated via mapping of the ablation treatment performed both inside the heart (endocardial) and out (epicardial). Substrate ablation may be effective in up to 50% of patients.

Table 29.2 Anticipated success rates of types of catheter ablation procedures

Ablation type	Anticipated success
Supraventricular tachycardia*	90% or greater
Atrial fibrillation	50–85%
Ventricular tachycardia from coronary artery disease	50–75%
Focal ventricular tachycardia	90% or greater

*Atrial flutter, Atrial tachycardia, AV node, AV node reentrant tachycardia, and Wolff-Parkinson-White syndrome
Source: Derived from T. J. Cohen, *Practical Electrophysiology,* Third Edition (Malvern, PA: HMP Communications, 2016), p. 107

Pacemakers and Implantable Defibrillators (Includes Leadless Pacemakers and Wearable and Subcutaneous Defibrillators)

30

Todd J. Cohen

Pacemakers (Standard and Leadless)

Pacemakers are useful in treating symptomatic bradycardias by electrically stimulating the heart muscle. These devices also can record events (such as tachycardias). A standard pacemaker is a device that is about the size of a half dollar and is typically implanted in the chest and attached to at least one wire, which is threaded to the heart through a vein in the chest. Alternatively, there is a leadless option that is inserted through a vein in the groin and wedged into the right heart ventricular muscle, toward the septum (Fig. 30.1). A doctor is likely to recommend a pacemaker for people who have symptoms such as fatigue, lightheadedness, dizziness, and syncope attributable to bradycardia.

In 2008, the American College of Cardiology, the American Heart Association, and the Heart Rhythm Society reported the indications for cardiac implantable devices like the pacemaker (pacemaker guidelines were updated in 2018 in "Guideline on the Evaluation and Management of Patients with Bradycardia and Cardiac Conduction Delay"). The indications for pacemaker therapy in general have not changed much over the years and are listed in Appendix B (see also Table 30.1). You may want to discuss this list with your doctor and ask him or her to explain why a pacemaker may be indicated. If you are not sure why a pacemaker has been recommended, ask questions and consider getting a second opinion.

Before the procedure, you will most likely be asked to be NPO (not eat or drink for 6–8 h prior to surgery). Prior to any procedure, inform your doctor of any medications you are taking, especially any blood thinners. A new pacemaker implant

T. J. Cohen (✉)
NYIT College of Osteopathic Medicine, New York, NY, USA
e-mail: tcohen03@nyit.edu

© The Author(s), under exclusive license to Springer Nature Switzerland AG 2025
T. J. Cohen, R. S. Blumenthal (eds.), *Surviving and Thriving With Heart Disease*,
Contemporary Cardiology, https://doi.org/10.1007/978-3-032-00579-3_30

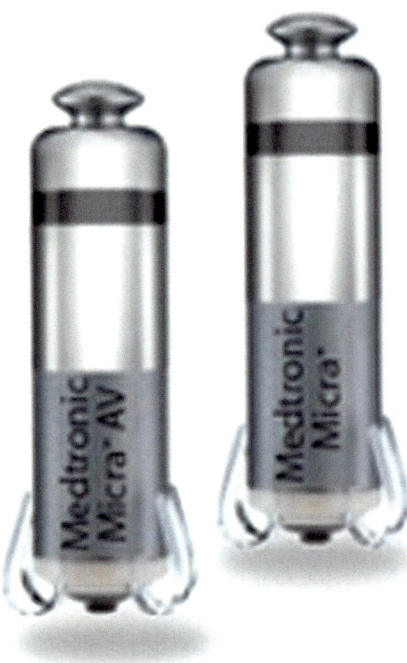

Fig. 30.1 A leadless pacemaker manufactured by Medtronic Inc. The author of this book, Dr. Todd Cohen, worked on a leadless pacemaker in the late 1970s under Dr. Victor Parsonnett, from Newark Beth Israel Medical Center, and was able to demonstrate proof of concept by eliminating a pacemaker lead and using a transmitter and receiver. The latest version of the device is a self-contained bullet-sized pacemaker, without a lead, that is fastened to the inside of the heart. The latter device comes in two varieties currently: a single chamber device, shown below, and another that can sense atrial activity (but cannot pace the atrium) and both sense and pace the ventricle. Future devices will eventually be able to sense and pace both the atrium and the ventricle. (Reproduced with permission from HMP Communications LLC from Practical Electrophysiology, Third Edition; Reproduced with permission of Medtronic, Inc.)

Table 30.1 When do you need a pacemaker?

If you have slow heart rhythms with symptoms
If you have an advanced heart block
To prevent or treat some rapid rhythms and vasovagal syncope
To treat heart failure by pacing the right and left ventricles synchronously (called biventricular pacing)

may require an overnight stay in the hospital to observe for any postoperative complications. Prophylactic antibiotics might be administered before the procedure and given for a few days afterward.

The traditional pacemaker (Fig. 30.2) is connected to a wire that may be attached to the heart with a screw or wedged into the heart with tiny, soft barbs (Fig. 30.3). During the procedure, the doctor will make a small incision (usually in the upper chest), and the lead(s) will be threaded down to the heart, where they will be able to sense your rhythm and pace if it is too slow. Your doctor will determine the number of leads required and discuss the procedural risks including clot formation, vascular damage or perforation, infection, lead dislodgement, and device malfunction.

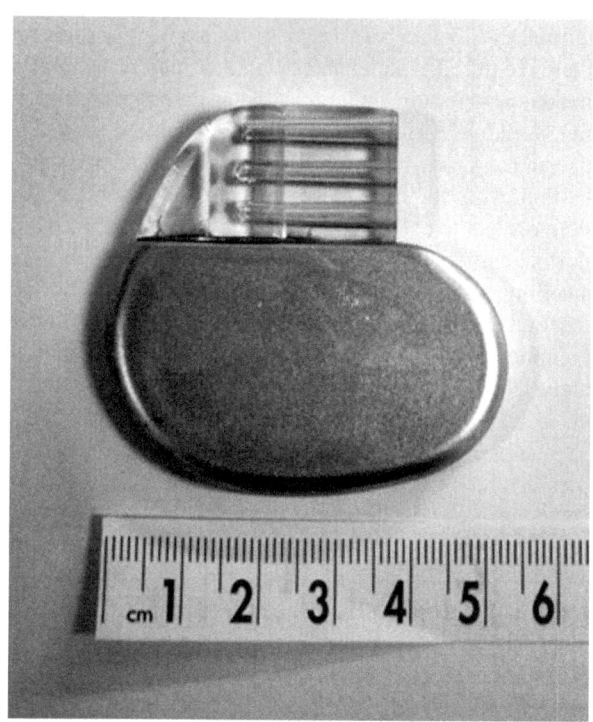

Fig. 30.2 A pacemaker pulse generator used to treat slow heart rhythms. One, two, or three leads may be attached to the device depending on the number of heart chambers that are required to receive pacing therapy. The generator shown has three places to connect pacing leads and may be used to help synchronize the right and left ventricles (biventricular pacing). (Adapted from T.J. Cohen, *A Patient's Guide to Heart Rhythm Problems* (Baltimore, MD: The Johns Hopkins University Press, 2010), p. 106)

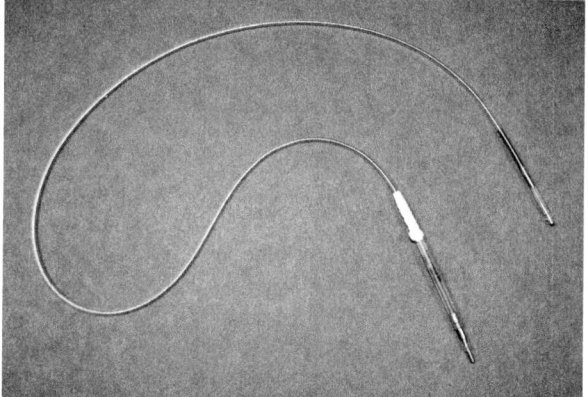

Fig. 30.3 A pacemaker wire, or lead, is inserted into a heart chamber and then connected to a pacemaker, which is usually implanted in the upper chest, underneath the skin. (Adapted from T.J. Cohen, *A Patient's Guide to Heart Rhythm Problems* (Baltimore, MD: The Johns Hopkins University Press, 2010), p. 107)

Depending on the technique used to implant the device, there may also be a risk of a collapsed lung. Major complications such as a heart attack, stroke, or death are rare. Although these risks may seem overwhelming, this procedure is relatively safe.

Alternatively, your doctor may decide that you are a candidate for a leadless pacemaker. This device is inserted through a large catheter in the groin, and the device is wedged into the right ventricular septum and attached by tiny barbs to the heart. The leadless variety has advantages and disadvantages over the standard leaded pacemaker. One advantage is the lack of a pacemaker pocket and leads. The latter can break due to movement, and if that occurs, it may need to be replaced. One current disadvantage of leadless pacemakers is their inability to pace the atrium. If that is required, a standard pacemaker may be necessary. Insertion of leadless pacemakers also requires a large catheter in the groin, and complications, such as bleeding, pseudoaneurysm, and perforation, may be more common. In the future, leadless pacemakers may become smaller and be capable of pacing both chambers.

Following the procedure, you may have some physical limitations for 6 weeks, with respect to exercise and lifting; but in general, you will be able to return to your normal daily activities. If you develop any fever, or notice any discolored discharge, swelling, excessive pain at the incision site (signs of infection for a standard chest-inserted pacemaker), or groin pain, swelling, or bleeding (signs of a groin/vessel complication from the leadless pacemaker), contact your doctor's office immediately. Normal follow-up includes a 2-week wound check and follow-up device checks at approximately 2 months, 6 months, and every 6 months thereafter. Typically, a pacemaker lasts about 8–14 years. For more details about pacemakers, please refer to Appendix B. If there are terms or concepts that you do not understand, ask your doctor about them.

Implantable Cardioverter Defibrillators (ICDs)

Question: True or false: You cannot use a microwave if you have an ICD (or defibrillator).

Answer: False. Patients with these devices can use a microwave safely.

Implantable cardioverter defibrillators (ICDs) were developed in the early 1980s and are useful to treat rapid rhythms. They are very similar to pacemakers and consist of a pulse generator and a lead or leads (Fig. 30.4). To treat rapid rhythms, these devices must be able to detect and terminate them (ventricular tachycardia and ventricular fibrillation). To do this, ICDs deliver high-voltage direct current energy, and therefore require more electrical circuitry and battery power than a pacemaker. They are also larger than pacemakers and roughly the size of a deck of cards, rather than the size of a half dollar. In general, the lead that is used in an ICD to cardiovert, or defibrillate, is slightly thicker and stiffer than a standard pacemaker lead (Fig. 30.4).

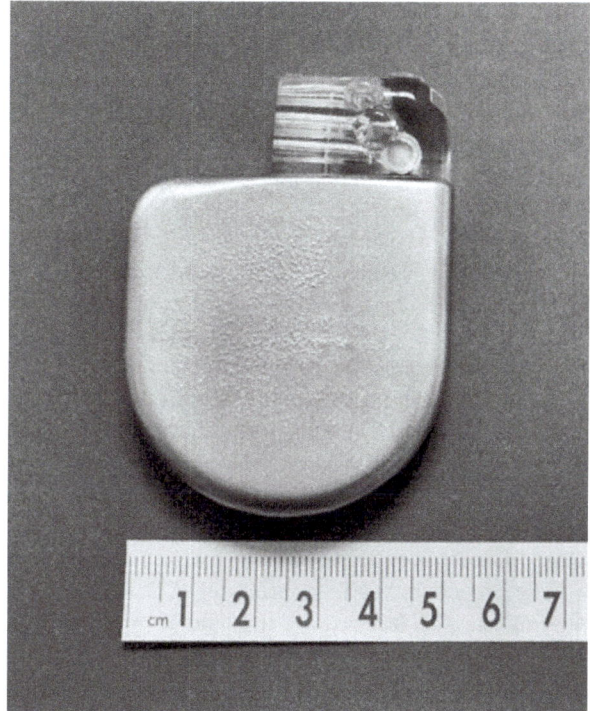

Fig. 30.4 An implantable cardioverter defibrillator (ICD) pulse generator, which is used to treat rapid rhythms from the lower chamber of the heart, called ventricular tachycardia or ventricular fibrillation. Note that the specific type of ICD shown in this figure is a biventricular device (see Chap. 31). (Adapted from T.J. Cohen, *A Patient's Guide to Heart Rhythm Problems* (Baltimore, MD: The Johns Hopkins University Press, 2010), p. 111)

Table 30.2 When do you need a defibrillator?

After cardiac arrest due to an arrhythmia
If you have symptomatic ventricular tachycardia or ventricular fibrillation
If you have ventricular tachycardia or ventricular fibrillation induced during an EP study
If you have loss of consciousness (syncope) and structural heart disease
If you have an EF of 35% or less and mild to moderate heart failure
If you have an EF of 30% or less and a prior heart attack
If you have a hereditary condition meeting criteria that places you at high risk for sudden death (Brugada syndrome, arrhythmogenic right ventricular cardiomyopathy/dysplasia, hypertrophic cardiomyopathy)

While the primary role of ICDs is to treat fast (tachycardia) or chaotic (fibrillation) rhythms, some also have pacemaker capabilities to help regulate slow rhythms (bradycardias). Simply put, ICDs monitor the heart rate, and if it is greater than a predetermined (or programmed) value, the ICD may deliver therapy to treat the arrhythmia. Ventricular tachycardia or ventricular fibrillation may be treated by the delivery of a shock (defibrillation) or rapid pacing (also called *anti-tachycardia pacing*). This ability to deliver a shock to the heart to terminate tachycardias is one important difference between an ICD and a simple pacemaker.

A patient may benefit from an ICD in various scenarios (see Table 30.2). These types of devices are indicated in patients who have experienced a sudden cardiac arrest, especially if the cause is not reversible. ICDs are also indicated in patients with ventricular tachycardia, whether spontaneous or induced during an EP study. In patients with unexplained loss of consciousness (syncope) and heart disease, an ICD is often very helpful. There are prophylactic indications for these devices (also called *primary prevention* because the person has not yet had an arrhythmic event), such as for patients with mild to moderate congestive heart failure and an ejection fraction of 35% or less.

Patients who have had a prior heart attack (myocardial infarction) and have an ejection fraction of 30% or less may also benefit from ICD therapy. If you have been referred for an ICD implant, you may want to discuss this list with your doctor and ask him or her to explain which ICD indication or indications you have. If you are not sure why an ICD has been recommended for you, you should ask questions and consider getting a second opinion. Typically, an ICD lasts about 6 years. For a more complete list of ICD indications derived in part from the American College of Cardiology, American Heart Association, and Heart Rhythm Society guidelines (defibrillator guidelines were updated in 2017 in "Guideline for Management of Patients with Ventricular Arrhythmias and the Prevention of Sudden Cardiac Death"), see Appendix C.

The procedure for implanting an ICD is very similar to that for implanting a pacemaker. The increase in size and complexity of the pulse generator and the increased size and stiffness of the high-voltage ICD lead carry a slightly higher risk of complications compared with implanting a pacemaker. Many of the risks involved in ICD surgery are the same, however, and include clot formation, vascular damage or perforation, infection, lead dislodgement, device malfunction, heart attack, stroke, and death. The ICD recovery period is also similar to that of a pacemaker.

Normal follow-up includes a 2-week wound check and device checks at approximately 2 months, 6 months, and every 6 months thereafter. People who receive an ICD are instructed to call their doctor's office if they receive one shock; if they receive two or more shocks, it is important that they be seen by a physician as soon as possible. Figure 30.5 shows an episode of ventricular tachycardia terminated by a shock from an ICD.

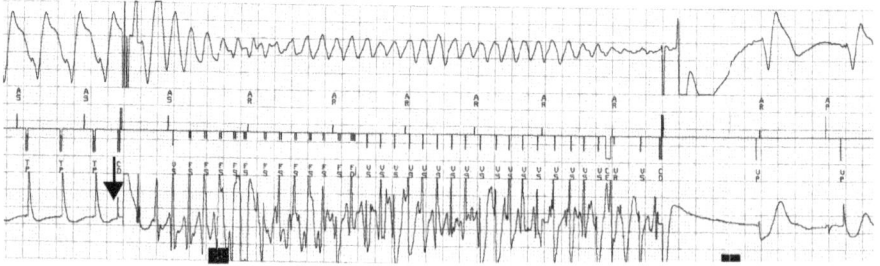

Fig. 30.5 This figure shows an episode of ventricular tachycardia requiring two shocks from an ICD in order to terminate the arrhythmia (Reproduced with permission from HMP Communications LLC from Practical Electrophysiology, Third Edition)

Wearable Cardioverter Defibrillator (WCD)

Patients who are at high risk for ventricular tachycardia, ventricular fibrillation, or sudden cardiac arrest, but are not candidates for a permanent implant of an implantable defibrillator, may benefit from a wearable cardioverter defibrillator (or WCD). Some examples are those with a recent heart attack and an ejection fraction of less than 30% that may improve over time. Another indication for a WCD is a patient with an infected ICD who requires removal of their implantable device and treatment with antibiotics in order to eradicate the infection. A WCD can protect these patients from sudden death (caused by ventricular tachycardia or fibrillation), during their antibiotic treatment period (when they do not have an ICD), thereby allowing their body to heal so they can eventually receive another device. Finally, those who may be at high risk for sudden death and are awaiting heart transplantation may benefit from a WCD as a bridge to transplantation.

Dr. Cohen utilized a WCD in one of his patients during the heart of the COVID-19 pandemic when the hospitals were on lockdown and unavailable for elective cardiac services. A patient had a long run of symptomatic non-sustained ventricular tachycardia (28 beats) and temporarily used a WCD until hospitals opened up again in New York for elective electrophysiology procedures. That patient eventually received an implantable defibrillator. Figure 30.6 shows a WCD in which the defibrillator is built into a vest and powered/controlled by a computerized harness. The patient is warned that a shock is coming by exploding gels and can abort the shock with the press of a button.

Subcutaneous ICD

Another variety of ICD is the subcutaneous ICD (or S-ICD). This variety is very helpful in those who do not require pacing for bradycardia or termination of their ventricular tachycardia. It avoids the placement of leads within the heart, which can break, get infected, and cause other problems. For those who need a defibrillator for primary prevention, i.e., have never had sudden death or ventricular tachycardia or fibrillation, are young and may require multiple ventricular lead replacements over their lifetime, and may be at risk for sudden death from an acquired or hereditary condition and just need a backup shocking box (defibrillator), the S-ICD may be a good option. Figure 30.7 shows an example of the S-ICD, which looks similar to a regular ICD but is positioned somewhat differently, and the leads are not implanted inside the heart, but rather underneath the skin (subcutaneously).

Case 6: A Memory of My Stepfather

On Sunday morning, I finished my usual morning swim at the local Y and headed down to the marina to clean my boat. The traffic was stop and go, so I lit another cigarette and sipped my coffee as I began the hour-long drive. Little did I know that on this day, my life would change forever.

Fig. 30.6 This figure shows a wearable cardioverter defibrillator (WCD), called a LifeVest (TM) manufactured by Zoll Medical Corp. (Chelmsford, MA). The patient usually wears this until it becomes clear that they either need or do not need an implantable defibrillator. This is a temporary protection from sudden death either because they do not yet qualify for an ICD or they cannot receive an ICD since they are being treated for an infection. It is also used as a bridge to heart transplantation (see Chap. 35). (Reproduced with permission from HMP Communications LLC from Practical Electrophysiology, Third Edition)

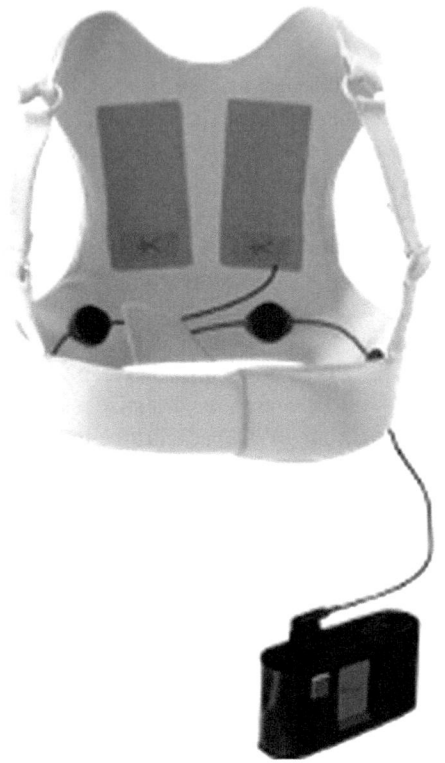

I had been working on the boat for several hours and was almost finished when I suddenly began to feel extremely tired. My hands were cramping up, and I felt tightness in my throat. I left the boat to lie down on the grass until I felt able to walk a few yards to a restaurant, where I drank a few glasses of orange juice. Still feeling weak, and totally clueless about what was happening, I left the marina and drove home. My hands were still cramping, and I was just not feeling right. I wondered if inhaling fumes from the acetone cleaner was making me feel sick. I arrived home exhausted. I showered and went to sleep, certain that I would be fine in the morning. But I wasn't. Next morning, I noticed that every time I climbed a flight of stairs, I felt tightness in my throat and was short of breath. Now I was frightened. Could I be having a heart attack?

I got into the car and drove the few blocks to my internist's office. He immediately arranged for a stress test, but a minute into the test, I was told I needed an angiogram. Then panic set in. "This can't be real," I thought, "I'm a healthy guy." But the angiogram revealed serious blockages in my coronary arteries, and I was told that I would have to have triple bypass surgery. I was shocked, scared, and angry. But then reality set in, and I knew I had had a heart attack.

I was relieved when my surgeon told me that the surgery had gone well. I would have a second chance. But I was also depressed. I had to change my lifestyle in so many ways. I was prescribed a heart-healthy diet and told that I had to stop smoking

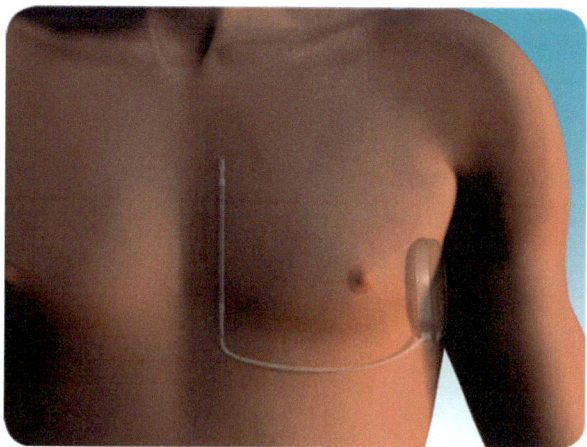

Fig. 30.7 A subcutaneous version of an ICD is shown (called a SICD) in which no intravascular leads are inserted into the heart, only subcutaneous wires/antennae that are tunneled under the skin and connected to the pulse generator that is shown. This is very helpful in those who are young, may not require many shocks, and may eventually require multiple devices and leads during their lifetime. This device does not offer pacing capabilities. (Reproduced with permission from HMP Communications LLC from Practical Electrophysiology, Third Edition; Image provided with courtesy of Boston Scientific. ©2020 Boston Scientific Corporation or its affiliates. All rights reserved)

cigarettes. I entered a cardiac rehab program and slowly regained my strength. But I couldn't kick the cigarette habit. I continued smoking in secret, hiding cigarettes in the trunk of my car and driving with the car windows open even in the coldest weather to conceal the odor of the smoke from my family. The doctor had said that I survived the heart attack because collateral blood vessels had formed from my daily swim. I started to swim again. I thought that I could continue smoking as long as I kept up the swimming. I was wrong.

Two years after my bypass surgery, I underwent a stress test and experienced a brief episode of ventricular tachycardia. After that, I went for an electrophysiology study, which showed that I needed an implantable defibrillator. Six weeks after I received the implant, I felt the device go off. It has gone off three more times since. Each time the defibrillator responded appropriately by shocking my heart back to its normal rhythm—thereby saving my life. I felt fine after each shock. There was no warning beforehand. I am grateful to my doctor and thankful for my defibrillator. It gives me hope that I can live to a ripe old age. After all, it saved my life four times. Oh yes, one more thing—I finally stopped smoking!

Implants for Heart Failure (Biventricular and Other "Optimizing" Devices)

31

Todd J. Cohen

The right and left heart chambers normally contract in synchrony to efficiently pump blood to the rest of the body. Patients with heart failure often have hearts that are out of synchrony, or dyssynchronous, meaning that the left and right ventricles contract out of sequence. This results in a less effective pumping mechanism and can lead to fluid buildup in the heart and lungs. Cardiac resynchronization therapy may restore synchrony by allowing the right and left sides of the heart to pump together more efficiently.

By placing a wire in both the left and right sides of the heart (the ventricles) and pacing both sides nearly simultaneously, doctors can improve the performance of the heart, including its ejection fraction. The biventricular approach can be used with a pacemaker or an ICD, and Dr. Todd Cohen was an investigator in the first study that coined the term biventricular pacing. In patients with weak heart muscles and heart failure, these biventricular devices offer cardiac resynchronization therapy (CRT), which can help alleviate heart failure symptoms.

Certain criteria must be present for a person to qualify for this type of device (see Table 31.1). These criteria include significant congestive heart failure (moderate to severe congestive heart failure, described as New York Heart Association class III or IV, despite treatment with optimal medical therapy), a low ejection fraction (35% or less), and the presence of a wide QRS complex on the ECG (see Chap. 16), such as that which is caused by an ECG finding indicating cardiac dyssynchrony called a bundle branch block. The MADIT-CRT study compared biventricular ICDs to

T. J. Cohen (✉)
NYIT College of Osteopathic Medicine, New York, NY, USA
e-mail: tcohen03@nyit.edu

Table 31.1 When do you need a biventricular device?

If you have moderate to severe heart failure despite being on optimal medical therapy, an EF of less than or equal to 35%, and a wide QRS duration on ECG.
If you have asymptomatic or mild heart failure with an EF of less than or equal to 30% with a wide QRS complex on ECG.
If you have a low EF and are likely to need a lot of right ventricular pacing.
After an AV node ablation (where you could require a lot of ventricular pacing).

regular ICDs in nearly 2000 patients who were asymptomatic or mildly symptomatic for heart failure (New York Heart Association class I and II) with an ejection fraction of 30% or less, and a wide QRS complex. The results demonstrated a significant improvement in both survival and heart failure with a biventricular ICD.

Some physicians believe that biventricular pacing is helpful following ablation of the AV node in patients with atrial fibrillation in which the heart rate remains rapid despite medications. Physician judgment may also play a part in determining whether a biventricular device is needed. Appendix D provides a list of indications for a biventricular device, such as a pacemaker or ICD. Discuss your indication with your physician (see also Chap. 30).

Patients with a biventricular device should be taking routine heart failure medicines, such as diuretics, beta-blockers, and an angiotensin-converting enzyme (ACE) inhibitor or an angiotensin II receptor blocker (ARB), or an angiotensin receptor-neprilysin inhibitor (ARNI; see Chap. 14).

A biventricular defibrillator (Fig. 31.1) uses an additional lead in the heart (referred to as the third lead). This additional lead is placed in the coronary sinus vein, which can pace the left ventricle. By pacing the left and right ventricles nearly simultaneously, pacemakers and ICDs improve heart function in approximately two out of three patients. The risks of this procedure are similar to those of other implantable devices placed in the chest through a vein. Although system problems are rare, patients should be aware that the more wires, leads, and parts involved, the greater the risk of system problems.

Figure 31.2 shows a fluoroscopic image of a left ventricular pacing wire inserted through the coronary sinus vein into a branch to pace the left ventricle. This wire is attached, along with a right ventricular pacing/defibrillator lead and a right atrial lead, into a biventricular pacing device. Figure 31.3 shows a measurement of transthoracic impedance that is used to detect fluid accumulation in the lungs. Dr. Todd Cohen developed the basis for these measurements and it was first utilized in a proprietary Medtronic algorithm called Optivol™ in their implantable defibrillators. Now, almost every defibrillator uses transthoracic impedance in order to detect heart failure.

There is now a newer device to treat heart failure that can pace during the vulnerable cycle of the electrocardiogram. This device is manufactured by Impulse Dynamics and is called the "Optimizer Smart System." This device delivers cardiac contractility modulation (CCM) and may help those with NYHA Class III heart failure, with a left ventricular ejection fraction from 25% to 45%, who do not

Fig. 31.1 A biventricular implantable cardioverter defibrillator (ICD) pulse generator used to treat people who have congestive heart failure and are at risk for sudden cardiac death. (Adapted from T.J. Cohen, *A Patient's Guide to Heart Rhythm Problems* (Baltimore, MD: The Johns Hopkins University Press, 2010), p. 115)

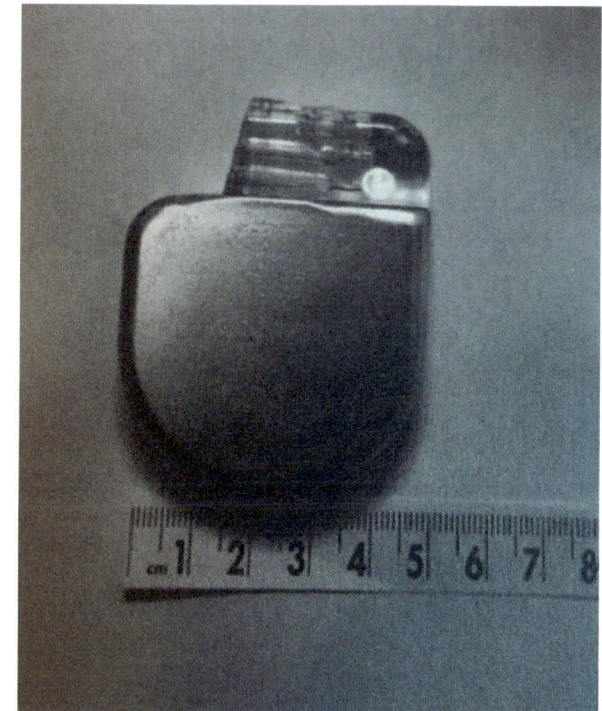

Fig. 31.2 A pacemaker lead inserted in a heart blood vessel called the coronary sinus vein intended to pace the left ventricle of the heart. Another wire is used to pace the right ventricle of the heart. Pacing both ventricles, in order to achieve cardiac resynchronization therapy, is an important treatment of congestive heart failure. This book's author, Dr. Todd Cohen, was part of the first study to coin the term "biventricular pacing." (Reproduced with permission from HMP Communications LLC from Practical Electrophysiology, Third Edition)

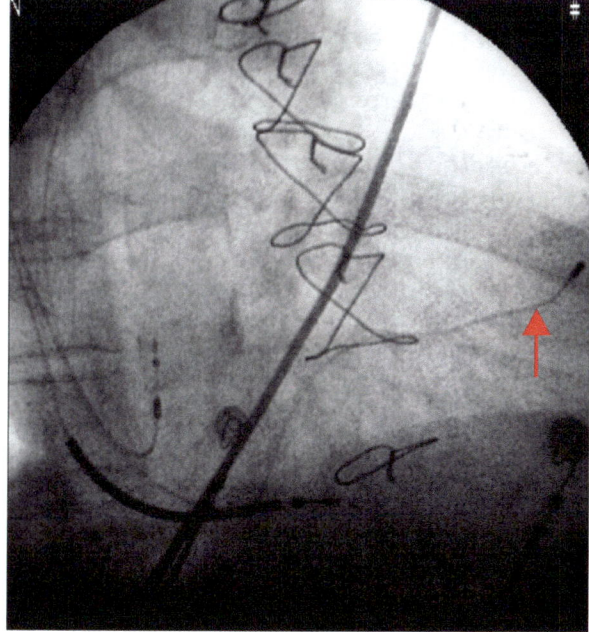

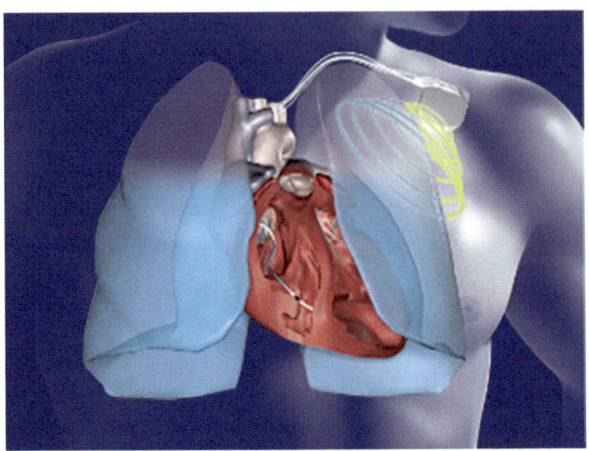

Fig. 31.3 An important feature now utilized in almost every implantable defibrillator, which is using transthoracic impedance to detect fluid accumulation in the lungs (heart failure). The basic concept and invention used in modern-day devices was developed by Dr. Todd Cohen. This figure shows Medtronic's version called the Optivol, which was the first defibrillator to incorporate transthoracic impedance and fluid accumulation detection into an implantable defibrillator. (Reproduced with permission from HMP Communications LLC from Practical Electrophysiology, Third Edition. Reproduced with permission of Medtronic, Inc.)

Table 31.2 When would you need an "optimizer" device?

If you have moderate heart failure despite being on optimal medical therapy, an EF of 25–45%, and a narrow QRS duration on ECG (don't qualify for a biventricular device).

qualify for cardiac resynchronization therapy (a biventricular implant). Table 31.2 shows when this type of "optimizing" device may be indicated.

Finally, a newer form of cardiac pacing may achieve many, if not all, of the effects of cardiac resynchronization by pacing within the conduction system. This newer modality is called conduction system pacing. In essence, pacing within the His-bundle or left bundle branch has been demonstrated to be more beneficial than right ventricular apical pacing over the long haul. This is because the electrical stimuli can hook into the normal conduction system, which results in a narrower, synchronized ventricular paced complex, without the necessity of two ventricular leads.

Conduction system pacing is often used in patients who need the criteria for cardiac resynchronization therapy but, for technical reasons, failed in an attempt at placing biventricular leads. In general, left-bundle branch pacing is easier and more stable in the long haul than His-bundle pacing. Please speak to your doctor regarding the risks, benefits, and alternatives to the above pacemaker treatment modalities.

Left Atrial Occlusive Devices

32

Davendra Mehta

Atrial fibrillation is the most common heart rhythm abnormality that originates in the upper chambers of the heart (left and right atrium). Its prevalence increases with age and about 8% of the population above the age of 70 years is likely to develop it at some stage. One of the most dreaded complications of atrial fibrillation is stroke. This is related to sluggish flow of blood in the upper chambers of the heart. As a result of sluggish flow and pooling of blood, clots form in a pouch called the left atrial appendage (LAA). Blood clots from LAA may then get dislodged and can block any artery in the body.

Dislodged blood clots from the heart can get stuck in arteries of the brain, ultimately leading to a stroke. Thus, stroke is the most disabling complication of atrial fibrillation and is associated with increased morbidity and mortality. The risk of stroke is highest in patients with atrial fibrillation who are above the age of 65 years and have diabetes mellitus, high blood pressure, heart failure, or had a previous stroke.

Blood thinners markedly reduce the incidence of stroke in high-risk populations by preventing and dissolving left atrial clots. One major limitation of the use of blood thinners is the risk of bleeding. Unfortunately, the risk of bleeding is even higher in patients with atrial fibrillation who are already at an increased risk of stroke. In patients who cannot tolerate blood thinners, surgical removal of the left atrial appendage can be performed by opening the chest and surgically tying off the left atrial appendage. Devices used to close the left atrial appendage are referred to

D. Mehta (✉)
Icahn School of Medicine at Mount Sinai, New York, NY, USA
e-mail: davendra.mehta@mountsinai.org

as LAA closure or occlusion devices. Systems have also been developed to close the LAA from outside the heart (such as the Lariat™ and the AtriClip™ by AtriCure, Inc. Mason, OH).

A simpler alternative to outside the heart LAA closure are the LAA occlusive devices placed from the groin (through a vein) into the heart. The Watchman™ (Boston Scientific Corp., Marlborough, MA) is an expandable umbrella-like LAA occlusive device that can be placed (from a groin vein into the heart at the opening of LAA in the left atrium (Fig. 32.1). It was first approved by the United States Food and Drug Administration (FDA) in 2015 for use in patients with atrial fibrillation who do not have any malfunction of their heart valves. An improved version was released in 2020 called the WatchmanFlex™. These devices are used only in patients who cannot tolerate blood thinners long-term due to bleeding or are at risk of bleeding (frequent falls or professional reasons). Occlusion devices are not considered for patients who have no problems with blood thinners. Table 32.1 shows the indications for implanting a LAA occlusion device.

Prior to implantation, a transesophageal echocardiogram is performed to confirm that there is no clot in LAA and that the size and shape are suitable for the occlusion device. This is performed by placing a probe through the back of the throat into the esophagus to look at the left atrium and appendage. The LAA occlusion procedure is undertaken if it is confirmed that there is no clot in the LAA. Most patients (95%) have a LAA that is suitable for the LAA occlusion device. The

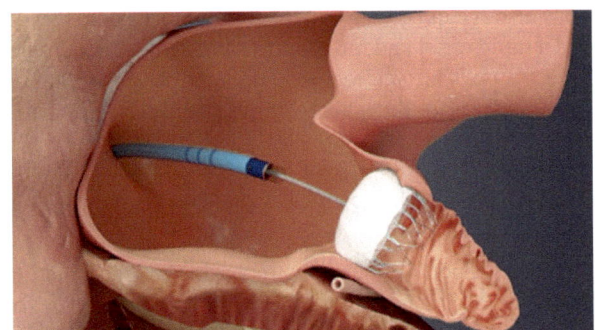

Fig. 32.1 The proper position of a left atrial appendage occlusion device (also called a left atrial closure device) in the left atrial appendage. (Image provided with courtesy of Boston Scientific. ©2020 Boston Scientific Corporation or its affiliates. All rights reserved)

Table 32.1 Indications for LAA occlusion/Watchman™ device

1. Atrial fibrillation and high risk of stroke (e.g., above age 65 years, diabetes, high blood pressure, or congestive heart failure)
AND
2. At least one of the following:
    (a) Recurrent bleeding from anywhere precluding long-term safe use of blood thinners (bleeding from the gastrointestinal tract and intracranial being the most common)
    (b) Persistent fall risk (such as old age and/or neurological conditions)
    (c) Lifestyle that increases the risk of trauma and bleeding
Shared decision-making is needed between the treating physician and the implanting physician.

procedure is done under anesthesia and is performed similarly to any cardiac catheterization, through the groin.

The femoral vein in the groin is cannulated, and a small tube is advanced into the heart under ECHO guidance (either intracardiac or transesophageal) and passed from the right atrium to the left atrium (transseptal procedure). Contrast dye is then injected into the LAA to confirm its size, and a folded LAA occlusion device is advanced in the tube to the LAA. The device is released into the opening of the LAA, where it opens like an umbrella when the sheath over it is withdrawn (Fig. 32.1). Once a good placement at the opening of LAA is confirmed, the device is then released and, if necessary, repositioned. The site of entry in the groin is closed by a temporary suture that is taken off the next morning. Patients are kept in the hospital overnight for observation and may return home the following day.

This is a relatively safe procedure with a very small (2–3%) risk of complications; the main ones being bleeding around the heart and device dislodgement. Following implantation, blood thinners are continued for 6 weeks. After that, an echocardiogram is repeated to confirm appropriate occlusion of the LAA. If good position is confirmed, blood thinners (warfarin or newer agents such as Xarelto or Eliquis) are replaced by aspirin and clopidogrel. Six months following implant, clopidogrel is stopped, and patients need to take only aspirin, which is continued indefinitely.

Long-term follow-up studies have shown that these devices are as effective as blood thinners in preventing stroke and are associated with about a 70% reduction in the risk of bleeding. As this implant procedure has become safer, its use has increased, with hundreds of thousands of these devices implanted worldwide.

To close the chapter, a more recently developed device, named the Amplatzer Amulet Left Atrial Occluder (Abbott, Santa Clara, CA), has also been approved for LAA occlusion. Like the Watchman, this device can be placed from the groin into the LAA appendage and used as an alternative to anticoagulants in those at risk for stroke with nonvalvular atrial fibrillation. Please talk to your doctor about the different devices and techniques for LAA occlusion, along with their implant experience, including the risks, benefits, and alternatives, before undergoing any of these procedures.

Coronary Artery Bypass Graft (CABG)

33

Daniel Kersten and Todd J. Cohen

Coronary artery bypass graft (CABG) surgery is another option for patients with advanced coronary artery disease in order to improve blood flow to the heart muscle (known as revascularization) when they have lifestyle-limiting angina or weakened heart muscle contractility. The procedure was first performed in the United States in the 1960s by physicians from the Albert Einstein College of Medicine in New York City. Since then, it has been shown to significantly improve survival rates in patients with coronary artery disease (CAD) and provide significant relief for CAD symptoms. For these reasons, CABG surgery is one of the most common major surgeries performed in the United States. Surgical advancements over the past decade have also introduced an alternative, less invasive procedure called percutaneous coronary intervention (PCI) (see Chap. 24).

The reasons to undergo either CABG surgery or PCI are similar. The most recent guidelines from the American College of Cardiology and the American Heart Association note two major reasons for a patient to undergo a procedure: (1) patients who continue to have CAD symptoms despite being on optimal medical therapy or (2) to reduce the risk of death in patients with extensive CAD. In rare circumstances, a procedure may be preferred over therapy with medications, but this option is generally reserved for patients in high-risk occupations (like airline pilots) who can only be permitted to resume their duties when they are completely revascularized.

Once it is decided that a patient needs some form of revascularization treatment, the choice of treatment must then be determined. This is usually decided after heart

D. Kersten
Department of Cardiology, NYU Langone Hospital – Long Island, Mineola, NY, USA

T. J. Cohen (✉)
NYIT College of Osteopathic Medicine, New York, NY, USA
e-mail: tcohen03@nyit.edu

© The Author(s), under exclusive license to Springer Nature Switzerland AG 2025
T. J. Cohen, R. S. Blumenthal (eds.), *Surviving and Thriving With Heart Disease*,
Contemporary Cardiology, https://doi.org/10.1007/978-3-032-00579-3_33

imaging is performed (see Chaps. 20 and 23) with either a computerized tomography angiogram (also called a cardiac CT angiogram) or with a coronary angiogram (a type of cardiac catheterization). The latter procedure is often preferred, especially if PCI (or stenting) is being considered, because the latter can be performed during the same procedure as the PCI.

Imaging allows physicians to see many important components, including blockages in any arteries, the layout of the heart's blood vessels, and the severity of the blockage. CABG surgery is the preferred intervention if there is severe disease in multiple vessels (generally more than three) or the blockage has certain characteristics, which would make PCI less successful. However, even if these conditions are present, a PCI may be preferred for elderly patients or patients with other severe medical problems, such as emphysema, as they may have a greater risk of complications from CABG surgery.

While CABG surgery is a relatively common procedure, it is also highly invasive. Prior to surgery, several tests need to be performed in order to assess a patient's ability to tolerate the procedure. This generally entails blood work, a chest X-ray, electrocardiography, echocardiography, and coronary catheterization. Some patients may require additional testing, such as pulmonary function testing, depending on other medical conditions they may have and how well they are controlled.

The procedure itself is performed in the operating room under sterile conditions by a cardiothoracic surgery team (including a heart surgeon) and requires monitoring of vital signs (such as blood pressure, breathing rate, oxygen saturation) by a cardiac anesthesiology team. It should be noted that during the operation, the heart is essentially stopped by cooling it, allowing the surgeons to operate more easily on this otherwise quite mobile organ. Patients are also placed on a heart-lung machine, with the help of a cardiac perfusionist, which both oxygenates and pumps blood throughout the body while the heart is arrested (kept still); occasionally, the surgery is performed while the heart is still beating. An incision is then performed down the center of the chest, followed by a sternotomy, in which the bone in the center of the chest, the sternum, is split in two. Then, a careful dissection of the chest structures is performed by the cardiothoracic (heart surgery) team in order to expose the heart.

Once the heart is properly exposed, a section—called a graft—is taken from one of the patient's blood vessels. This graft typically comes from an artery inside the chest wall, called the internal mammary artery, or from a vein in the leg, called the great saphenous vein. The decision on which area to take the graft depends on several variables but generally, the internal mammary artery is preferred due to its location, which is closer to the heart, and better graft survival. Whichever graft is selected, it is placed by creating an opening into the coronary artery in an area after the blockage, and the graft is connected to this opening; this is called the distal anastomosis (or connection). Then, as the heart is rewarmed, another opening is placed into the aorta, and the unconnected end of the graft is connected to this opening; this is called the proximal anastomosis. Once connected, the blocked coronary artery has been bypassed.

The final results of CABG surgery may be visualized in Fig. 33.1. This figure shows a saphenous vein graft (to the left) and an internal mammary graft (to the right). This procedure is repeated for each of the required grafts, depending on the

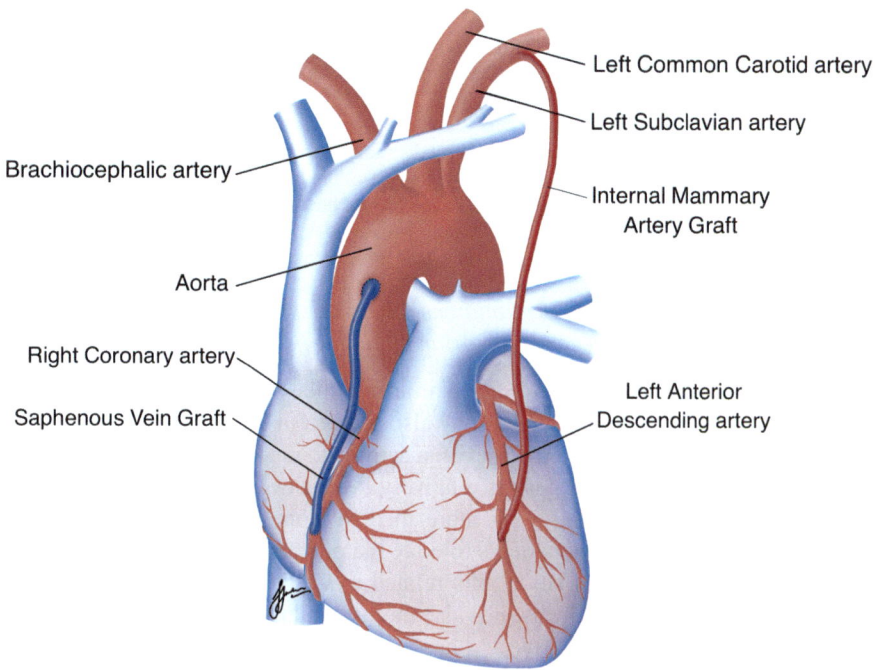

Fig. 33.1 Two types of grafts (saphenous vein graft to the left and internal mammary graft to the right). This graft typically comes from an artery in the chest wall called the mammary artery or a vein in the leg called the saphenous vein. The internal mammary artery is taken down from the chest wall but remains attached to its original blood vessel and only just bypasses the coronary artery. A saphenous vein graft has to be completely removed and reattached to the aorta and then the coronary artery. This drawing is for illustration purposes only. (Figure drawn by Jerry Jose, DO)

number of blockages in the heart. If a patient requires two grafts, it is called a double bypass graft procedure; three grafts are called a triple bypass; four, a quadruple bypass; and so on. Once the procedure is completed, the patient is slowly weaned off the heart-lung machine, and the incisions through the chest are closed.

Once the patient is stable postoperatively, he or she is admitted to the surgical intensive care unit for close monitoring. However, if the patient continues to be stable, he or she may be transferred to a regular hospital bed. Most patients should expect to spend about a week in the hospital following a routine CABG, and complete recovery may take several weeks. As with any surgical procedure, the major risks related to CABG surgery are infection, excessive bleeding or clotting (including deep venous thrombosis and stroke), and adverse effects of anesthesia (confusion, breathing problems, etc.). In addition, there is a risk of acute kidney failure and neurological problems (such as stroke), and these could portend a poor outcome. Lastly, there are cardiac risks—likely as a result of the heart being subjected to a large operation—which include new damage to the heart muscle (a new heart attack) and arrhythmias. The latter occurs in upwards of 30 percent of patients and can vary in severity.

Table 33.1 Key points for coronary artery bypass graft (CABG) surgery

One of the most common surgeries performed in the United States of America.
Invasive, open-chest procedure performed in an operating room by a cardiothoracic surgery team with an anesthesia team.
Usually performed for patients with extensive coronary disease (usually more than one blockage) or those who fail management with medications.
Procedure entails taking a blood vessel graft, typically from either the chest or leg. The graft is then attached to an area after the blockage to restore blood flow to previously blocked areas of the heart.
Requires hospitalization for about a week and a longer recovery time (unlike coronary stenting) but is, overall, a well-tolerated procedure.

Atrial fibrillation is much more common following open chest heart surgery such as CABG, as compared to PCI. Ventricular arrhythmias, such as ventricular tachycardia and/or ventricular fibrillation, may also be seen in the immediate postoperative period and should be treated acutely via cardioversion and/or defibrillation. The rate of death from CABG surgery is relatively low, between one and five percent, and is more likely in patients with more medical comorbidities (problems) and advanced age; however, most patients tolerate the procedure well.

Table 33.1 reviews some key points related to CABG. In general, PCI is less invasive and has fewer side effects. It is also more useful in less severe CAD. CABG, on the other hand, is more invasive and has more side effects (as mentioned above). It is useful with more complicated coronary artery disease, if PCI fails, or if an emergent complication (such as coronary artery dissection) occurs during the stenting procedure.

Valve Repair and Replacement

34

Daniel Kersten and Todd J. Cohen

Valvular heart disease is a relatively common form of structural heart disease in the United States. An estimated 2.5 percent of the population has moderate to severe valvular disease, with the risk of development increasing with age. In 2017, the US Centers for Disease Control and Prevention (CDC) reported that approximately 27,000 Americans died as a result of valve disease. Heart valve replacement surgery is one of the more common cardiac surgeries performed in the United States, as over 182,000 procedures occur each year. Since valvular heart disease is often a consequence of aging, especially aortic stenosis (AS; a narrowing of the aortic valve), these numbers are expected to increase dramatically in the coming years.

Before exploring the topic of valve replacement, there should be a brief review of the heart's valvular system (see Chap. 1). There are four valves in the heart, two on the right side (tricuspid and pulmonic valves) and two on the left side (mitral and aortic valves). Valves open and close depending on their location and the time during the cardiac cycle (heart contraction or relaxation). Valves allow for blood to flow forward when open and prevent reverse blood flow when closed. If there is poor blood flow through a valve due to swelling and/or scarring, this is referred to as stenosis.

When valves allow for the reversal of blood flow, this is known as regurgitation. Depending on the type of valve disease and its severity, valvular replacement may be required. There are two portions of valve anatomy: the leaflets are the actual pieces of tissue that move, and the ring (or annulus) that the leaflets connect to and secure the valve inside the heart.

D. Kersten
Department of Cardiology, NYU Langone Hospital – Long Island, Mineola, NY, USA

T. J. Cohen (✉)
NYIT College of Osteopathic Medicine, New York, NY, USA
e-mail: tcohen03@nyit.edu

Aortic Valve

There are two approaches to replacing the aortic valve: via a surgical approach or a catheter. Table 34.1 compares the two approaches to aortic valve replacement. Currently, the catheter approach is approved only for the replacement of stenotic aortic valves. This procedure is called transcatheter aortic valve replacement (TAVR; see Chap. 27). Transcatheter procedures are much less invasive and can be performed by an interventional cardiologist in a manner similar to cardiac catheterization. Initially, this procedure was reserved for patients with AS who could not tolerate the classical, more invasive surgical approach, but in recent years, it has been approved for more widespread use in patients with AS.

A small incision is made into an artery (typically in the groin), and a catheter is introduced into the vessel and advanced to the aortic valve. This catheter has a valve loaded on a balloon (see Fig. 27.1). When at the appropriate area, the balloon is inflated and the valve expands inside and over the old valve. The balloon is then deflated, and the new valve remains in place, providing a functional valve for the patient.

The original, invasive method of valvular replacement is surgical valve replacement. This is an open-heart procedure and requires a cardiothoracic surgery team. The heart must be slowed or stopped using cooling, while a heart-lung machine allows for blood to continue circulating throughout the body. An incision is typically performed along the middle of the chest, and the heart is accessed. To replace the aortic valve, the valve is completely removed from the heart, and a new heart valve is sewn into place. The valve can also simply be repaired, although replacement is the more common approach. Repair is usually reserved for those with a dilated aortic root or annulus but intact valve, and the root is repaired and the original aortic valve reimplanted.

The rationale behind using a transcatheter or surgical approach generally depends on the type of disease. AS is more commonly corrected with TAVR, and aortic regurgitation (AR) is corrected using the surgical approach. The major exception to this rule is patients undergoing replacement of a stenotic aortic valve who also need to undergo another open-heart operation, such as coronary artery bypass grafting (CABG, see Chap. 33). Generally, these patients will undergo the surgical approach to replace the diseased valve at the same time as the other procedure. The majority

Table 34.1 Methods of aortic valve replacement

Transcatheter aortic valve replacement (TAVR)
    Less invasive
    Catheter places the valve inside the heart
    For aortic stenosis only
Surgical aortic valve replacement (SAVR)
    Open-heart procedure
    Surgeon removes the diseased valve from the heart and replaces it with an artificial valve
    Either for aortic regurgitation or for aortic stenosis if the patient is also undergoing other open-heart procedures simultaneously (i.e., CABG)

of patients with aortic regurgitation will be treated with medications, as opposed to surgery, until there is worsening heart function or the patient becomes symptomatic. However, since TAVR has had expanded indications due to its minimally invasive nature and good patient outcomes, AS patients often undergo valve replacement in earlier stages of disease compared to those with aortic regurgitation.

Mitral Valve

The mitral valve has several approaches for repair or replacement. It should be noted that, unlike the aortic valve—which is typically replaced—the mitral valve is usually repaired. It should also be noted that the cause of a patient's mitral valve disease is important in selecting the type of surgical approach, specifically in patients with mitral stenosis (MS). In developed nations, such as the United States, MS is most commonly caused by calcification of the valve and prevents the valve from moving properly; this is called calcific MS. However, in the rest of the world, MS is typically caused by infection with Strep throat. Infection causes inflammation and scarring of the valve, which causes poor valve movement, a condition called rheumatic MS. This condition has become much less common in developed nations due to greater access to antibiotics. The approaches to mitral valve repair or replacement are listed in Table 34.2.

One approach to valve repair for those with MS is percutaneous balloon valvuloplasty, which can be performed in a manner similar to TAVR. A catheter is introduced into a blood vessel in the groin and advanced to the mitral valve. On the tip of the catheter is a balloon, and—when the balloon section is inside the valve—it is inflated and then deflated. This process causes the valve's opening to increase in size and is repeated as necessary to ensure adequate opening. This procedure is used for rheumatic mitral disease only.

Table 34.2 Methods for mitral valve repair or replacement

Percutaneous balloon valvuloplasty
   Minimally invasive
   Balloon expands mitral valve
   For rheumatic mitral stenosis (MS)
Commissurotomy
   Typically invasive
   Cuts to commissure of the mitral valve
   For rheumatic MS
Repair
   Typically invasive, although clipping can be done less invasively with a catheter (TMVr such as the MitraClip™)
   The preferred initial method for mitral valve surgery
   May entail repair of the annulus, leaflets, or chordae tendineae
Replacement
   Invasive
   Not the preferred initial management of mitral valve disease
   Valve is removed from the heart and replaced with an artificial valve

In a commissurotomy, cuts are made to the commissures of the mitral valve to allow for greater valve motion. Commissures are the two furthest meeting points of the leaflets of the mitral valve; leaflets are the portions of the valve that open and close and allow blood to flow. In MS, these commissures become fused and do not permit adequate valve motion; therefore, by cutting the commissures, there is better valve motion. Many centers have opted to perform balloon valvuloplasty as opposed to commissurotomy because of shorter hospital stays, quicker recovery, and lower risk of complications.

Like the aortic valve, the mitral valve can malfunction by being stenosed. Still, it can also leak as a result of damage or disease to the valve apparatus or dilation of the heart muscle. Mitral valve repair may be preferable to mitral valve replacement if mitral valve surgery is required. There are numerous techniques by which surgeons can repair the mitral valve, depending on what issues are noted with the valve before and during surgery, but in general, surgeons will remove and repair diseased sections of the valve. They may also repair structures outside of the valve itself, such as the base (also known as the annulus) of the valve, because this could contribute to poor valve movement. Repair of this ring is called an annuloplasty. Repair may also focus on the chordae tendineae, which are small muscles that help open the mitral valve.

Mitral valve replacement is not a preferred initial option for surgical repair of the mitral valve, but certain patients with advanced disease may require it. This procedure is performed in a similar manner to surgical aortic valve replacement. The valve will be removed from the heart, and a new valve will be sewn into place. Valve replacement is not the preferred initial approach to mitral valve disease as it is highly invasive and has a higher risk of death during operation, between two and six percent. Overall, the 5-year survival rate is 65 to 70 percent.

Commissurotomy, valve repair, and valve replacement typically require an open-heart procedure performed by a cardiothoracic surgery team. Much like surgical aortic valve repair, the heart must be cooled to slow or stop the heart, and a heart-lung machine is used to continue blood flow to the body. It should be noted, however, that some centers are using approaches similar to TAVR in the repair or replacement of the mitral valve. There is a percutaneous approach to repair the mitral valve (in those with significant mitral regurgitation or MR), in which a catheter-based approach, as opposed to a surgical approach, is used to improve the leaking of the valve. This procedure is called transcatheter mitral valve repair (TMVr) and is discussed in Chap. 27. The MitraClip™ is one such device that has been proven to be relatively safe and effective in the treatment of severe MR in those who qualify for this procedure. Please speak to your cardiologist about which of these techniques may be best suited for you.

Tricuspid and Pulmonic Valve

Disease of the tricuspid and pulmonic valves are rarer than a disease of the aortic and mitral valves. Typically, the disease of these valves, especially the tricuspid, is due to either lung disease or left heart stiffness or failure. Therefore, treatment of these conditions may rely on treating the underlying problem. However, sometimes the problem is so severe that it requires repair or replacement of the valve.

The tricuspid valve can either be repaired or replaced. In general, if a tricuspid valve has severe enough stenosis, surgery is performed. However, it is a little more complicated for tricuspid regurgitation (TR) as the underlying cause of the problem determines the surgery type. If the disease is functional TR, this suggests that the reason for the valve problem is due to the ring that surrounds the valve (the annulus). Organic TR, on the other hand, means that the valve problems are due to the valve itself.

Both tricuspid repair and replacement are open-heart, surgical procedures. Therefore, the heart must be cooled to slow or stop it, a heart-lung machine to allow for oxygenated blood to flow to the body, and the chest must be opened. This procedure is performed by a cardiothoracic surgery team under anesthesia. Much like disease of the mitral valve, the mainstay of tricuspid valve surgery is valve repair and not replacement. The approaches to tricuspid repair are similar to mitral repair as well. A repair could entail valvuloplasty, commissurotomy, or annuloplasty (an especially useful approach for functional TR); these techniques were previously described in this chapter. It could also involve repairing the leaflets of the valve or the muscles that open the valve (chordae tendineae). Again, the type of disease and severity typically dictate the approach to treatment.

Replacement of the tricuspid valve is usually not the mainstay of tricuspid disease. The valve may be removed and replaced with another valve, although some techniques allow for replacements to be attached to the existing valve leaflets, avoiding the need to remove the entire valve. The latter approach is useful for the tricuspid valve due to its proximity to major sections of the heart's electrical system, which can be damaged during removal of the entire valve. Tricuspid valve replacement is an invasive and intensive procedure, with mortality during operations being reported as up to 20 percent. However, much of this data is from older studies, and newer investigations should be performed as surgical technique has greatly improved. Simpler percutaneous methods, similar to TAVR, TMVr, and the MitraClip can be used to treat severe TR. This includes the EVOQUE (Edwards Lifesciences; similar to TAVR/TMVr) and the TriClip (Abbott; similar to the MitraClip)

The pulmonic valve is rarely subject to surgical intervention. Pulmonic regurgitation (PR) is generally not due to problems with the valve but some other problem in the body, such as pulmonary hypertension. Therefore, the treatment of TR relies on controlling the underlying problem. Pulmonic stenosis (PS) is usually managed with valvuloplasty, which was previously described in the mitral valve section. In this procedure, a balloon inflates inside of the valve opening and widens the area of the valve so there can be more effective blood flow across the valve.

Types of Replacement Valves

The final section of this chapter pertains to patients who undergo valve replacement. There are two types of valves that can be implanted: mechanical and bioprosthetic valves. Table 34.3 compares these two types of valves and their pros and cons.

Table 34.3 Mechanical versus bioprosthetic valves

Mechanical
First developed
Use metals and plastics
Durable, less likely to require repeat operation later in life
Requires life-long anticoagulation with warfarin
Bioprosthetic
Newer
Use animal tissue, from cows or pigs
Do not require lifelong anticoagulation
Can require reoperation decades later

Mechanical valves are made from non-organic substances such as metals and plastics. Bioprosthetic valves, however, are relatively newer than mechanical valves and are usually made from animal structures, either from cows or pigs. Neither type of valve has been found to improve survival, and both have their unique benefits and risks. In recent years, bioprosthetic valves have become the dominant type of selection.

Mechanical valves require lifelong anticoagulation, which means patients have an increased risk of bleeding. Currently, newer oral anticoagulation drugs that do not require routine lab work, such as Xarelto®, have not been approved for use in patients with mechanical heart valves, because they are much less effective. Therefore, patients must use drugs, such as warfarin, which require routine lab work to monitor the effectiveness of the medications and dietary modifications. Bioprosthetic valves do not require lifelong anticoagulation but are not as durable as mechanical valves and may eventually weaken (damage) over time, ultimately requiring reoperation and replacement. Please talk to your cardiologist and cardiac interventionalist/surgeon to determine which valve is best for you.

Heart Assist Devices, Artificial Hearts, and Heart Transplantation Surgery

35

Daniel Kersten and Todd J. Cohen

When the heart becomes too weak to pump blood throughout the body, patients may require either assist devices or a new heart altogether to restore adequate blood flow to the body. While heart transplantation is currently the best method for long-term survival with a failing heart, new devices have become approved to help prolong the quality and duration of life—along with adequate medical management—and often serve as a bridge to heart transplantation.

Heart Assist Devices

Assist devices (also known as mechanical circulatory support) are pumps that can be installed inside of the heart and aid the patient in properly pumping blood from the heart. There are two types of assist devices: those for short-term use and ones for long-term use. Short-term use devices are for patients who need cardiac support emergently such as patients with active infection of the heart muscle (myocarditis), severe heart failure exacerbation, or post-cardiac surgery, for instance. This mechanical support may come from a few options and have varying insertional techniques (either via catheter or surgery). One catheter-implanted device is known as an intra-aortic balloon pump and is placed outside of the heart in a region of the major artery that carries blood away from the heart, the aorta. This device inflates a balloon during heart relaxation (diastole) and deflates during contraction (systole); making it

D. Kersten
Department of Cardiology, NYU Langone Hospital – Long Island, Mineola, NY, USA

T. J. Cohen (✉)
NYIT College of Osteopathic Medicine, New York, NY, USA
e-mail: tcohen03@nyit.edu

easier for the pumping of blood to the rest of the body. This is often considered the first option for short-term mechanical support.

Another type of short-term catheter-implanted device may also be placed inside of the heart in the left ventricle (for instance, the Impella®, Abiomed, Danvers, MA; see Fig. 35.1). These devices function by taking blood from the left ventricle and then ejecting the blood into the aorta. A final method uses tubing to remove blood from a leg vein, oxygenate it, and then return it to a leg artery (TandemHeart®

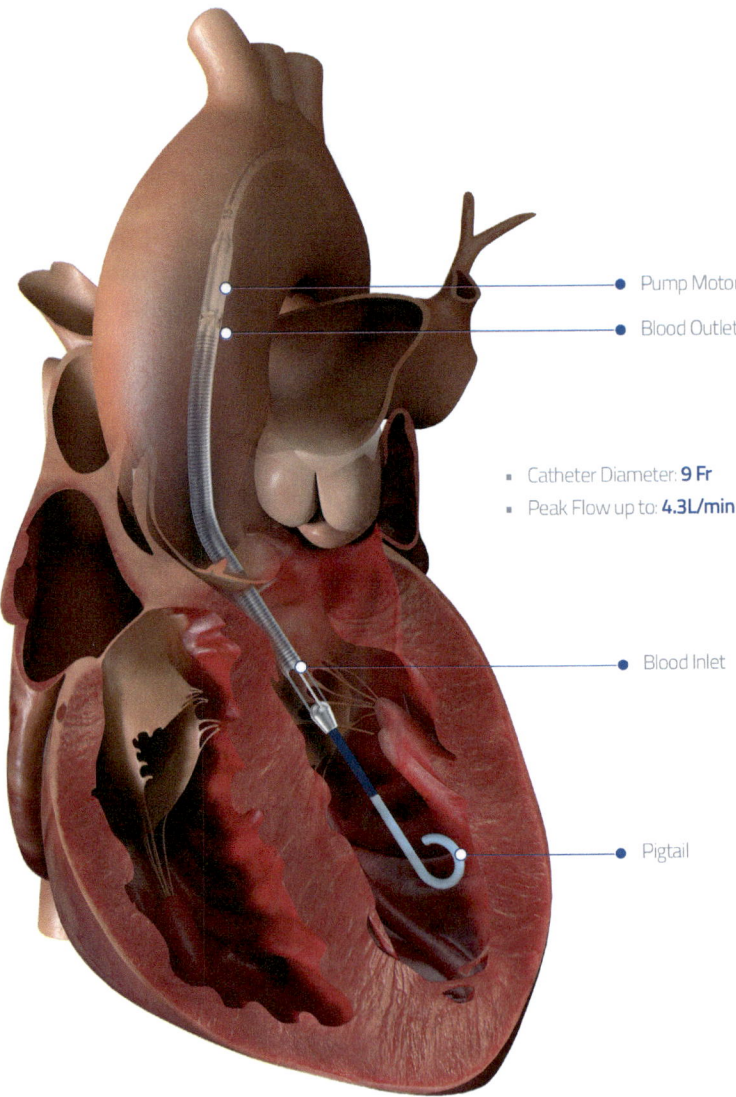

- Pump Motor
- Blood Outlet

- Catheter Diameter: **9 Fr**
- Peak Flow up to: **4.3L/min**

- Blood Inlet

- Pigtail

Fig. 35.1 The Impella Heart Assist Device by Abiomed. The Impella is a short-term catheter device that can be placed in the left ventricle to assist with heart contraction by ejecting blood from the left ventricle into the aorta. (Reproduced with permission of ABIOMED, Inc.)

systems, CardiacAssist, Pittsburg, PA). In the Impella® system®, the pump is inside the catheter, while the pump for the TandemHeart® system is outside of the body (usually strapped to a leg). The advantage of these devices is that they can quickly be applied to help resuscitate acutely ill patients.

There are also surgically implanted short-term assist devices. These options are usually reserved for patients who have just undergone cardiac surgery and need temporary assistance with their cardiac function. These devices essentially consist of tubes (called cannulas) that are implanted inside the heart and pump outside of the body. The tubes carry blood from one section of the heart to another, thus moving blood. These systems may be connected to extracorporeal membrane oxygenation (ECMO) machines, which put oxygen into the blood. A third method of providing support can be simply using ECMO alone by inserting catheters into the venous (deoxygenated) and arterial (oxygenated) systems of the body. Deoxygenated blood is drawn from the venous system, passed through the machine for oxygenation, and then returned to the arterial system.

Long-term cardiac assist devices, such as left ventricular assist devices (LVADs), are typically used to bridge patients with end-stage heart failure to heart transplantation and are usually implanted in the left ventricle. Examples include the HeartMate (Abbott Laboratories, Chicago, IL) and the HeartWare HVAD (Medtronic PLC., Dublin, Ireland). These devices usually consist of an inflow tube, which takes blood from the ventricle and into a pump, which then pushes the blood to an outflow tube that is inserted into the aorta. These devices are typically powered by an external battery pack connected to an apparatus that the patient must wear. In general, these devices require the patient to be on anticoagulation and antiplatelet therapies to prevent blood clots from forming, require monitoring of blood pressure typically via ultrasound or intra-arterial monitoring (as the traditional blood pressure cuff is no longer accurate), and can lead to valve issues and arrhythmias.

Table 35.1 summarizes both short-term (both percutaneous and surgical) and long-term assist devices.

Table 35.1 Key points for short-term (percutaneous and surgical) heart assist devices and long-term heart assist devices

Short-term, percutaneous devices
    Intra-aortic balloon devices or catheter-inserted pump devices
    Quicker to install using a catheter that is inserted into a blood vessel
    Often used in acutely ill patients who need urgent stabilization (i.e., shock)
Short-term, surgical devices
    Installed after open-heart procedures
    Use tubing systems and/or ECMO to move blood through the heart or the body
    Temporary assistance after cardiac surgery
Long-term devices
    Typically, a bridge between severe heart failure and heart transplantation
    Inflow tubing takes blood (usually in the ventricle) and pushes it into an outflow tube (usually in the aorta) using a pump installed near the heart (see Fig. 35.2)
    Must wear an external battery pack
    Requires anticoagulation and antiplatelet therapy
    Need blood pressure monitoring via ultrasound or intraarterial catheters
    Associated with valve abnormalities and arrhythmia

Fig. 35.2 An illustration of an artificial heart by Dr. Jerry Jose, DO. The device shows a wearable power supply tethered to an implantable heart pump

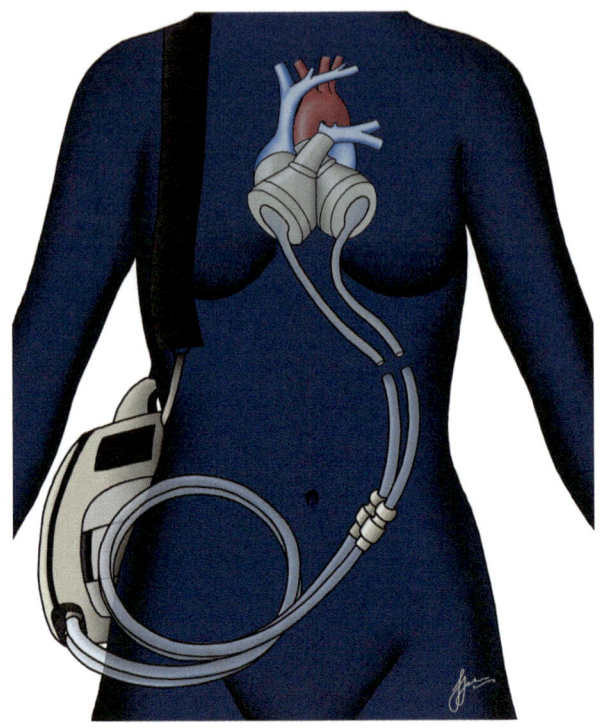

Artificial Hearts

Artificial hearts have become an interesting prospect for cardiology, especially with the proliferation of three-dimensional printing technology. Figure 35.2 shows one embodiment of an artificial heart as illustrated by artist Dr. Jerry Jose. Several prototypes have been developed over the past few decades but currently, there is only one commercially available artificial heart called the SynCardia Total Artificial Heart (SynCardia Systems, Tucson, Arizona). This device is used as a bridge to heart transplantation. It uses artificial ventricles, which replace the failing heart tissue, and a driver system, worn by the patient, to pump the blood from the ventricles. There are currently other devices in development as potential new therapies that could be used in lieu of heart transplantation, especially for patients who are poor candidates for transplant surgery.

Heart Transplantation

Heart transplantation is a highly invasive operation and is reserved for patients who have heart problems that have either failed other treatments or been deemed not treatable with either medical or surgical management. These heart problems can include end-stage heart failure, certain congenital heart defects (defects present at birth), intractable ventricular arrhythmias, and certain cardiac tumors. Surgical candidates need to demonstrate a likelihood of survival after the operation, minimal medical comorbidities, and have a reasonable life expectancy. Therefore, transplant is usually reserved for the younger (typically less than 70 years old) and healthier patients. Heart transplants are performed at heart transplant centers, which specialize in this type of surgery.

When a patient is declared suitable for transplant, they are placed on a list and will be contacted if a heart becomes available. Ideally, the transplant team will handle logistical arrangements to coordinate the donor and recipient surgeries, which will minimize the time between heart removal and implantation, and thereby will reduce the period during which the heart has no blood flow. The donor heart is first stopped and removed from the donor's body. While this is happening, the recipient undergoes a large incision down the center of the chest, and their heart is exposed. The old heart is then removed, and the new heart muscle reimplanted; the methods by which this occurs are beyond the scope of this book.

Immediately after surgery, patients are monitored closely in the surgical intensive care unit. Patients may require certain medications or temporary pacemakers so that the heart can pump effectively. Certain patients may even require a permanent pacemaker to be implanted, approximately 10–20 percent of patients. However, many patients are out of the hospital about seven to ten days after the surgery. Additionally, since the new heart is not the patient's original heart, patients require immunosuppression therapy so that the body does not reject the organ. Immunosuppression is required for the remainder of the patient's life, although the dosage can be lowered about 1 year after the procedure.

One major problem with immunosuppressive drugs is that they may interact with other drugs a patient may be taking, such as statins to lower cholesterol, and alter levels of certain drugs in the body, which can cause serious side effects. Additionally, a major concern is an increased risk of infection as the patient's immune system is suppressed in order to prevent organ rejection. Patients may then require prophylactic medications, such as antibiotics, antivirals, and vaccinations, to prevent infection. These patients must be closely monitored, as immunosuppressants can blunt symptoms of infection. Patients on immunosuppressive therapy also have an increased risk of cancer and may require routine screening. Lastly, posttransplantation patients have an increased risk of certain medical problems, such as high blood pressure, high cholesterol, diabetes, kidney problems, and joint pain; therefore, routine visits with your primary care doctor are essential after the procedure.

The length of survival time after transplantation surgery has risen dramatically over the past several decades. A recent large study from the International Society of Heart and Lung Transplantation registry noted that the median life expectancy after transplantation is 12.5 years. For patients who live at least 1 year after transplant, the median survival is nearly 15 years. Most patients also demonstrate a much-improved quality of life after the procedure. Nearly three-fourths of patients reported

Table 35.2 Key points for heart transplantation

Usually reserved for younger patients with few medical problems and good life expectancy.
Generally used for end-stage heart failure which has failed medical and/or surgical management, among other reasons.
Must be performed at specialized centers.
Open-heart procedure in which old heart muscle is replaced with the heart muscle from a recently deceased donor.
Requires immunosuppression after the procedure to prevent rejection of new heart by the body.
Immunosuppressive drugs increase the risk of infections and certain cancers.
Careful monitoring is required for immunosuppressive drugs to prevent interactions with other drugs.
Most patients report significant improvements in lifestyle after the procedure.

either a normal lifestyle or few heart disease symptoms, while only 10% of patients reported greater limitations. Notable long-term complications reported are fatigue, sexual dysfunction, problems with memory, easier bruising, and abdominal cramping.

Key points regarding cardiac transplantation are summarized in Table 35.2.

Alcohol Septal Ablation for Hypertrophic Cardiomyopathy and Repair of Atrial Septal Defects

36

Srihari Naidu and Amer Sayed

Septal Ablation for Hypertrophic Cardiomyopathy

Hypertrophic cardiomyopathy (HCM) is a genetic condition that runs in families. The disorder causes the heart to become thick and stiff, resulting in a decreased amount of blood going out of the heart to the rest of the body. In addition, the heart can be irritable and lead to fast heart rhythms (such as atrial fibrillation and ventricular tachycardia). Symptoms of this condition can be shortness of breath, tiredness, dizziness and lightheadedness (presyncope), chest pain, ankles or leg swelling, or even fainting (syncope), and sometimes, although rare, sudden death.

This thick muscle condition can cause those symptoms in two ways; first, the heart loses the ability to relax and hold the necessary amount of blood in the lower chamber of the heart (the ventricles) in order to pump it out of the body. The treatment of this problem is medications, including those that help the heart muscle relax (such as verapamil and beta blockers), as well as water pills (diuretics). Secondly, the thick muscle gets in the way of the exit door to the heart (known as the aortic valve), where the septum is located, and causes "obstruction." It is this area causing the obstruction that can be treated by removing the "extra" muscle either physically

S. Naidu (✉)
Department of Cardiology, Westchester Medical Center, Valhalla, NY, USA
e-mail: srihari.naidu@wmchealth.org

A. Sayed
Department of Cardiology, Adams County Regional Medical Center, Cincinnati, OH, USA

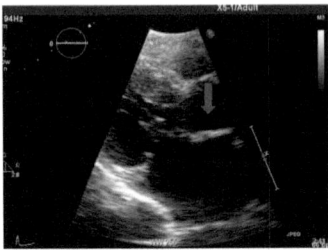 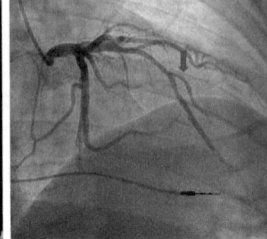 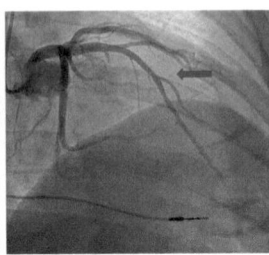

Fig. 36.1 Left: HCM with thick septum (arrow). Middle: The target artery for ablation that gives blood to the muscle (arrow). Right: The target is "ablated" after alcohol septal ablation procedure (arrow) and is no longer present

by surgery (simply by "shaving" the muscle) or through catheters reaching into the heart by alcohol septal ablation.

Alcohol septal ablation occurs by injecting some pure alcohol (a toxic substance for the heart) into the coronary artery supplying blood to the "problematic" thick heart muscle, which results in a "controlled heart attack" or ablation. The ablated muscle then shrinks over the next few months, eliminating the obstruction and the symptoms. Although the procedure takes an hour, the shrinking of the septum takes up to 6 months, during which the patient continues to feel better.

Evaluation of HCM can be performed in specialized centers (also called "centers of excellence" or "comprehensive HCM centers") that have options for surgery and alcohol ablation, and then a team of doctors discusses each case individually to determine the most appropriate course of action for each patient. Only hospitals that perform more than ten to twenty of these procedures per year are generally considered expert centers, so patients should ask this question prior to proceeding.

Each patient usually receives a full medical history and physical exam during their visit, lab work, ECG, continuous heart monitor, stress test, heart catheterization (angiogram), and imaging with an echocardiogram (Fig. 36.1) or cardiac magnetic resonance imaging (MRI). The echocardiogram is essential to see how thick the heart muscle is and if it is causing an obstruction. Since hypertrophic cardiomyopathy runs in families, your doctor might suggest testing your family members for the disorder.

Treatment of HCM starts with medicine, which can be adjusted, if necessary, over weeks, to assess symptom improvement. Medication can also be given if there is an abnormal heart rhythm (arrhythmias). Some rhythm-controlling medicines include those used to treat atrial fibrillation (anticoagulants, rate-controlling medications, and antiarrhythmics; see Chap. 25). In some patients, an implantable loop recorder (ILR) may help monitor the patient's heart rhythm. If there are any dangerous arrhythmias (such as ventricular tachycardia or fibrillation) or the patient is considered at higher risk for sudden death, an implantable cardioverter-defibrillator (ICD) should be considered. Finally, if symptoms continue, the doctor may consider procedures to decrease the thickness of the heart muscle with either surgery or alcohol septal ablation.

Preparation for Alcohol Septal Ablation

Before the ablation procedure, the doctor usually performs a right and left heart catheterization (angiogram) to measure the pressure in the right and left sides of the heart, respectively. The catheterization is performed by entering the groin vessel (femoral vein) and placing small flexible tubes (called catheters) into the right atrium, right ventricle, and pulmonary artery. Additionally, another groin vessel (femoral artery) is accessed, and a catheter is positioned around the aorta into the left ventricle in order to confirm high pressures inside the heart as well as the "outflow tract" obstruction.

A variety of catheters are used to access the heart and coronary arteries to measure pressures. In addition, a specialized catheter is used to access the specific coronary artery branch (septal perforator) that supplies blood flow to the thick heart muscle, causing the outflow tract obstruction. Once a suitable septal coronary artery is identified and confirmed, alcohol can then be carefully delivered in order to ablate the septum. Although it sounds very invasive, most patients don't feel anything, and very light sedation is all that is required.

Alcohol septal ablation (Fig. 36.1) is a non-surgical procedure done in the cath lab, as well with a similar catheter entering the groin artery as described above. A temporary pacemaker is usually inserted before the ablation, in the same setting, as a precaution due to a small potential risk of heart block (electrical conduction problem). This is usually placed in the left neck under sedation. A small tube with a balloon at the tip can then be delivered to the targeted artery that supplies blood to the thick muscle, and a small amount of alcohol (roughly one to two milliliters) is injected into that vessel, causing a "controlled infarction." The muscle causing the obstruction dies and shrinks, which makes it easier for the blood to leave the heart and flow to the rest of the body. The procedure typically takes around 1 to 2 hours, and the hospital stay can vary between 2 and 4 days, depending on when the temporary pacemaker can be removed. During most of this time, the patient can walk around and is already starting to feel better.

Table 36.1 shows some of the risks of an alcohol septal ablation. Please note that in about ten percent of patients, no benefits are achieved from the procedure. In an additional 5 to 10 percent of patients, heart block can develop following the procedure, and a pacemaker may be indicated. Bleeding can occur in less than 3 percent of patients. Additionally, fluid can build up around the heart (pericardial effusion), and further heart attacks and/or blood clotting can occur (each occurring less than

Table 36.1 Risks of alcohol septal ablation (ASA)

Infection < 1%
Bleeding < 2–3%
Blood clots < 1%
Heart attack in another area of the heart < 1%
Fluid around the heart < 1%
Heart block (damaging the electrical conduction in the heart from the upper chambers to the lower chambers) 5–10%
Failure of the procedure to help ~10%

one percent incidence). Because of this, after the ablation, the patient should be monitored in the intensive care unit, or the telemetry floor for any possible complications.

If a heart block develops, a permanent pacemaker should be placed. Otherwise, the temporary pacemaker is removed, and the patient can be discharged home. The results of the ablation procedure can take up to three to six months to fully show the benefit and improvement in symptoms. Your doctor may ask for another echocardiogram to assess the degree of improvement before discharge and again in 3-months. In almost all patients, medications can be reduced or eliminated as the patient starts to feel normal again and remain symptom free.

Repair of Atrial Septal Defects

An atrial septal defect (ASD) is a "hole" in the wall that separates the top two chambers of the heart. Every child is born with an opening between the upper heart chambers, called a fossa ovalis; this is a normal fetal opening that allows blood to detour away from the lungs before birth. After birth, the opening is no longer needed and usually closes or becomes very small within several weeks or months. Sometimes, the opening is larger than normal and doesn't close after birth, and these are called patent foramen ovale (PFO).

A PFO can cause problems in two ways. First, it allows deoxygenated blood to leak from the right side of the heart to the left side, and that will decrease the oxygen level going to the rest of the body. Second, clots can pass from the right side of the heart to the left side and then to the rest of the body, which can cause multiple problems, including strokes in the brain.

In contrast, ASD has a few types, and they are mostly present from birth. Even though some of those "holes" can cause problems and need to be addressed, most of them are small and do not cause any known harm. Often, they are found unexpectedly and do not require any treatment. If a large or medium-sized ASD is not found and treated, however, it can cause symptoms as a person gets older, usually by age 40. This is because a large ASD causes oxygenated blood to leak from the left side of the heart to the right side, which over time puts extra strain on the lungs. This can lead to elevated lung pressures and increased resistance, making it harder for blood oxygenation.

Common symptoms caused by ASD are shortness of breath, tiredness, abnormal heartbeats or arrhythmias, and, in severe cases, the skin can turn blue while exerting yourself. Another way this "hole" can be diagnosed is by testing after a stroke occurs without a known reason, especially at a young age. Similar to the PFO, an ASD can cause some blood to go from the right side of the heart to the left side, including any clots formed in the legs.

Tests that can be ordered to look for and evaluate either an ASD or a PFO include:

1. ECG: The test shows the electrical activity of the heart and any potential rhythm problem, but also can help uncover some types of ASD as parts of the heart enlarge.

2. Chest X-ray: This test shows the lungs and heart, including what the heart looks like and if there is any fluid in the lungs or signs of high blood pressure in the lungs. This can be helpful for the evaluation of heart problems.
3. Echocardiogram: The test shows the anatomy, structure, and function of your heart. The echo can be done with a "bubble" study, where a sterile salt solution is shaken until tiny bubbles form and then injected into a vein. The bubbles travel to the right side of your heart and appear on the echocardiogram. Seeing those bubbles in the left side of the heart can help in finding the ASD.
4. Transesophageal Echocardiogram: The test is similar to the regular echocardiogram, but is done under sedation and through your mouth while you sleep. This gets much better pictures of any potential holes in the heart and can also be done with the same bubble study to confirm whether either an ASD or a PFO is present.

If your ASD is large or medium-sized or causing symptoms, you will most likely need a procedure to close it. This can be done in different ways: surgery which simply closes the hole with a patch sutured on top of it, or by catheter without surgery, by something called "transcatheter closure." Nowadays, almost all of these holes (over 90%) are closed through a catheter while the patient is awake.

Transcatheter closure can be described as a less-invasive surgical procedure that is used to treat patients with atrial septal defect (ASD) or patent foramen ovale (PFO), which are the most common two holes between the upper heart chambers. The "plug" that closes the hole is a septal repair device and consists of two connected patches that are permanently placed in the hole to cover both the left and right atrial sides. Within the first 3 months after placement, the lining of the heart wall grows over the patch and seals the hole completely. This device that closes the hole (Fig. 36.2) can be delivered from the groin vessel (vein) with the guide of an

Fig. 36.2 The device that closed the atrial septal defect under x-ray (arrow)

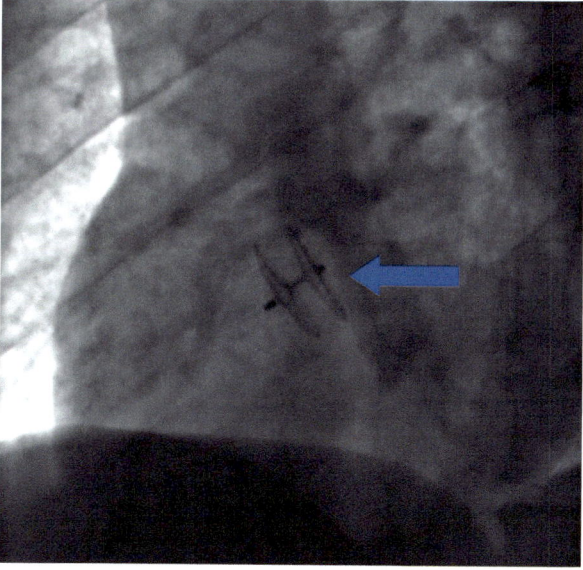

x-ray machine called "fluoroscopy" and also an ultrasound machine device. In expert hands, the procedure takes no more than 30–40 minutes, and the patient remains awake with mild sedation only.

Although complications are uncommon with this procedure, a tear of the heart or blood vessels, dislodgement of the device, or the development of irregular heartbeats may occur. These arrhythmias or palpitations are almost always minor and usually resolve within the first month.

Many unique procedures in cardiology can be done with minimal sedation and through catheters from the groin. Two of them are described in this chapter. You can find references related to these topics in the bibliography by looking for the terms "hypertrophic cardiomyopathy" or "atrial septal defect." Patients should make sure they are being seen by qualified physicians who perform at least ten of these invasive procedures per year, in order to make sure they get the best possible outcomes. In experienced hands, these procedures have been a major advance in cardiology and have helped thousands of patients.

Part VI

Treatments: Cardiac Risk Factors and Lifestyle Modifications (Thriving)

When I see a patient in consultation, I first formulate an assessment of their cardiac risk factors. Of course, there are irreversible contributors such as age and gender. The older you get, the more likely you are to develop heart disease, and men develop heart disease on average seven to ten years earlier than women. Family history of early heart disease and hereditary risk factors are also very important. If you have a first-degree relative (mother, father, sibling, or child) under the age of 65 who develops heart disease, their condition may have a genetic component, which means your risk may increase. If that is the case, you should do everything possible to prevent yourself from getting heart disease.

For example, if your mother or father had coronary artery disease at a young age, you should optimize the risk factors that we are about to discuss. This includes being active (not sedentary) and addressing high cholesterol (Chap. 37), high blood pressure (Chap. 38), obesity (Chap. 39), cigarette smoking (Chap. 40), and diabetes (Chap. 41). These five chapters focus on manageable, reversible, and treatable risk factors of heart disease. Read them carefully.

As you read them, focus on: (1) understanding the problem; (2) knowing your numbers (your cholesterol levels, blood pressure, weight, and blood sugar); (3) ways you can treat your problem first without medications, and if necessary, with medications; and (4) addressing all the things you can change, including your diet, level of physical activity (exercise), reducing stress, stopping smoking, excessive drinking of alcohol (more than one drink per day), and avoiding substance abuse. Your heart disease risks should be found in this book, but if not, please ask your healthcare provider where you can get more information. Research your problem, ask questions, and get the answers!

Figure 5.1 reviews five heart disease risks that you can modify to improve your quality and quantity of life. Look at this figure and use it as a guide so you can become healthier! Imagine yourself becoming healthier as you get your cholesterol under control. You can rein in your high blood pressure. And, if you are overweight or obese, you can make a big dent in that as well. Stopping smoking is tough, but you can do it with the help of your doctor. Finally, to prevent diabetes, you need to control the sugar in your diet, watch your weight, exercise, treat prediabetes (and prevent its progression to diabetes), and manage diabetes if you have it.

Many of you will need medications to treat the above risk factors. The chapters in this section will help you understand those too. But first, we are going to review the three pillars of managing heart disease risks: a heart-healthy diet, regular exercise, and knowing your numbers.

What Is a Heart Healthy Diet?

This is a diet that is low in saturated fats (less than 6%), avoids trans-fats, and limits the intake of high-fat dairy products and red meats. It means making smart choices—fish and poultry over red meats, grilled foods over fried foods, and skim or partly skim milk over whole milk. It is also high in fruit and vegetable consumption and favors whole grains and nuts (high-fiber diet), as well as cooking with vegetable oils such as olive oil instead of butter and lard. It also includes moderating salt and sugar intake (the sweets and sodas).

Chapter 37 (High Cholesterol), Chap. 38 (High Blood Pressure), and Chap. 39 (Obesity) not only discuss these key heart disease risk factors but also focus heavily on the benefits of diet and exercise. These chapters will give you helpful information regarding heart-healthy diets. Chapter 38 discusses the DASH (Dietary Approach to Stop Hypertension) diet. It is a good way to help three bad risks (high cholesterol, high blood pressure, and obesity). Appendix K lists some diets that should be considered for those with heart disease. It includes types of food that can be consumed as part of each specific diet, along with a "Food Journal" to track your diet and compliance over a four-week period.

Exercise Regularly

Everyone should exercise at least 150 minutes every week. This could include a brisk walk, jogging, biking (including a stationary bike), or using an elliptical. You feel better when you exercise, and regular aerobic exercise can help curb anxiety and make you feel better. It can help you achieve your target weight, improve your blood pressure, and minimize your stress. Using an app is a great way to track your progress. I recommend exercising for 30–50 minutes, five times per week. Wear a good pair of walking shoes or sneakers and go for a brisk walk around your neighborhood, on the beach, or along the boardwalk. Or go for a bike ride or a swim.

Check out the chapters in this book on wearable technology and fitness so you can do what you enjoy and keep track of your progress. If you have a heart condition, begin your exercise regimen by first talking to your doctor. If you have heart failure, or have had a heart attack, stent, or bypass surgery, they may want you to have a stress test before giving you a prescription, or they may start you in cardiac rehabilitation and then transition to home and outside exercise activities. Ask your doctor about any restrictions related to having sex or the use of drugs for erectile dysfunction, such as the phosphodiesterase-5 inhibitors including sildenafil (Viagra), tadalafil (Cialis), and vardenafil (Levitra). Appendix L lists some recommended exercises that may be considered for those with heart disease (or for preventing heart disease). Remember to start with a low workload and duration, and build this up very slowly under the guidance of your physician. This appendix also gives you a method for tracking your exercise progress on a weekly basis.

"Know Your Numbers" and Calculate Your Framingham Risk Score

In the next few chapters, you will learn the target numbers for cholesterol, normal blood pressure, and body weight, and its related value, body mass index (BMI). We will also identify ideal values for fasting blood sugar and something called A1C, or hemoglobin A1C These last two numbers tell us whether you are at risk for developing diabetes or have prediabetes.

There are many other numbers that may pertain to you. For example, I tell my heart disease and heart failure patients that they should know their last ejection fraction (EF), an indicator of how well the heart is contracting. A normal EF is between 50% and 70%. It is important to realize that you can have a normal EF and still have heart failure (see Chap. 14). Your EF could determine whether you qualify for an implantable defibrillator or heart failure treatment device. Appendix J gives you your "Surviving and Thriving" card, where you can track these numbers and also keep essential "backup" medical information ("Plan B") available in your purse, wallet, or another convenient spot.

There is a nice survey created by the Cleveland Clinic which will help you estimate your 10-year risk of coronary heart disease, based on information from the National Institutes of Health. So, gather your blood pressure and cholesterol numbers (you'll need your total cholesterol and HDL), and you can access the link here and calculate your 10-year risk of coronary heart disease.

https://my.clevelandclinic.org/ccf/media/Files/heart/Framingham-Risk-Tool-Men-Women.pdf? *A More recent ASCVD risk score has incorporated race and diabetes into the estimation of 10-year cardiovascular disease risk. The latest tool for risk assessment is called the PREVENT equations, which is an online calculator that provides personalized risk estimates by combining assessments of heart, renal, and metabolic health. The PREVENT calculator estimates both 10- and 30-year risks for cardiovascular disease risk, ASCVD, heart failure, and stroke.*

So, calculate your risk and try to make these important changes so you can live a full, fun, and active life.

High Cholesterol

37

Roger Kersten and Todd J. Cohen

A very important component of the treatment of heart disease (and vascular disease or stroke) is addressing cholesterol. Cholesterol, a fat in your blood, is not all bad. Some cholesterol is required to make certain hormones that help regulate the flow of nutrients and waste products in and out of our body's cells. Cholesterol may be broken down into different types (also called fractions). The total cholesterol reflects all of the fractions put together but does not indicate how much bad cholesterol (low-density lipoprotein or LDL), good cholesterol (high-density lipoprotein or HDL), or triglycerides are in the mix. *A healthy total cholesterol level is less than 200 mg/dl.* Borderline total cholesterol is 200 to 239 mg/dl, and high total cholesterol is 240 mg/dl or more. Other cholesterol components include intermediate-density lipoproteins (IDL), chylomicrons, and very low-density lipoproteins (VLDL).

Apolipoproteins are another type of particle that carries cholesterol particles in blood and influences how cholesterol particles are cleared from tissues and blood. They may be associated with the development of vascular disease (and eventually heart disease). It can be overwhelming to try to understand everything about these particles, but it is important to focus on a few details in understanding how cholesterol should be approached.

R. Kersten (Retired)
Department of Cardiology, St. Francis Hospital & Heart Center, Roslyn, NY, USA

T. J. Cohen (✉)
NYIT College of Osteopathic Medicine, New York, NY, USA
e-mail: tcohen03@nyit.edu

© The Author(s), under exclusive license to Springer Nature Switzerland AG 2025
T. J. Cohen, R. S. Blumenthal (eds.), *Surviving and Thriving With Heart Disease*,
Contemporary Cardiology, https://doi.org/10.1007/978-3-032-00579-3_37

Cholesterol-Related Components

HDL

HDL has a role in protecting our blood vessels and is referred to as "the good cholesterol." This fraction of cholesterol helps to remove cholesterol deposits from within the walls of arteries. Men and women should have an HDL ideally 60 mg/dl or more; however, men are at risk if their HDL is less than 40 mg/dl and women if their HDL is less than 50 mg/dl. *In general, a good target level for your HDL level is 60 mg/dl or more if you are a woman and 50 mg/dL or above if you are a man.*

This particle, when elevated, is often protective against the development of coronary artery disease though its protection may be variable. Some people with higher HDLs develop vascular disease if they have other cardiac risk factors, while others with low HDLs do not. HDL levels in men are on average 10 points lower than in women. Men typically have HDL levels between 35 to 45 mg/dl. There is a particular group in Milan that has very low HDL levels and elevated triglycerides; however, the development of vascular disease in this group is rare. The Milan group has a protective substance in their blood referred to as apo-A Milano that seems to exert a protective effect that overcomes the hazard associated with low HDL. Some drugs can raise HDL levels, though the results of these medications in decreasing coronary artery and vascular disease have been disappointing. A low HDL can best be managed by weight management, exercise, moderating alcohol consumption, and smoking cessation.

LDL

LDL, "the bad cholesterol", is associated with depositing cholesterol in blood vessels. It essentially does the opposite of HDL (which removes excess cholesterol). Not only does LDL build plaque and thereby cause blood vessels to narrow, it also increases inflammation inside the blood vessel wall. The inflammation seems to make the plaque less stable and more likely to rupture. If a plaque ruptures, it can trigger the formation of a clot within the blood vessel itself. Even small size plaques can be dangerous for this reason. If a small-sized plaque ruptures, it can cause a clot to form, which can block off the artery within seconds. When this happens in a coronary artery, it can cause a heart attack. When this occurs in a cerebral artery or blood vessel in the brain, it can cause a stroke.

It is recommended that the LDL level be less than 100 mg/dl in healthy patients and less than 70 mg/dl in patients with heart disease (such as coronary artery disease). A level of 55 mg/dl or less is preferable for those with diabetes and a history of acute coronary syndrome (a condition in which there is an abrupt reduction of blood flow to the heart muscle, as occurs with a heart attack).

Elevated LDL levels are initially managed with diet and exercise; however, medications are often required to achieve recommended LDL levels to reduce the risk of heart attack and stroke.

Triglycerides

Triglycerides are a combination of glycerol and three molecules of fat, hence the name triglyceride. *In general, triglycerides should be less than 150 mg/dl.* Borderline triglycerides are 150 to 199 mg/dl. Levels of triglycerides between 200 mg/dl and 499 mg/dl are considered high. High levels of triglycerides (greater than 400 mg/dl) are possibly associated with cardiovascular disease. When triglycerides are very elevated (greater than 1000 mg/dl), there is a risk of developing inflammation of the pancreas (pancreatitis). There are medications that can lower triglycerides, but it is not clear if these decrease the risk of heart attack or stroke.

Lipoprotein (a) [Lp(a)]

High levels of Lp(a) in the blood have been linked to the development of vascular and some types of valvular disease. The amount of Lp(a) that we produce is largely determined by genetics. It is also not yet known if lowering levels of Lp(a) with medications will result in a decrease in heart attacks or strokes. Currently, there is ongoing research to see if medications that lower Lp(a) will also decrease cardiovascular risk without causing other side effects.

Homocysteine

Homocysteine is a substance that results from our bodies breaking down some nutrients. High levels of homocysteine have been associated with an increase in cardiovascular events. Patients who have an elevated risk of cardiovascular disease and elevated levels of homocysteine may require treatment with folic acid (folate) and/or vitamin B-12. It is not recommended to take any supplements without the recommendation of a healthcare provider.

Managing Your Cholesterol with Diet and Exercise

Risk factor modification begins with knowing your numbers, calculating your risk of a coronary event over the next 10 years, and then tackling those risks with diet and exercise. A heart-healthy diet and exercise can have an important effect on your cholesterol numbers and can help to lower your LDL by achieving an ideal weight, and even raise your HDL, and help control triglycerides. If your numbers are borderline, your doctor may have you try to modify your diet, refer you to some resources, track your weight, and may even send you to a nutritionist or dietician in order to get you on the right track. If diet and exercise are not sufficient, medications will also be necessary.

Medications

Statins

In regard to the treatment of cholesterol in people with coronary artery and vascular disease, *anyone who can be on a statin should be*. Statin medications include atorvastatin (Lipitor), rosuvastatin (Crestor), pravastatin (Pravachol), and simvastatin (Zocor) to name a few. These medications not only lower LDL cholesterol but also decrease the risk of heart attack and stroke. Statins decrease inflammation and may lower the risk of plaque rupture. They work by inhibiting the synthesis of cholesterol in the liver, which reduces overall cholesterol levels in the body. As a result, cells have no choice but to take cholesterol from the blood, thereby lowering the amount of cholesterol inside blood vessels, slowing plaque formation and atherosclerosis.

There have been a number of concerns regarding side effects from these drugs, though most are mild and can be reversed by stopping the medication. Sometimes, switching from one statin to another is all that is needed. Statins are usually well tolerated. However, some people complain of muscle aches. Very rarely, patients can develop a condition called rhabdomyolysis in which the muscle fibers themselves break down and can lead to acute kidney failure. People with this condition often experience muscle pain, severe fatigue and weakness, decreased ability to produce urine, and dark urine.

When statins are taken concomitantly with a fibrate known as gemfibrozil (see below), the risk of muscle aches or damage increases. Liver damage is another very rare side effect of statins, as is the presence of elevated blood glucose. In general, if liver enzymes elevate significantly, stopping the medication or reducing its dose is usually all that is needed.

Nonstatins

Aside from statins, there are many other agents that lower LDL cholesterol and even Lp(a). The following is a list of some of these secondary medications.

Bile Acid Resins

Bile acid resins are a class of drugs that bind to fats, specifically bile acids. Bile acids are high cholesterol fats produced in the body that help absorb fat from digested food. Bile acid resins stop the absorption of these high-cholesterol fats back into the body. This facilitates their excretion and thus reduces cholesterol. Because certain vitamins are fat soluble, vitamin A, D, E, and K deficiencies may occur. Due to lower absorption of bile acids, there are lower levels of cholesterol in the body, and thus, more cholesterol is used for essential cell function and less contributes to atherosclerosis. Cholestyramine, one of these drugs, can also reduce blood glucose and may have some additional benefit in patients with diabetes. Furthermore, bile acid resins may cause gastrointestinal upset and should *be used with caution in patients with high triglycerides.*

Ezetimibe and Bempedoic Acid

If a statin is unable to be tolerated or cholesterol remains elevated, other medications (both oral and injectable) can be used. Ezetimibe is similar to bile acid resins, except it prevents cholesterol absorption in the small intestine from food, as opposed to the former, which prevents bile acid reabsorption in the small intestine. Ezetimibe may be used alone or together with a statin in order to produce additional cholesterol-lowering effects. These medications include ezetimibe (Zetia or Ezetrol) and bempedoic acid (Nexletol and Nexlizet, the latter being a combination of bempedoic acid and ezetimibe). Ezetimibe reduces cholesterol absorption from the gastrointestinal tract, while bempedoic acid blocks cholesterol synthesis. When statins don't achieve the targeted cholesterol-lowering effects, both of the above drugs can be used to get additional LDL lowering. Recently, a large study (CLEAR-OUTCOMES) showed a significant decrease in cardiovascular events in statin-intolerant patients who were randomized to bempedoic acid rather than placebo.

PCSK9 Inhibitors (Evolocumab, Alirocumab Are the Generic Names)

LDL receptors are cellular proteins that are responsible for taking LDL from the blood and bringing it inside the cell for use. Evolocumab stops LDL receptor destruction, thereby increasing the number of receptors present on the cell surface. With more receptors present, more cholesterol is removed from the blood, which can help slow down the atherosclerosis process. The PCSK9 inhibitors (Praluent or Repatha) are injectable medications that can also help decrease cardiovascular events. These drugs can be used alone or in combination with other cholesterol-lowering medications. Side effects include flu-like symptoms, muscle pain, soreness at the injection site, and high blood glucose levels (diabetes). This drug is recommended for those with a history of heart attack or stroke, and/or a persistently elevated cholesterol despite the use of a statin.

Fibrates

These oral medications decrease triglycerides. Examples include fenofibrate or gemfibrozil. These drugs may have some effect on lowering LDL and raising HDL as well. These drugs work by helping the body use fatty acids for energy instead of depositing them into atherosclerotic plaques. Unlike statins, PCSK9 inhibitors, and Vascepa, the fibrates have no clear benefit in reducing cardiovascular events. Drug interactions need to be considered before these medications are prescribed, as cholesterol gallstones can occur and *concomitant use of gemfibrozil with statins raises the risk of muscle aches and rhabdomyolysis.*

Fish Oil

Fish oil, a combination of docosahexaenoic acid (DHA) and eicosapentaenoic acid (EPA), is useful in decreasing triglyceride levels. There are some claims that these oils may help skin health, brain function, and joint pain. When it comes to heart health, with the exception of lowering triglycerides, the other advantages of fish oil have not been fully proven. Pure EPA (also called Vascepa) has been shown in one large trial to lower cardiovascular events (heart attack and stroke) by about 25 percent when used with a statin in those with vascular disease. Other types of fish oil (both prescription and over-the-counter) have provided mixed results as to benefits in treating cardiovascular disease. However, Vascepa has also been shown to increase risk of atrial fibrillation, atrial flutter, and bleeding. The most commonly reported side effects are musculoskeletal pain, swelling of the hands and feet, arrhythmias, and joint pain.

Supplements and Over-the-Counter Medications (OTCs)

Many people choose to take OTCs because they are natural substances, and they believe these will have less of a chance of causing harm. In fact, anything that you take, natural or manufactured, is a drug. There is no proof that natural cholesterol-lowering agents are any safer or better than prescription medications. Near all OTCs are not put through the same intense testing that prescription drugs are. The Food and Drug Administration (FDA) does not require OTCs to have studies that prove that they work. The labels on all supplements have a statement that says that they have not been evaluated by the FDA. There is generally another sentence on the label, that says that the product is not intended to diagnose, cure, or prevent any disease.

While impurities can be found in all drugs at times, there is close monitoring that is required by the FDA for prescription medications. The FDA does not monitor supplements unless there is a suspicion that it is causing harm. There have been cases of illness and even deaths from impurities found in supplements. There is also some evidence that some supplement manufacturers do not produce consistent batches of their products, causing variations from buying one bottle to the next.

Niacin or vitamin B3 can have a modest effect in lowering LDL, can slightly raise HDL, and improve triglycerides. It is available as an OTC as well as in pharmaceutical preparations. It is hard to tolerate due to flushing. Niacin in either form can cause elevation in liver function tests (hepatitis), gout exacerbations, increased glucose (hyperglycemia), increased uric acid, and flushing. There has not been any

Table 37.1   High cholesterol facts

High cholesterol (greater than 200 mg/dl) is a significant risk factor for heart disease.
Considered a modifiable risk factor that can be controlled through diet, exercise, and
medications.
LDL is "bad cholesterol" and should be less than 100 mg/dl; less than 70 mg/dl if you have
coronary artery disease.
HDL is "good cholesterol" and should ideally be 60 mg/dl or more.
Triglycerides may be linked to heart disease, especially when greater than 400 mg/dl.
Statins are the cornerstone of medical treatment, especially if you already have coronary artery
disease.

convincing benefit in decreasing vascular risk with niacin on top of a statin. It is for
this reason why it is not medically recommended at this time.

Red yeast rice, an OTC, has been shown to lower LDL cholesterol. The wiser
choice is to take a prescription statin, as there is quality control by the FDA, and you
know what product you are getting.

Garlic may have some effect on the reduction of cholesterol, though no formal
studies have conclusively shown a decrease in heart attacks or strokes. Aged garlic
was found to help small blood vessel circulation in skin that may be helpful in
wound healing.

Table 37.1 reviews some key facts regarding high cholesterol. *Please note there
are guidelines that address the target levels of each of the cholesterol particles. The
guidelines are revised when new information and studies become available. As is
the case with guidelines for the treatment of hypertension, the guidelines for treating cholesterol are based on the research available at the time they were written. In
areas of cholesterol treatment where there is limited availability of convincing
research, a panel of experts will make recommendations regarding these topics. It is
for this reason that some of the opinion-based recommendations in guidelines may
differ between different medical societies. A word of caution when reviewing lab
results: it is not enough to use the normal values that are indicated by the lab.
Adjustment in medications may still be needed even if the values fall in the "normal" range reported by the lab. The normal values supplied by the lab do not
address the guidelines for treatment for each person with various clinical conditions.*

High Blood Pressure or Hypertension

38

Roger Kersten and Todd J. Cohen

Blood pressure that is consistently elevated is referred to as high blood pressure or hypertension. While anyone can have an occasional elevation in blood pressure, consistently elevated blood pressure can have a negative impact on health. Hypertension increases the risk of heart attack, stroke, kidney failure, and heart failure. In the most recent guideline update for the treatment of hypertension, the level at which blood pressure elevations should be treated was lowered. Based on a careful review of the available research, the guidelines stated that treating blood pressure more intensely at lower levels than previously recommended resulted in fewer strokes and cardiovascular deaths. There are differences in opinions on the treatment of hypertension in some settings, and there are also differences in the guidelines within the United States versus those developed by our European colleagues.

Figure 38.1 shows a nurse (Jill Cohen, R.N.) taking blood pressure in the Long Island Heart Rhythm Center located at the New York Institute of Technology's Riland Health Center in Old Westbury, New York. Blood pressure is reported as two separate numbers. The systolic pressure, the top number, that measures the pressure while the heart muscle contracts and pushes blood out into the arteries. The diastolic pressure, the bottom number, measures the pressure after the heart has finished contracting and is relaxing. Both levels are important to consider in the treatment of hypertension.

Table 38.1 shows the facts related to your blood pressure and the different levels that are measured. Blood pressure levels are considered elevated at readings above

R. Kersten (Retired)
Department of Cardiology, St. Francis Hospital & Heart Center, Roslyn, NY, USA

T. J. Cohen (✉)
NYIT College of Osteopathic Medicine, New York, NY, USA
e-mail: tcohen03@nyit.edu

© The Author(s), under exclusive license to Springer Nature Switzerland AG 2025
T. J. Cohen, R. S. Blumenthal (eds.), *Surviving and Thriving With Heart Disease*,
Contemporary Cardiology, https://doi.org/10.1007/978-3-032-00579-3_38

Fig. 38.1 Jill Cohen R.N. taking a patient's blood pressure in the Long Island Heart Rhythm Center on the New York Institute of Technology campus in Old Westbury, New York

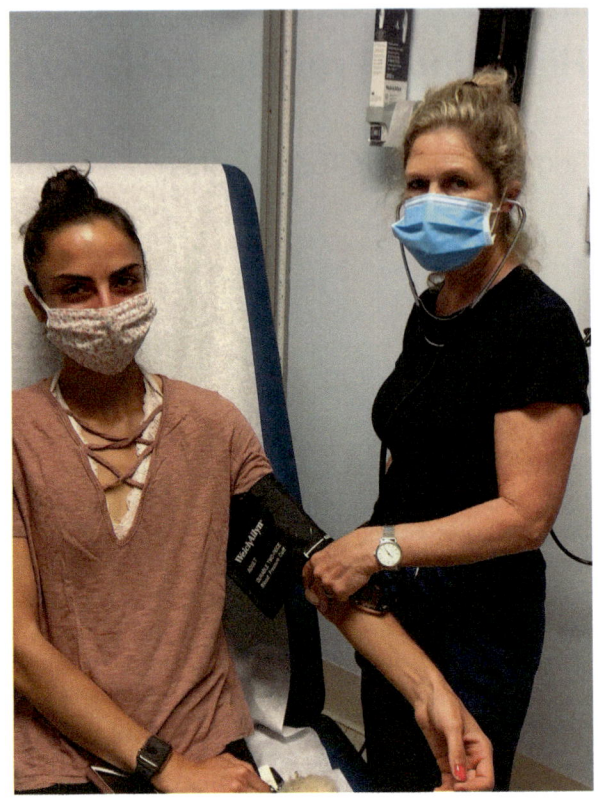

Table 38.1 High blood pressure facts

High blood pressure is a modifiable risk factor for heart disease.
Risk factors include heart attack and stroke.
Blood pressure is recorded as 120/80 mmHg (the first or top number is the systolic and the second or bottom number is the diastolic).
Normal blood pressure is less than 120/80 mmHg.
Above 120/80 mmHg is elevated.
130 to 139 mmHg systolic or 80 to 89 mmHg diastolic is stage 1 high blood pressure and should be treated by lifestyle modification and possibly medications.
140 mmHg or more systolic or 90 mmHg or more diastolic is stage 2 high blood pressure and requires both lifestyle modification and medications.
Above 180 mmHg systolic or 120 mmHg diastolic is considered a hypertensive crisis and requires immediate attention.

120/80 mmHg. Hypertension is diagnosed if blood pressure is repeatedly above 130/80 mmHg. This level is often called stage 1 hypertension and requires lifestyle modification and possibly medications. Above 140/90 mmHg is called stage 2 hypertension and usually requires both lifestyle modification and medications. Above 180/120 mmHg is called hypertensive crisis, and your healthcare provider should be contacted immediately since this could be an emergency.

Blood pressures that are too low can be dangerous as well. Low blood pressure, referred to as hypotension, can cause dizziness, lightheadedness (presyncope), and increase the risk of passing out (fainting or syncope). The blood pressure at which someone experiences symptoms may vary by individual. Some feel dizzy with systolic blood pressures of 90 mmHg, while others have no symptoms with readings as low as 80 mmHg.

Before giving someone the diagnosis of high blood pressure (hypertension), it is important to take the blood pressure on multiple days, in calm, non-medical settings. This is because your blood pressure may be elevated by the stress of seeing a doctor (also called "white coat syndrome"). Many people have reactive blood pressures, and the elevation related to stress can best be managed by stress reduction exercises such as deep breathing, visualization, biofeedback, mindfulness, and yoga.

The most common type of high blood pressure is called *essential hypertension* and does not have a single identifiable cause. It may be related to genetics, poor nutrition, obesity, and inadequate regular exercise. Hypertension may have a genetic basis, meaning that it can run in families. In rare situations, elevated blood pressure may be due to a distinct cause, called secondary hypertension. Sometimes hypertension can be due to a narrowed blood vessel that goes to the kidney or due to an excess in epinephrine, norepinephrine, or cortisol production. There are tumors that can also result in elevation in blood pressure. In some studies, keeping blood pressure too low has been associated with an increase in health risks as well. While there is a lot known about treating blood pressure, there is still much yet to learn.

Treating High Blood Pressure

Lifestyle Modifications

This gets back to the three pillars described in the section opener, in which we talk about a heart-healthy diet and exercise. This, together with stress reduction, reaching your ideal body weight, and decreasing alcohol and salt intake, can help lower your blood pressure. About half of the people with hypertension are salt responders. If a person is responsive to salt, decreasing its intake will result in a lower blood pressure. *The DASH (Dietary Approaches to Stop Hypertension) diet* has been shown to be the most effective method in lowering blood pressure as well and is recommended by the National Heart, Lung, and Blood Institute. Table 38.2 shows the components of the DASH diet, which includes fruits and vegetables, grains and nuts, and fish and poultry. In general, it calls for a low-saturated fat diet with less than 2300 mg of sodium per day. The DASH diet is the first one listed in Appendix

Table 38.2 DASH diet

Fruits and vegetables
Some nuts and grains
Fish/poultry (very little red meat)
 Low sodium (< 2300mg of sodium per day); low saturated fats

K (with some sample foods), and the "Food Journal" allows you to track your progress with this diet.

More About Sodium

Naturally, there is sodium or salt in unprocessed foods such as fish, meats, and vegetables. Salt can be used as a preservative and can enhance the flavor of foods. Processed foods are those that have been modified in some way by the food industry, either for taste or to extend shelf life. Frequently, salt is an ingredient in processed and prepared foods. Foods that are pickled or preserved often have a lot of salt. The labels that are on the packaging of foods are required to reveal how much salt, fat, carbohydrates, sugar, protein, and vitamins are contained in a serving. The typical American diet contains too much salt.

On average, Americans consume 3.4 grams (3400 mg) of sodium a day. *It is recommended that less than 2.3 grams (2300 mg) be consumed per day but ideally less than 1.5 grams (1500 mg).* Be careful to pay close attention to the serving size on the labels, as it can be misleading. For example, some soups cans give the amount of sodium in a serving size for only 1/3 of the can. If you eat the full contents of the can, you will be consuming three times the amount indicated in a single serving!

Salt tastes good, and everyone in the food industry knows this. If you get food from a restaurant, you can bet that there is a higher amount of sodium in the food since it will enhance the taste. When ordering out, most restaurants will accommodate a request for no added salt, though the ingredients may still be salty (i.e., cured meats, anchovies, olives, pickles, etc.). A study published in JAMA in 2023 demonstrated that reducing salt consumption lowered blood pressure significantly in most participants. The investigators found *a low-salt diet was equally as effective as a first-line blood pressure medication.*

Know Your Body Mass Index (BMI)

Most Americans are either overweight or obese. Read Chap. 39 to understand more about this, and learn what you can do about it. When you go to the doctor, they typically weigh you and calculate your BMI. A normal BMI should be under 25. What can you do about it?—Talk to your doctor! Managing your BMI begins with a heart-healthy diet (such as the DASH diet discussed above) and exercise (see the section opener).

Alcohol Consumption Matters

Alcohol consumption in any form has been associated with elevations in blood pressure and with causing arrhythmias, such as premature atrial and ventricular contractions, and atrial fibrillation. The ideal amount of alcohol intake has been debated for several years. Some studies suggest that alcohol intake in moderate quantities (one serving daily for women and up to two servings daily for men) may modestly decrease cardiovascular events, though this is not entirely clear. It is *not recommended* that those who do not consume alcohol start in order to decrease their cardiovascular risk. Alcohol is both directly and indirectly toxic to the heart. Think of the direct effects as having the potential to damage your heart muscle, while the indirect effects are linked to increased blood pressure and hormone changes that make the heart work harder. There are other negative effects on health that can be caused by alcohol, which need to be considered when thinking about drinking. If you do consume alcohol at all, it is best to drink in moderation.

Medications

Medications are often needed to control blood pressure when lifestyle modifications (diet, exercise, and stress management) are not effective enough. It is not unusual that more than one medication is needed. There is no shortage of medications used to treat blood pressure. There are several major classes of blood pressure medications that can be grouped according to how they each work. These include beta-blockers, diuretics, renin-angiotensin system blockers, calcium channel blockers, alpha blockers, and hydralazine. Below is a list of these medications, their main effects, and some common side effects.

Diuretics are medications that can decrease blood pressure by decreasing sodium and fluid in the body. Diuretics lead to the elimination of water as well as electrolytes such as sodium, potassium, and magnesium, to name a few. This may lead to rare side effects such as arrhythmias, and kidney function should be periodically assessed with a common blood test. Different types of diuretics work on different kidney components and can be combined to assist in treating people with too much body fluid or swelling (edema).

There are essentially three types of diuretics, which are defined by the part of the kidney where they act. These include the thiazide diuretics that work on the distal convoluted tubule, loop diuretics that work on the loop of Henle, and mineralocorticoid receptor antagonists that work via the renin-angiotensin system and block aldosterone.

Typically, *thiazide diuretics* (hydrochlorothiazide) are often a first-line medication in the treatment of high blood pressure. Patients on this medication may experience a slight increase in their frequency of urination. This medication is often used in combination with an ACE inhibitor or ARB (see below), and is sometimes combined in a single pill formulation for simplicity. Other *loop diuretics*, such as furosemide (Lasix), bumetanide (Bumex), and torsemide (Demadex), work on a different part of the kidney and are more useful in removing excess fluid in heart failure, as opposed to controlling blood pressure.

Mineralocorticoid receptor antagonists are a group of diuretics that work in the kidney to lower blood pressure by stopping reabsorption of fluid and electrolytes. They do this at the final step of the renin-angiotensin-aldosterone system by blocking the effects of aldosterone. Aldosterone is responsible for the absorption of water and sodium and the secretion of potassium. Because aldosterone is blocked, water and sodium are excreted, and blood volume and blood pressure are lowered. These medicines have been shown to help treat heart failure, leg swelling, and even cirrhosis of the liver. Some common mineralocorticoid receptor antagonists include eplerenone (Inspira) and spironolactone (Aldactone). These medications should be used with caution in patients with kidney disease, and potassium levels should be assessed periodically to ensure they are not elevated. Some of these drugs may also have testosterone-lowering effects and may lead to breast tissue enlargement in males (gynecomastia). Low doses of these medications can reduce these problems, and one more expensive version (eplerenone) largely eliminates this problem.

ACE Inhibitors, also known as angiotensin-converting enzyme inhibitors, block a chemical reaction in the body, resulting in a lowered blood pressure. They affect the renin-angiotensin system by blocking the formation of angiotensin II (the active form of angiotensin). This class of medication can help facilitate heart restructuring (after a heart attack or from prolonged hypertension), block the reabsorption of water from the kidney, and block blood vessel constriction, thereby lowering blood pressure. These drugs may also be useful in preventing heart attacks, treating heart failure, and offering protection of the kidneys in diabetic patients. Some common types of ACE inhibitors include benazepril (Lotensin), captopril, enalapril (Vasotec), lisinopril (Prinivil or Zestril), quinapril (Accupril), and ramipril.

There are some patients (approximately five to ten percent) who may develop a bothersome cough, which is not dangerous. The medication can be changed if this becomes an issue. Rarely, ACE inhibitors may cause dangerous swelling of the face and airway, a deadly side effect known as angioedema. This may close the airway and prevent breathing and is an emergency. Anyone experiencing this must immediately call 911. ACE inhibitors may also cause an increase in potassium and need to be used with caution in patients with kidney problems. Furthermore, these medications must not be used in people with renal artery stenosis of both kidneys, as this may lead to kidney failure. Finally, these medications are toxic to the fetus and must be avoided in pregnancy.

ARBs are angiotensin II receptor blockers and work on the same renin-angiotensin system as the ACE inhibitor drugs. In general, ARBs and ACE inhibitors should not be used together. Like ACE inhibitors, ARBs may be used to lower blood pressure, decrease hospitalization and death from heart failure, and protect the kidneys from the effects of diabetes. Some common ARBs include azilsartan (Edarbi), candesartan (Atacand), irbesartan (Avapro), losartan potassium (Cozaar), telmisartan (Micardis), and valsartan (Diovan). Caution needs to be used in patients with kidney problems, and the potassium levels should be monitored periodically. ARBs are also contraindicated in pregnancy and may lead to a benign cough (though less frequently than an ACE inhibitor) or the more dangerous angioedema.

Beta-blockers are medications that lower blood pressure by blocking beta receptors where adrenaline works; a hormone that is involved in fight or flight. *In addition to lowering blood pressure, these medicines are useful in decreasing heart rate and extra heartbeats (arrhythmias) as well.* There are many different types of beta-blockers; some are even useful in treating congestive heart failure. Some common beta-blockers include atenolol (Tenormin), bisoprolol (Zebeta), carvedilol (Coreg), labetalol (Normodyne), and metoprolol (Lopressor or Toprol). Caution needs to be taken in patients with slower heart rates, lower blood pressures, and those with certain circulatory and lung problems, such as chronic obstructive pulmonary disease (COPD) or asthma.

Two other beta-blockers that have unique properties, called intrinsic sympathomimetic activity (ISA), may have less effect on slowing heart rates and lowering blood pressure and may be useful in those who syncopize from an overactive vagus nerve (a condition called vasovagal syncope). They include pindolol (Visken) and acebutolol (Sectral). Beta-blockers may also hide some reactions (such as a fast heartbeat) that people can get with low blood sugar (hypoglycemia). These agents should be used with caution in patients who are on medicines to lower their blood sugar, as they may be unaware that they are hypoglycemic.

Calcium channel blockers are a class of drugs that block calcium channels, slowing the heart rate and relaxing smooth muscle in blood vessels and heart. By relaxing these muscles, blood vessels widen (vasodilate), and blood pressure falls. Additionally, the heart rate may also slow. There are different types of calcium channel blockers: some lower heart rate by slowing electrical conduction through the heart—verapamil (Calan, Covera, Isoptin, or Verelan) and diltiazem (Cardizem or Tiazac)—while others act predominantly on relaxing the smooth muscle in blood vessels—nifedipine (Procardia or Adalat) and amlodipine (Norvasc). Verapamil and diltiazem work similarly to beta-blockers by slowing conduction in the SA and AV nodes, but they should be used cautiously, if at all, in those with congestive heart failure. Nifedipine and amlodipine help expand blood vessels.

Verapamil and diltiazem are more likely to cause heart rate slowing (bradycardia), whereas drugs like nifedipine and amlodipine are more likely to cause swelling of the hands and feet, flushing, and dizziness. In general, calcium channel blockers should usually be avoided (except in specific instances) in those with heart failure and a reduced ejection fraction. Both groups of calcium channel blockers have the ability to cause constipation. When starting these medications, increasing fiber (whole grains, fruits, and vegetables) and water intake (hydration) is recommended to prevent constipation.

Alpha receptor blockers can either work peripherally on the blood vessels or centrally in the brain. Those that work peripherally help the blood vessels to relax, thereby decreasing blood pressure. These include prazosin (Minipress, Vasoflex, Lentopres), doxazosin (Cardura), and tamsulosin (Flowmax) and are also useful in helping facilitate urination in men with prostate symptoms. The central alpha blockers, such as clonidine (Catapress), lower blood pressure and may cause a decrease in heart rate. They may cause drowsiness at first and have also been shown to help people with drug withdrawal symptoms.

Hydralazine (Apresoline) is a direct vasodilator that relaxes blood vessels. This drug may cause an increase in heart rate but can be used in patients with advanced kidney disease. It is used for acute severe hypertension. Hydralazine, when combined with isosorbide dinitrate (Isordil), has also been shown to be effective in treating heart failure when an ACE inhibitor or ARB cannot be used, especially in the African American population. Hydralazine may rarely cause drug-induced lupus (a systemic inflammatory response) and fluid around the heart (pericardial effusion). Both conditions generally resolve by stopping the drug. Because hydralazine may cause an increase in heart rate to compensate for the decrease in blood pressure, it is contraindicated in people who experience angina or have coronary artery disease. These people have narrowed heart vessels, and the muscle cannot meet the blood and oxygen demand requirement from elevated heart rates.

Supplements Some supplements have been advertised to lower blood pressure and include garlic, cocoa, flaxseed, and fish oil. Be careful taking these supplements. There is no great study that shows that they work, and it is better to eat a healthy balanced diet rich in fruit, vegetables, and nuts (like the DASH diet) while *watching salt intake*.

Obesity

39

Roger Kersten and Todd J. Cohen

When visiting your doctor, the first thing they will usually do is take your height and weight and calculate your body mass index (BMI). Your BMI is a measure of your body fat based on your height and weight. It is your weight in kilograms divided by your height in meters squared. This is a number you should know, along with your blood pressure and cholesterol measurements. A normal BMI is 18.5 to 24.9. Obesity is defined as a BMI of 30 or more. Overweight is defined as a BMI of 25 or more. Over 40 percent of adult Americans are obese, and approximately another 30 percent are overweight. Obesity is associated with an increased risk of heart disease and stroke. Additionally, it is associated with an increased risk of type 2 diabetes and even some types of cancers. Obesity may also be associated with an increased inflammatory response.

When obese and overweight patients lose weight, many positive effects result. Weight loss is associated with a drop in blood pressure, improved insulin sensitivity, and a decrease in inflammation. The goal of treating obesity is not simply dieting but includes a long-term plan of behavioral modification to maintain a healthy weight and improve one's fitness level.

The Role of Exercise and Diet in Maintaining a Healthy Weight (Todd Cohen MD)

Table 39.1 *reviews some important facts regarding obesity.*

R. Kersten (Retired)
Department of Cardiology, St. Francis Hospital & Heart Center, Roslyn, NY, USA

T. J. Cohen (✉)
NYIT College of Osteopathic Medicine, New York, NY, USA
e-mail: tcohen03@nyit.edu

Table 39.1 Obesity facts

BMI stands for body mass index.
Defined as a BMI greater than 30 kg/m^2 body surface area.
Has over a 40 percent prevalence in the United States.
Associated with increased inflammation and cancer risk.
Increases blood pressure and makes one more prone to type 2 diabetes.
Increases the risk of stroke and heart disease.
Is best treated with behavioral modification.

Table 39.2 Benefits of Different Forms of Exercise

Exercise	Benefits
Aerobic (running, jogging, walking, swimming)	Burns fat Increases endurance Lowers blood pressure
Strength training (lifting weights, body weight exercises)	Builds muscle Slows decline of muscle mass with age Increases bone density
Stretching (yoga, warming up) Balance (yoga, tai chi)	Improves flexibility Improves balance Improves stability Improves ranges of motion

The treatment of obesity is more effective when an exercise program (see Chap. 37 and Table 39.2) *is combined with a heart-healthy diet that is sustainable and tolerable* (see Chaps. 37 and 38). *The key is sustainable and tolerable, and that goes for the diet and the exercise! In* Table 39.2, *we see the different types of exercise broken into categories. Appendix L also lists a variety of aerobic exercises and provides you with a fitness tracker that may be helpful as you start and/or follow an exercise program. Before starting any fitness program, please consult your doctor. Aerobic exercise is often referred to as cardio and is intended to get your heart rate up, get your heart pumping, and enhance circulation. Even if you can't get your heart rate up, the heart can respond by increasing the amount of blood pumped out with every beat or stroke (stroke volume).*

My favorite aerobic exercises include those of low impact which includes the elliptical, biking, and swimming. A brisk walk is also gentler on the joints than the pounding that occurs with running. Jogging and running are great too, but over time may take a toll on your joints, especially if you have a BMI on the heavier side. Make sure you wear a good pair of running shoes (sneakers) and gradually build up your activity level to avoid injury (i.e., pulling a muscle, tearing your Achilles tendon, or putting an untoward strain on your cardiovascular system). Aerobic exercise should never be started all of a sudden, at a high energy level, and for a long duration. You need to build up to it. Aerobic exercise needs to be combined with stretching and warm-up exercises to prevent muscular strain and cramping.

Warming up and cooling down can be accomplished by sitting on the floor with your feet and legs extended straight out and holding your toes either with your hand

Table 39.3 Diet regimes for heart health

Diet	Specifications
DASH diet (**D**ietary **A**pproaches to **S**top **H**ypertension)	Eat more fruits, vegetables, beans, nuts, low-fat/non-fat dairy
	Eat less sugar, fatty meat, sugar, sweets, sodium, and full-fat dairy
Mediterranean diet	Eat mostly fruits, vegetables, nuts, herbs, whole grains, beans, and plant-based foods
	Eat moderate amounts of poultry, dairy, and eggs
	Avoid refined grains, oils, foods with added sugars, and processed foods
Ornish diet	Eat mainly fruits, vegetables, whole grains, legumes, seeds, and nuts
	Avoid meat, poultry, fish, egg yolks, refined carbohydrates, saturated fats, excessive dairy products, alcohol, and caffeine
	Limit fat intake to only fats from plant-based foods
Weight watchers	Foods are assigned different point values based on their calorie, fat, and protein contents
	Social accountability component
Sugar busters	Avoid all added sugar and processed foods
	Eat vegetables, whole grains, lean meats, fruits, and healthy fats
American Heart Association Diet	Eat a variety of fruit and vegetables, whole grain products, high fiber foods, fish
	Incorporate physical activity
	Avoid foods with saturated and trans fats

or with a strap. Standing up and holding onto a chair with one hand and pulling your other foot backward with your free hand while bending your knee is also helpful. Core strengthening with sit-ups can also help. Yoga and Tai Chi can help with stretching and balance. These practices can help both physically and mentally. Lastly, strength training with weights specifically guided by an experienced fitness training program can help reverse the effects of aging and gravity.

Table 39.3 lists some diets that I think are worthy to look at as a long-term solution depending on your personal situation. This information again appears in another format in Appendix K along with some typical meals followed by a "Food Journal" to help track your progress with your selected diet. Please note, fad diets may advertise rapid weight loss, though continued weight loss may not be as successful. The initial weight loss of most diets is, in fact, water loss. There is no one diet that is optimal for every patient. Plus, there is a lot of overlap between the DASH diet, the Mediterranean diet, the American Heart Association diet, and Sugar Busters. These diets favor more whole unprocessed grains, fruits and vegetables, less saturated fats, and less sugar.

The Ornish diet is a mostly plant-based low-fat diet (fats are limited to plants), which has been claimed to stop the progression of coronary artery disease and even reverse it in some. It is a very strict diet, and one has to be very motivated to maintain compliance with this diet over the long haul. The Weight Watchers program is a very regimented calorie-counting program and has helped many people lose weight. Sugar Busters is a diet invented by a heart surgeon and is one my family has used at *one time or another. Many of my family members are still busting sugar, and even one of them has become a vegan (vegetarian including no dairy or meat). See* Chaps. 37 and 38 *to learn more about a heart-healthy diet and the DASH diet as a means to get better control over your blood pressure (as well as other risk factors).*

Each of these diets has its advantages and disadvantages. Your doctor may steer you to a weight management program or a licensed dietician. I believe that it is important to realize that calorie counting may not be as important as restricting certain types of food. You should also realize that any diet that you cannot follow long-term is not likely going to work long-term. That is why I am not in favor of very strict diets that are essentially impossible to follow long-term.

Medications

Medications for weight loss have been used for several years, though not without serious concerns such as heart valve disease, arrhythmias, high blood pressure, and even cancers. Many of these drugs work by decreasing appetite (Lomaira, naltrexone) and/or preventing fat reabsorption in the intestines (orlistat; Alli, Xenical). Medications used to promote weight loss in type 2 diabetes are also useful in those with a higher BMI.

Please talk to your primary care physician and your heart doctor before contemplating or trying a medication. No matter the drug used, none are meant as long-term solutions for maintaining a healthy weight. In patients who have been unsuccessful with diets and lifestyle modification and are at risk of serious diseases such as heart disease and diabetes, surgical procedures (*bariatric surgery*) may be considered. Of note, a diabetes medication, semaglutide, is being marketed in a weight loss formulation known as Wegovy, and there is great optimism about this medication. This medication is a weekly injectable medication (GLP-1 receptor agonist) that slows gastric emptying and increases satiety. The medication can cause low blood pressure but may be useful in those with a BMI of 30 or more. For optimal results, these weight loss medications should be taken in conjunction with a well-balanced diet, adequate hydration, and proper exercise. Adverse effects of these medications include hypoglycemia, nausea, vomiting, constipation, and diarrhea. Make sure to speak with your doctor if you experience any adverse effects. For more information, see Chap. 41.

Surgical Intervention

If lifestyle changes are not enough, surgical intervention can be used to promote weight loss. One type is called *gastric banding* surgery, in which a sleeve is inserted around the stomach to make the patient feel full after eating smaller food portions. Any bariatric surgical procedure contemplation should only be considered after you have been unsuccessful in your attempts with weight loss and, again, must be discussed with your primary physician and cardiologist, not just your bariatric surgeon. Any surgical procedure should not be taken lightly. Even after a successful procedure, dietary changes and exercise are necessary.

In closing, obesity is an important risk factor that needs to be addressed in patients who are at risk of, or have, heart disease. Diet and exercise are the cornerstones for treating patients who are overweight or obese. Medications and surgery are last resorts, and not generally recommended. It is much better to address this problem early, before it gets out of control. So, please discuss your specific BMI with your doctor and discuss what you should do to gain better control over your risks for heart disease. It will likely include a mixture of a heart-healthy diet and regular exercise. Start today, and take the first step toward living a productive and active life.

Smoking

40

Roger Kersten and Todd J. Cohen

It is well known that smoking causes many health conditions including cardiovascular disease. Tobacco use, either chewing or smoking, can increase the risk of cancer, heart attack, stroke, and vascular disease. Cigars, cigarettes, pipe smoking, chewing tobacco, and even second-hand smoke (the smoke inhaled by someone in the vicinity of a smoke) have all been shown to increase risk. Exposing others to cigarette smoke (even nonsmokers) has been shown to cause an increase in asthma attacks and other lung conditions, such as emphysema or chronic obstructive pulmonary disease (COPD). Tobacco use in any form can increase the risk of many cancers, including lung, head, and neck. Third-hand smoke is caused by smoke particles that fall onto food and are then eaten. Even third-hand smoke can cause health issues. By stopping smoking, a person may improve their health and the health of the entire family.

How to Stop Smoking

Quitting smoking is something that most people dread, but there are many things that may make it easier. It sometimes requires a combination of things, such as medications and acupuncture, for example. Some people have achieved success by gradually reducing the number of cigarettes smoked in a day until there is no longer a craving. Other people have quit by using nicotine products like a nicotine patch or nicotine-infused gum to overcome the addiction. A certain medication, called bupropion (Wellbutrin or Zyban), was noted to be helpful in achieving smoking

R. Kersten (Retired)
Department of Cardiology, St. Francis Hospital & Heart Center, Roslyn, NY, USA

T. J. Cohen (✉)
NYIT College of Osteopathic Medicine, New York, NY, USA
e-mail: tcohen03@nyit.edu

© The Author(s), under exclusive license to Springer Nature Switzerland AG 2025
T. J. Cohen, R. S. Blumenthal (eds.), *Surviving and Thriving With Heart Disease*,
Contemporary Cardiology, https://doi.org/10.1007/978-3-032-00579-3_40

cessation while it was being studied as an antidepressant. Another medication, called varenicline (Chantix), blocks the ability of nicotine to bind to certain receptors in the body and has been found to be highly effective in treating tobacco addiction when used correctly.

Whatever method you use, it is important not to give up. Discuss your plans with your healthcare provider so that additional support can be given. Once someone is successful at quitting tobacco use, they should try to never take another puff again. Tobacco is so addicting that even an innocent drag on a cigarette can end up triggering the craving all over again.

Some people are afraid of weight gain that may occur with quitting. There is a small amount of weight gain, about five pounds, that has been associated with stopping smoking. It may be that those who notice a significantly larger weight gain when they quit smoking have transferred their addiction from nicotine to food. Starting an exercise program along with quitting tobacco may be very helpful in preventing additional weight gain. Exercise has even been shown to increase the likelihood of being successful at quitting. Vaping nicotine has also been used to break the habit of smoking cigarettes. However, significant concerns about potential lung damage from vaping have led us to recommend avoiding it altogether.

Commentary by Dr. Todd Cohen

Table 40.1 lists some smoking facts for you to consider as you help yourself and your loved ones try to break this bad habit. First, it is an independent risk for heart disease and is associated with a variety of cancers, including those that affect the lungs, esophagus, pancreas, and bladder. It is the leading preventable cause of worldwide mortality. Although it is a modifiable risk, I, as a cardiologist, acknowledge that it is extremely difficult to stop smoking. My stepfather, who had lung cancer and coronary artery disease, including coronary bypass surgery, was still sneaking cigarettes long after those life-changing events. To stop smoking, you need to pull out all the stops and work with your healthcare provider and use all the tricks of the trade, including behavioral modification, patches, gums, medication, meditation, and everything it takes to break this deadly habit.

Table 40.1 Smoking facts

Smoking is an independent risk factor for heart disease (heart attacks, stroke, and vascular disease).

Smoking is associated with a variety of cancers including lung, larynx, esophageal, pancreas, bladder, and endometrial cancer.

These risks are modifiable (meaning if you stop smoking, the risk decreases).

The leading cause of preventable worldwide mortality is smoking.

Stopping smoking is very hard.

Techniques to stop smoking include behavior modification, hypnosis, nicotine patches and gum, and medications such as buspirone.

Smoking cessation can have a big impact on your future health.

Diabetes

41

Roger Kersten and Todd J. Cohen

Diabetes mellitus is a condition associated with an elevation in blood sugar (glucose) and is a major risk factor for the development of cardiovascular disease. Chronically elevated glucose can cause damage to the heart and blood vessels (cardiovascular system), kidneys, nerves, and eyes. Often, before one develops diabetes, their blood glucose levels may become elevated, but not high enough to meet the criteria for diabetes. This condition is called prediabetes, and often can progress to diabetes unless steps are taken (such as diet and exercise) to prevent the progression.

When we talk about knowing your numbers, it is important to know your fasting blood sugar and your hemoglobin A1C level. Diabetes can be diagnosed with these numbers in the following manner. First, a fasting blood sugar can be obtained by taking a sample of your blood after you have had nothing to eat or drink for eight hours. The levels of glucose and the A1C in your blood are measured. A normal fasting blood sugar is less than 100 mg/dl. A fasting sugar of 100 to 125 mg/dl is called prediabetes, and 126 mg/dl or above is diabetic. Additionally, a hemoglobin A1C level (or A1C blood test) can tell how your blood sugar has been over the past three months. A normal A1C is less than 5.7 percent; 5.7 to 6.4 percent is prediabetic; and 6.5 percent or more is diabetic.

An oral glucose tolerance test can be administered and measures your blood sugar 2 hours after drinking a sugary drink. A glucose level of less than 140 mg/dl is normal, 140 to 199 mg/dl is prediabetes, and 200 mg/dl or more is diabetic.

R. Kersten (✉) (Retired)
Department of Cardiology, St. Francis Hospital & Heart Center, Roslyn, NY, USA
e-mail: rkerstenm@yahoo.com

T. J. Cohen
NYIT College of Osteopathic Medicine, New York, NY, USA
e-mail: tcohen03@nyit.edu

© The Author(s), under exclusive license to Springer Nature Switzerland AG 2025
T. J. Cohen, R. S. Blumenthal (eds.), *Surviving and Thriving With Heart Disease*,
Contemporary Cardiology, https://doi.org/10.1007/978-3-032-00579-3_41

Table 41.1 Diabetes facts

A leading cause of death in the United States and worldwide.
An independent risk factor of cardiovascular disease and stroke.
Patients with diabetes are predisposed to developing chronic kidney disease.
90 percent of all patients with diabetes have adult onset (type 2).
Over the past two decades, the number of patients with diabetes has doubled.
Hispanic and Latin Americans, African Americans, and Native American Indians have a higher risk of developing prediabetes or diabetes.
Risks for type 2 diabetes include obesity, age over 45 years, sedentary lifestyle, and a history of gestational diabetes.

Finally, a random blood glucose with symptoms of diabetes and a glucose level of 200 mg/dl or more may be diagnostic.

There are two types of diabetes. In type 1 diabetes, a person does not produce enough insulin and is dependent on taking insulin in order to live. People with the more common type 2 diabetes may need insulin to help control their blood sugars, though this is not always the case. Very often, type 2 diabetes can be helped, if not controlled completely, with lifestyle changes and/or oral medications. Patients with type 2 diabetes make insulin in their body, though it is not adequate to control blood sugar. There are also some additional injectable medications, other than insulin, that are useful in controlling blood sugar.

The problems caused by diabetes go beyond just an elevation in blood sugar levels. Diabetes is associated with an increased risk of heart attack, stroke, kidney disease, peripheral arterial disease, and congestive heart failure. It is the leading cause of preventable death in the United States. African Americans, Native American Indians, and Hispanic and Latin Americans are more prone to prediabetes and type 2 diabetes.

Approximately 90 percent of all diabetics have type 2 diabetes, and more than one in three adult Americans have prediabetes. As stated above, patients with type 2 diabetes make insulin, though it is not adequate to control blood sugar. Type 2 diabetes can often be managed solely with lifestyle modification, whereas type 1 diabetics will always need medication. If lifestyle modification is not enough to lower blood sugar to appropriate levels, oral and injectable medications can be used. Some risk factors for developing type 2 diabetes include obesity, age greater than 45 years, sedentary lifestyle, and a history of gestational diabetes. Table 41.1 lists some important facts related to diabetes.

Lifestyle Modifications

Diet and Exercise

It is important for people with diabetes to try to maintain a healthy weight. Obesity and being overweight have been associated with glucose (sugar) intolerance that will cause higher blood sugars (see Chap. 39). Decreasing your caloric intake helps with weight loss, but not all calories are the same.

A diet lower in sugar and carbohydrates will help to reduce blood sugar values in diabetic patients. Simple carbohydrates like white bread and pasta tend to break down more quickly than complex carbohydrates like whole grains, though both will increase blood sugar. A food that has a *high glycemic index* can raise blood sugar higher and more quickly than one with a low glycemic index. A diet that is lower in carbohydrates and sugars may help to lower blood sugar. Weight management and control of blood sugars have made low-carb diets popular. These diets, sometimes called ketogenic or "keto" diets, recommend that carbohydrate and sugar intake be kept low. As a result of lowering the intake of carbohydrates, there is an increase in proteins and healthier fats that go into these diets. To learn more about diets, see Chaps. 37 and 38, as well as Appendix K.

It is important to discuss diet improvements with your healthcare provider, as a low-carbohydrate diet may decrease blood sugar levels. If successful, a low-carbohydrate diet may allow your doctor to lower and/or discontinue certain sugar-lowering medications. This is a positive situation but needs to be monitored to avoid low blood sugar, a condition known as hypoglycemia. Hypoglycemia can be dangerous if not recognized and treated.

Exercise is also very important in all patients with cardiovascular disease with or without diabetes. Exercise provides many benefits, including helping in weight management, reducing blood sugar, reducing inflammation, improving fitness, improving sleep, decreasing fatigue, and even decreasing depression and memory loss. Exercising for 30 minutes per day, 5 to 7 days per week, with aerobic exercises such as using a stationary bike, treadmill, swimming, or elliptical, combined with the use of light weights (resistance training), fits the bill (see Chap. 39 and Appendix L). Before starting an exercise program, check with your healthcare provider for any specific restrictions or recommendations.

Medications

If lifestyle modification does not result in you achieving the goals of treatment of diabetes, or if you have type 1 diabetes, medications will be needed. There are so many different medications that are useful in treating blood sugar levels in diabetes, and some are even helpful in decreasing heart attacks and heart failure. Some of these medications are in pill form, and others are injectable.

Insulin

Not all diabetic patients need insulin. Insulin is naturally produced in the pancreas and signals your body's cells to take up blood sugar. Insulin causes the level of sugar in the blood to fall as it pushes it into cells in order to provide cellular energy. In type 1 diabetes, where there is not enough insulin produced by the pancreas, blood sugar levels can become very high. At the same time, there is no insulin to push the sugar into the cells where it is needed to make energy. In this situation, the blood sugar is quite high and the cells are starving for fuel. If the cells cannot get enough sugar, lactic acid builds up in the bloodstream and ketones can be detected in the urine.

As a result of a lack of insulin, our bodies will break down fats and protein for energy, resulting in a buildup of ketones that may lead to a condition called diabetic ketoacidosis. This condition is deadly if not treated promptly in the hospital with insulin. Diabetic ketoacidosis should not be confused with harmless benign dietary ketosis. It is often recommended that while people are on low-carb diets, they use a type of dipstick to check to see if they have ketones in the urine. If a person successfully gets ketones in the urine, it indicates that they are using their own fat stores to power their cells. As the process continues, the fat stores of the body will be burned, and weight loss will result.

Insulin is injectable either by needle, pen, or pump under the skin (subcutaneously), and is available in both short- and long-acting forms. A combination of short- and long-acting insulins is frequently used to mimic how our bodies release insulin throughout the day and in response to eating.

A Note of Caution (Hypoglycemia)

Taking too much insulin for someone's needs can result in hypoglycemia (low blood sugar). Low blood sugar can occur if someone suddenly eats less than usual without adjusting their medications, or if kidney or liver function decreases, which may cause some medications to remain active longer. If low blood sugar is not recognized and treated quickly, it can be fatal. Symptoms of hypoglycemia include sweating, a fast heart rate, slurring of words, fatigue, weakness, passing out (syncope), coma, and even death. In patients suffering from a hypoglycemic event, it is important to get sugar into their body as quickly as possible. In a conscious patient, orange juice or candy with sugar is recommended. In patients who cannot swallow or are too weak to swallow, glucose paste, available at the pharmacy, can be placed inside the cheek, where it will absorb fairly quickly. Intravenous glucose can be given directly into the bloodstream in hospitals or by emergency medical personnel. Once the blood sugar starts to increase and the patient begins to improve, it is important to continue monitoring as the blood sugar may drop again.

Sulfonylureas

These oral medications, which have been used for many years, help control blood sugar by increasing insulin production from the pancreas and improving the body's sensitivity to insulin. Like insulin, they can cause low blood sugar and weight gain. These medications should be used with caution in patients with reduced kidney function, as impaired clearance can cause the drugs to accumulate in the body, increasing the risk of dangerously low blood sugar (hypoglycemia). Sulfonylureas can be short- or long-acting. There has been some concern that these medicines may cause heart attacks, though other studies have not shown this finding. While not a complete list, examples of these medications include glipizide, glimepiride, and repaglinide (Glucotrol, Amaryl, and Prandin, respectively).

Biguanides

This is a very frequently used oral drug that helps to control blood sugar by decreasing the absorption of sugar from the intestines, decreasing the liver's production of glucose, and improving our cells' sensitivity to insulin. These drugs may help with weight loss. Unfortunately, some people experience stomach upset, such as nausea and diarrhea, when taking biguanides. These medicines need to be used carefully in patients with kidney impairment, as they can result in lactic acidosis. Patients undergoing tests that require intravenous contrast should follow the advice of their healthcare provider and hold the medication for a short period of time before the procedure. Metformin is a commonly used biguanide that may be useful in other non-diabetic conditions as well. This medication may even decrease the risk of some cancers.

Glucagon-Like Peptide 1 Receptor Agonists (GLP-1 Receptor Agonists)

This type of drug is injectable and works like a substance that exists naturally in our body known as glucagon-like peptide 1. GLP-1 is made in the small intestine and, among other things, may cause the pancreas to release insulin. Glucagon is a hormone also produced in the pancreas that balances the effects of insulin by increasing blood sugar. This medication may be useful in decreasing the release of glucagon and delaying the stomach from emptying. The GLP-1 receptor agonists may even help the pancreas to make more insulin by making cells known as pancreatic beta cells. This class of drug includes exenatide (Byetta), dulaglutide (Trulicity), semaglutide (Ozempic), tirzepatide (Mounjaro), and liraglutide (Victoza), all of which are injectable. Both semaglutide and liraglutide have been shown to decrease cardiovascular events, such as heart attack and stroke, in these patients. Semaglutide and tirzepatide are especially effective in reducing weight and are approved for the treatment of obesity in the Wegovy and Zepbound formulations (see Chap. 39).

DPP-4 Inhibitors (Dipeptidyl Peptidase IV Inhibitors)

These medications are oral and may have multiple effects, including preventing the breakdown of GLP-1 by inhibiting DPP-4. By blocking the enzyme DPP-4, the blood sugars will fall by keeping GLP-1 around longer, as described above in the discussion of GLP-1 receptor agonists. Examples of these medications include sitagliptin (Januvia), saxagliptin (Onglyza), linagliptin (Tradjenta), and alogliptin (Nesina). So far, none of these drugs have been found to have a clear benefit in the treatment of cardiovascular disease and have no significant effect on weight. These medications may cause other side effects, including elevation in liver function tests, muscle and joint pain, and inflammation of the pancreas (pancreatitis). In general, the side effects are uncommon, and these drugs are well tolerated.

Thiazolidinediones (Glitazones)

The thiazolidinediones (glitazones) are peroxisome proliferator-activated receptor agonists (or PPARs). These medications, including rosiglitazone (Avandia) and pioglitazone (Actos), work by reducing glucose production and improving cellular insulin sensitivity. There are different PPARs in our body. PPAR gamma seems to have the effect of lowering blood sugars. These medications are generally not a first choice for patients with heart disease since they may increase body weight and even some cardiac events. These drugs should not be used in patients with heart failure or a history of bladder cancer.

Sodium-Glucose Transport Inhibitors (SGLT2 Inhibitors).

These oral medications are the newest on the scene in the treatment of diabetes. These drugs have caught the attention of cardiologists, as they seem to cause a decrease in cardiovascular events, especially in heart failure hospitalizations. These drugs work in the kidneys and allow more sugar to pass into the urine, where it is eliminated from the body. Members of the SGLT2 inhibitors include canagliflozin (Invokana), empagliflozin (Jardiance), and dapagliflozin (Farxiga). These agents have been shown to cause a mild amount of weight loss and a decrease in the risk of hospitalization for heart failure. Dapaglifozin, empagliflozin and canagliflozin have been shown to decrease cardiovascular events. Importantly, this class of medications (and empagliflozin specifically) can be helpful in the treatment of heart failure due to diastolic dysfunction (see Chap. 14).

All of these drugs should be avoided in patients with very poor kidney function. The side effects of these medications can include lower blood pressure and dehydration. Canagliflozin should be used with caution in patients with circulation problems and foot ulcers, as it may increase the need for amputation. Dapagliflozin may increase the risk of bladder cancer and should be avoided in patients with or at risk for this condition.

Since these medications put more sugar in the urine, their use can increase the risk of urinary tract infections as well as both bacterial and fungal skin infections of the genitals. The infections, especially those of the skin, are not too common; however, they can be very dangerous. In some circumstances, the infections can rapidly progress, and surgery may be required to control the infection. Any suspicion of infection, either of the urinary tract or the skin, needs to be evaluated and treated quickly by a healthcare provider.

Alpha-Glucosidase Inhibitors

Alpha-glucosidase inhibitors include acarbose (Precose) and miglitol (Glyset). They work by stopping enzymes that break down carbohydrates in the small intestine. This slows the breakdown of carbohydrates, allowing them to enter the bloodstream more gradually from the digestive tract. Blood glucose levels are therefore elevated slowly, and high blood sugar is prevented. This is helpful for people who tend to get hyperglycemic right after they eat. These drugs also raise GLP-1, mentioned above, which also delays digestion and helps regulate blood sugar. It is very helpful in those with obesity and can be helpful as a weight loss treatment in this group (see Chap. 39). Side effects include gastrointestinal upset and low blood sugar.

Yoga and Meditation

42

Jean Aronoff and Todd J. Cohen

This chapter is dedicated to the "Grace of the Guru" and bringer of light—BKS Iyengar, Master Yogi.

The heart is the center of yoga and the still point of meditation. Yoga and meditation are now emerging as a scientific system of health and well-being. They are suitable for the common man and woman living amidst the challenges, difficulties, and dilemmas of modern life. Yoga and meditation practices create rejuvenation, rehabilitation, and recovery from degenerative and debilitating diseases, such as heart disease. Disease, or *dis-ease*, is slowed as the technological advances of modern medicine are integrated with the yogic understanding of the mind-body complex, known as *psychophysiology*.

People today are more aware of yoga *asanas* (postures), meditation, relaxation, and the psychological benefits that these practices impart. Yoga and meditation are

---

Jean Aronoff is a founding member and former staff teacher at the Iyengar Yoga Institute of Greater New York. She has taught a varied yoga curriculum at colleges and adult education courses throughout NYC and Long Island. These included yoga for children, seniors, pregnancy, stress reduction, individuals with special needs, and private instruction. She has hosted and taught an annual yoga retreat at an ashram in Pennsylvania. She taught Iyengar Yoga at Om Sweet Om Yoga in Port Washington, NY. She notes that she has made five trips to India, three on pilgrimage to Pune to study yoga directly with B.K.S. Iyengar, his daughter Geeta, and son Prashant.

J. Aronoff
Yoga Instructor at Om Sweet Om, Port Washington, NY, USA

T. J. Cohen (✉)
NYIT College of Osteopathic Medicine, New York, NY, USA
e-mail: tcohen03@nyit.edu

© The Author(s), under exclusive license to Springer Nature Switzerland AG 2025
T. J. Cohen, R. S. Blumenthal (eds.), *Surviving and Thriving With Heart Disease*,
Contemporary Cardiology, https://doi.org/10.1007/978-3-032-00579-3_42

experiential and are inseparable. Yoga is meditation in movement. Meditation is a specific type of mindfulness, which will be discussed in Chap. 43. Yoga, meditation, and relaxation are preventative medicine. They can awaken and balance your physical and mental (emotional and spiritual) energies. Any ordinary person can have the extraordinary experience of yoga and meditation.

The heart acts as a translator between mystical experience and intelligence —Rumi

Commentary by Dr. Todd Cohen:

Iyengar Yoga is a particularly rewarding type of yoga that takes you through a series of poses called asanas. Unlike the more fluid Hatha yoga, Iyengar is slower and geared more towards stretching, meditation, and relaxation. I have taken many of Jean's yoga classes at Om Sweet Om together with my wife, Jill (who is the cardiology nurse in my medical practice), and we have found them particularly useful in keeping us grounded as individuals, as a couple, and with our work and devotion to medicine. Jean's yoga class is an hour long, with a focus on a part of the body or an emotion, typically suggested in advance by a yoga classmate. Some poses may be seen in Fig. 42.1.

We begin by inverted stretching against a wall (pose 6) and proceed to her opening chant in which we sit in a cross-legged yoga pose on a mat and Jean chants, "Bow to the light within, Bow to BKS Iyengar for his teaching, Bow to Mother Earth, Bow to Patchy Mamma India." Then, we take three slow deep breaths in and out, followed by an inhalation and exhalation of "Om" three times. Figure. 42.1 shows some of the Iyengar poses, including downward dog (pose 3), tree pose (pose 9), warrior 1 (pose 10), warrior 2 (pose 11), and triangle pose (pose 12). Iyengar yoga is less fluid than the more typical Hatha yoga, and each pose lasts between one and two minutes long. There are some inversions, but the entire routine is modifiable based on one's own injuries and flexibility. For example, I participated in her class after breaking my elbow and did not do any weight-bearing exercises or stretches with that arm.

The class ends with her classic Shavasana, or corpse pose meditation (pose 8), in which each one of us lies supine in a comfortable position on the yoga mat with props for our head or our legs (such as blankets or a bolster). During this, we listen to the instructor's relaxation/meditation chant. Shavasana (see below) is the culmination of her excellent class and has helped us achieve a significant degree of relaxation. I have used yoga and massage for relaxation, and find Jean's Iyengar class to be even more restorative and more helpful than a routine massage.

Jean's Shavasana chant (20 step relaxation/medication technique)

This technique can be practiced sitting or lying down:

1. Take a long, slow, deep inhalation and a long, slow, deep exhalation.
2. Relax your scalp.
3. Relax your forehead, cheeks, and skin on your face.
4. Relax your eyelids and let your eyes sink deeper and deeper into cooling pools of water.

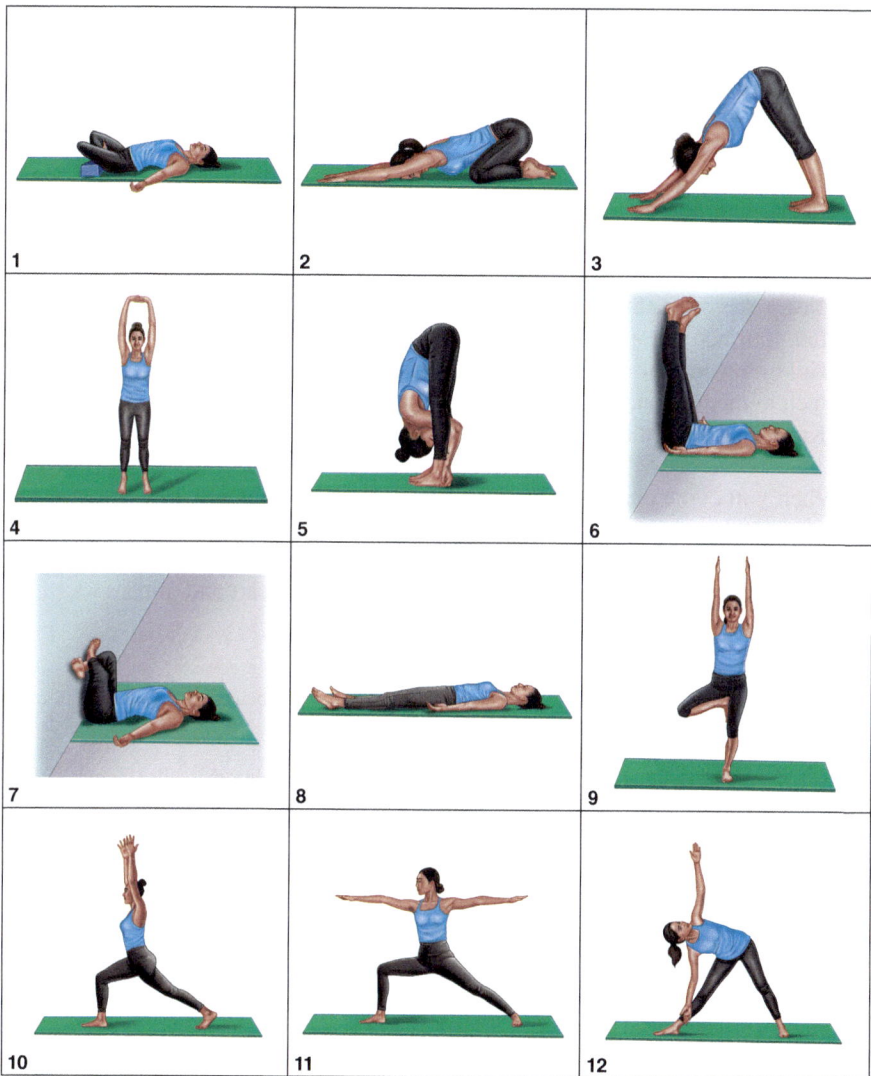

Fig. 42.1 Classic yoga poses including downward dog (pose 3), tree pose (pose 9), warrior 1 (pose 10), and warrior 2 (pose 11)

5. Relax your jaw muscles, lips, teeth, gums, and let the tongue rest in the bottom of the mouth (when the tongue is touching the roof of the mouth, it creates tension).
6. Relax your entire face.
7. Relax your throat muscles.
8. Relax your lungs and feel the cooling breath going in and the warm breath going out.
9. Relax your heart and breathe in love and breathe out love.
10. Relax your belly and breathe.

11. Relax your arms, wrists, hands, and fingertips, feeling them as hollow cylinders empty and void.
12. Relax your legs, feet, toes feel them as hollow cylinders empty and void.
13. Relax your upper back, shoulders, and neck.
14. Relax your entire spine from head to toe, letting it sink deeper and deeper into the floor.
15. Relax your mind.
16. Re-check the tension areas of your eyes, tongue, back of your neck, belly, and breathing.
17. Now relax your entire body.
18. Let your body drop down, back, and into the floor.
19. Going beyond the words into the silence, into the oneness, quietly begin your mental meditation.
20. Know that relaxation is not the ending but the beginning…

When you come out of meditation, do not move too quickly. Move slowly and gently, and take a few minutes to come back to your normal self. Feel the effects on your body and mind. The effect of the 20-step relaxation/meditation technique is to produce a state of silence, peace, and a still point in the heart and mind.

Om Shanti, Shanti, Shanti,
  Om Peace, Peace, Peace
  Jean has provided the following heart affirmation that she believes will be helpful to those with heart disease.
  I Love My Heart Affirmation
  My heart lovingly carries joy throughout my body, nourishing the cells. Joyous new ideas are now circulating freely within me. I am the joy of life expressing and receiving. I now choose the thoughts that create an ever-joyous now. It is safe to be alive at every age. I radiate love in every direction, and my whole life is a joy. I love with my heart. I love and appreciate my beautiful heart! —Louise Hay

The benefits of Iyengar Yoga according to Jean Aronoff:

- Reduces disease-causing inflammation
- Increases lung capacity
- Enhances cardiovagal function
- Boosts beneficial HDL cholesterol
- Improves respiratory function and heart rate
- Lowers blood pressure
- Improves circulation and boosts muscle tone
- May decrease depressive symptoms associated with CV disease and heart failure

Commentary by Dr. Todd Cohen
Although I could not find scientific data to document conclusively all of the above reported benefits noted by "Yoga Jean," Table 42.1 documents established benefits listed at the National Institute of Health's National Center of Complementary and

Table 42.1 Yoga facts (according to the National Center for Complementary and Integrative Health)

Relieves stress and supports mental and emotional health.
Relieves lower back and neck pain.
Relieves symptoms of menopause.
Helps manage anxiety and depression.
Helps with smoking cessation and weight control.
Helps with sleep and balance.

Integrative Health. More concrete benefits could not be established as of yet because of the type and size of the trials that evaluated the benefits of Yoga.

Benefits of Yoga and Meditation

The following are real-life experiences of health care professionals, yoga teachers, yoga students, and cardiac patients who have practiced yoga and meditation throughout their lives. These are firsthand accounts of how yoga and meditation have changed and enhanced the lives of real people.

Lisa Bondy, Director of Yoga at the Center for Wellness and Integrative Medicine, Katz Institute for Women's Health at Northwell Health

I am a practicing yogi of 35 years and have been teaching for 20 years. As a practicing yogi, I have gained a deep personal understanding through my study and experience of the transformative and healing powers of yoga practices. These practices include *asana* (the practice of the postures), *pranayama* (the practice of breath work), and meditation (the practice of stilling the mind and senses), as well as lifestyle and diet. As a teacher, I have the privilege of sharing these powerful healing practices with people of all ages and conditions. The transformation I witness is across the board profound.

I am certified in Cardiac/Medical Yoga and have taught two sections of Medical/Chair Yoga weekly since 2016. I also teach the yoga portion of the Heart Healthy Program at the Center for Wellness and Integrative Medicine. This is a six-week program that educates people with heart disease about how to take the necessary steps to live healthy lives. The program is based on *Heart Smart for Women: Six S.T.E.P.S. in Six Weeks to Heart-Healthy Living*, by Stacey Rosen, MD, and Jennifer Mieres, MD. Each author has over 25 years of medical experience in the field of cardiology.

A yoga-based program can have preventative effects on heart disease as well as facilitate recovery from cardiac procedures. According to Ina Stephens, MD, RYT, C-IAYT, FAAP, who is an Associate Professor of Pediatrics and the Pediatric Infectious Diseases and Medical Education Director at University of Virginia's Pediatric Medical Yoga and Integrative Health, "Yogic practices, specifically Medical/Chair yoga for this population, interrupts different inflammatory events along this cascade."

Additionally, the Cardiac/Medical Chair-based yoga practice is often recommended to people with heart disease, as it makes yoga accessible to those who cannot stand steadily or lack the mobility to move easily. It is a gentle and modified form of yoga that provides assistance and aids in physical, mental, and emotional healing, rehabilitation, and prevention of disease. It helps with managing stress and in developing lifestyle choices that promote health and vitality physically, emotionally, and spiritually.

What I have seen from teaching individuals with heart disease after they graduate from cardiac rehabilitation programs is that, because of their trauma, they may experience both physical and emotional manifestations. They may have aches and pains or feel unsteady, which subsequently can affect their balance, coordination, and breathing. Some patients may feel frightened, alone, frustrated, and depressed. The yoga that I teach them has a profound effect in a relatively short time, usually in only one or two classes. Their aches and pains start to diminish, their coloring improves, they smile, talk more, and appear overall happier and more relaxed.

Many of these patients often begin feeling more like they used to after three months of attending a weekly class. With their fears greatly diminished and newly found senses of relaxation, they feel encouraged to make healthier lifestyle choices, practice gratitude and acceptance, and enjoy being alive. As their teacher, I feel inspired and grateful to know that the yoga that I have taught them has made a positive impact on their lives.

Netti Jonth, 93-year-old cardiac patient and yoga student
In response to the question "How has the practice of yoga affected my life," I would sum it up by saying "in a most positive way." I am 93 ½ years old and was introduced to yoga more than 30 years ago by a teacher friend. At that time, I was still working and attending a class once a week after school. It was held at the home of a lovely lady who was a retired nurse trained as a yoga instructor. I came to the class as a complete novice, knowing very little about yoga practice, and I was not a practitioner of exercise or even of any sports. I soon learned of the benefits of my weekly sessions. Yoga made me feel energized after a day's work teaching, yet at the same time, more relaxed and comfortable. Unfortunately, the yoga practice did not prevent me from having a heart attack in 1998, which was diagnosed as mild and congenital. I had elevated cholesterol, but I did not smoke and was not overweight; however, both of my parents and two siblings had heart-related medical histories and deaths.

After the heart attack, I received stents and made a quick and good recovery with the medications and my cardiologist's recommendation to attend St. Francis Hospital's cardiac rehabilitation program at the De Matteis Center. I took his advice and have been attending that exercise program three days a week ever since 1998. In addition, I've continued the yoga class and increased my attendance to twice a week after retirement. I am convinced that the yoga classes have helped me remain healthy at my age as well as given me great pleasure. The breathing skills, stretching, leg lifts, and balance practice help me feel more secure as I go about my daily routines. I hope I can continue to live independently and continue to practice yoga for a long time to come.

Agnes Dickson, RN (retired)

Yoga has been an integral part of my life for over 45 years. I believe that yoga benefits the mind, the body, and the soul. Regarding the physical benefits, I am 73 years old (soon to be 74) and can still touch my toes and stand on my head. Participating in a yoga class makes my mind feel significantly calmer and more focused.

The most significant aspect of yoga has been the strong and constant sense of community one derives from attending classes regularly. The bonds of friendship that I have formed have sustained and enriched my life in a myriad of ways. I've had a number of outstanding teachers throughout the years who have served as both guides through the process and mentors through life outside the classroom. They have encouraged my progress, helped to develop my skills, and kept me motivated throughout my journey. They have been essential to both my practice and my life. Each class is like an oasis in the hubbub of everyday life. Yoga class is like a mini-retreat and a blessing to be able to attend. I am grateful to be a part of the yoga community and to have it be such an important part of my life.

Mindfulness

43

Anu Raj

Cardiovascular Disease (CVD) continues to be the primary cause of human mortality. Factors such as obesity, blood pressure, substance use, diabetes, and a sedentary lifestyle are often associated with CVD risk. An integrated, comprehensive treatment approach includes medical and psychological intervention. In recent years, psychological interventions have attracted attention due to several factors: they are not medically invasive, they can be generalized to other aspects of lifestyle, and they target other underlying psychological ailments. Mindfulness-based psychological interventions have emerged as one such area of application for physiological pain and physical illnesses.

What is mindfulness? Mindfulness is described as "the awareness that emerges through paying attention, on purpose, in the present moment, nonjudgmentally to the unfolding of experience moment to moment." Meditation, as discussed in Chap. 42, can be thought of as a specific type of mindfulness. There is a link between mindfulness practice and heart disease. In particular, this practice helps with stress reduction as a means to reduce the risks of getting heart disease. It can also be a beneficial complement to other treatment modalities in those with heart disease. For more information on mindfulness, you can find an article in the bibliography of this book by looking for the term "mindfulness."

A. Raj (✉)
Department of Family Medicine, New York Institute of Technology College of Osteopathic Medicine, Old Westbury, NY, USA
e-mail: anu.raj@nyit.edu

Several practitioners propose a two-part approach to mindfulness. The first part involves attention to immediate experiences. These interventions improve self-regulation (understanding and managing the reactions to feelings) and give a sense of control. Sensations and thoughts are acknowledged without any corresponding action. In other words, mindfulness allows a person to remove themselves from their immediate thoughts, sensations, and emotions while still acknowledging them. This results in increased self-awareness. The second portion of this approach focuses on an appraisal of one's attention to the current experiences. In other words, approach current experiences through the lens of curiosity, acceptance, and non-judgment.

What is the purpose of assessing one's experience from a neutral stance? A neutral stance is nonjudgemental and therefore reduces any guilt or shaming that often accompanies lifestyle behaviors. For example, an obese person having a craving for ice cream might focus on the sensation of the craving, and pass judgment or blame themselves for their obesity. Removal of such judgment in mindfulness exercises reduces the chance of comorbidity of depression or anxiety. Mindfulness-based treatments focus on increasing self-reliance, as well as increasing one's sense of self-control. Being kind and compassionate to oneself increases self-confidence and increases one's ability to return to more challenging tasks in self-regulation.

Depression and anxiety tend to be comorbidities in CVD. Depression is often correlated with lack of self-control, expectation of poor health outcomes, and a sense of guilt associated with the CVD ailment. Mindfulness training targets the judgmental assessment and teaches self-forgiveness. Anxiety is often correlated with the expected negative outcome of CVD. Mindfulness addresses the immediate and current experiences without projecting into the future, which helps to reduce anxiety.

Let's take the case of a smoker with CVD. Mindfulness teaches the person to engage in focused attention on the bodily cravings for a smoke. If that person assesses their craving with curiosity instead of a need, then they might allow the sensation of craving to pass (remember, you can think it, you can feel it, but you cannot do it). Once it passes, the person may attend to the happy feeling and positive thoughts associated with not smoking (you notice feeling happy about not smoking in this instance). This increases self-satisfaction and self-control. The chance for that person to allow the subsequent craving to pass without actually smoking is higher.

Commentary by Dr. Todd Cohen

I have personally used mindfulness myself and in my practice. Fig. 43.1 shows a painting of my two children (Justin and Brittany) when they were young, created by my mother, Marilyn Vasen. The painting was a present from my mother, who always said, "the present is a present." So, visualize yourself being present in the present. I have used that line many times in my life and have used a mindfulness and meditation app called Buddhify, which can be downloaded to your smartphone (Apple- or Google-based). You can also explore it on your computer at www.buddhify.com. This is an inexpensive application, and in particular, one of the mindfulness exercises that I have used is called "RAIN." When you download the app, there is a rainbow-shaped wheel called what is happening. If you select "Stress and Difficult Emotion

Fig. 43.1 This is a figure that was a present from Dr. Cohen's mom to him. It illustrates Dr Cohen's son (Justin) and daughter (Brittany) when they were young. Dr Cohen's mom always said their presence is a present. This is the essence of mindfulness and being present. He always remembers the presence of the painting as being present in the moment and also as being a present

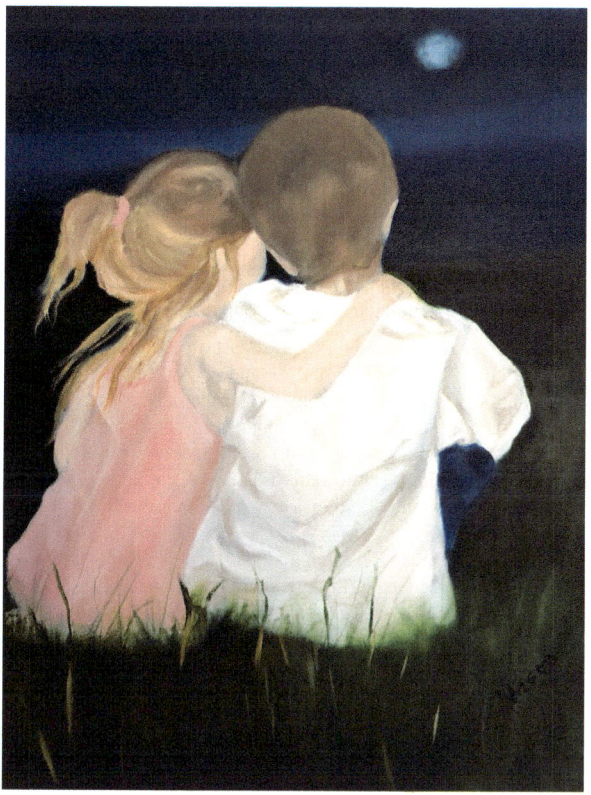

1" in orange from the wheel, you get the "Stress and Difficult Emotion 1" wheel with a myriad of choices. If you choose **RAIN**, there is a 12-minute, four-stage mindfulness. Meditation geared to creating space in the stress (or storm) of life.

The four stages are **R**ecognizing, **A**llowing, **I**nvestigating, and **N**onidentifying. The first stage is **"recognizing"** what is happening in your mind right now and giving it a name such as "fear" or "anxiety." This is "fear," this is "anxiety," recognizing it along with its physical sensations (tension, palpitations, etc.) and giving it a name. This is "tension," this is "palpitations." The second stage is **"allowing."** When experiencing a difficult emotion, one tends to push that experience away. Don't do that, rather allow and accept it. The third stage is **"investigating,"** noticing the experience and what is grabbing your present attention, and not pushing it away. Also, investigate what your body is presently experiencing. . The fourth and final stage is **"nonidentifying."** In this stage, relax your mind, and visualize the following: consider yourself as the sky, and what you are experiencing as a storm or clouds passing by. Just let this (stress or experience) pass as if it is a storm.

Remember to use all the tools that you can to improve your mental health and minimize stress. As my internist from the past (Dr. Burton Gillette) once said, "it is not what you are eating, it's what's eating you." Table 43.1 reviews the facts presented above and gives tips on using mindfulness to deal with life's stresses.

Table 43.1 Mindfulness facts

Mindfulness is the awareness that emerges from being present and experiencing the moment.
It is a multistage approach that brings attention to one's experiences and accepts them.
Remember Dr. Cohen's mom's statement: "the present is a present."
Remember Dr. Gillette's words of advice, "it's not what you're eating, it's what's eating you."
Use RAIN in the Buddhify App (www.buddhify.com) to help you deal with stress.
Use all the tools that you have available to help minimize stress and improve your mental health.

Children and Heart Disease

44

Thomas Chan

You don't think of kids having cardiac disease, and luckily for the most part they don't go together. This chapter will focus on some of the most common cardiac issues, some conditions that need to be thought about when suspected, and when to seek specialized help.

Cardiac disease in the young is a relatively rare occurrence, but since the heart and its function are so vital, it can be serious when it does happen. That being said, there are a few complaints that may be present and might bring a cardiac problem to light. First, Table 44.1 shows signs and symptoms that should be brought to your doctor's attention during infancy. If your baby or infant turns pale or blue, is not gaining appropriate weight, and seems to be "failing to thrive," you should seek medical attention. Additionally, if the baby has weak pulses, trouble breathing, or any form of distress, immediate medical attention should be sought. Finally, your doctor may hear a heart murmur (an unusual heart sound heard with a stethoscope) that may need further medical workup.

When a murmur is heard, it is important to distinguish whether the murmur is an innocent or functional murmur (a normal heart sound caused by rapid flow across a normal heart and valve) or a pathologic murmur (something as a result of a birth defect, or inherited or congenital heart defect such as a hole in the heart [septal defect], or valve disorder, see Chaps. 15 and 36). There are clinical features based

T. Chan (✉)
New York Institute of Technology College of Osteopathic Medicine, Old Westbury, NY, USA
e-mail: tchan02@nyit.edu

Table 44.1 Heart-related signs and symptoms in infants and young children	Pale or blue color skin changes Persistent poor weight gain or failure to thrive Weak pulses Trouble breathing or distress Cardiac murmur

Table 44.2 Heart-related signs and symptoms in older children	Chest pain Palpitations Syncope Cardiac murmur

on the quality of the heart sounds that may be useful in distinguishing the two (such as the type, grade, quality, duration, and harshness of the murmur). An echocardiogram, described in Chap. 18, is extremely helpful in distinguishing between the two. An innocent or functional murmur is very common in childhood and not clinically important. A pathologic or abnormal heart murmur may be of significance and will warrant clinical follow-up.

Table 44.2 shows a few examples of cardiac symptoms to be aware of as your baby becomes older. The appearance of a murmur should be investigated again with a noninvasive echocardiogram. Chest pain or discomfort are very infrequent complaints, but should also be evaluated. Heart rhythm problems are uncommon, but not rare, and may present with any of those symptoms and/or along with palpitations, lightheadedness or dizziness (presyncope), or complete loss of consciousness (syncope). In particular, the presence of an extra connection between the upper and lower chambers of the heart (a condition called Wolff-Parkinson-White syndrome) can be a cause of these problems in children. It is not uncommon for infants to have these conditions, but most extra or accessory pathways disappear as the child gets older. If not, and the child is symptomatic, they may need treatment with medications, or potentially a cardiac catheter ablation procedure (see Chap. 29).

Chest pain, palpitations, and syncope don't mean there is necessarily a heart problem, but as a general rule, if these symptoms are happening while the child is active, and especially during vigorous activities, this should be addressed. During physical activity, the heart will be working harder as it is under stress. If these issues (chest pain, palpitations, or syncope) occur during these times, it could be a cry for help and should be investigated.

Chest Pain

Chest pain in children (as opposed to in adults) is usually not related to the heart. Many of us think of chest pain always as a heart attack, in which your coronary vessels are blocked and starved of oxygen. Classic symptoms associated with heart attacks are crushing chest pain and chest pain that radiates to the left arm and jaw. While a pediatrician may still consider a coronary artery problem as the source of chest pain, after a thorough history, physical exam, and ECG, the origin of chest pain in children is very rarely determined to be from the heart. More commonly, the complaint is caused by muscle or bone pain from the chest wall, the lungs, or even the esophagus (such as gastroesophageal or acid reflux).

Costochondritis is a common musculoskeletal cause of chest pain. There is cartilage that connects the ribs to the sternum or chest bone. Childhood is often a very active time and a period of rapid growth. Due to this, the musculoskeletal system can be stretched, and tender points can ensue, which manifest as chest pain. The hallmark of this condition is that when pressing on the chest, at certain points or costochondral junctions (the sides of the sternum), you can reproduce the chest pain. This is a reassuring sign that points to the bones and cartilage as the likely origin, rather than the heart.

The lungs can also be the source of chest pain. We all know of a cough or difficulty breathing as lung issues, but due to its proximity to the heart and location in the chest, if there is an issue with the lungs, it can manifest as chest pain. This is why if your child is seen for chest pain, he or she is just as likely to get a chest X-ray as an ECG. Conditions such as pneumonia or an infection of the lung may be the culprit. Cough, difficulty breathing, and fever are also common symptoms of pneumonia. A chest X-ray will often diagnose pneumonia, but it can also be diagnosed with a good lung exam. Pneumonia itself is one of the most common causes of childhood chest pain. If you think of the lungs as two complex balloons (which, essentially, they are!), if that balloon pops a little or develops a small leak, it may manifest as chest pain. This is called a pneumothorax (collapsed lung) and may be associated with trouble breathing and can also be picked up on a chest X-ray.

We think of acid reflux (also called gastroesophageal reflux) as a condition that occurs when we get older, stressed, or keep a poor diet, and for the most part we are right. It is so common in middle age that you will be hard-pressed to find an adult who hasn't at least taken an antacid at some point. However, children can develop this as well. We all know babies spit up and overall outgrow this, but it will still occur on occasion. Children are overall resilient because the acid coming up is not a usual occurrence. The classic story will be about chest pain when lying or sitting down. It usually goes away on its own, and oftentimes you may even get the symptoms after eating, which helps to diagnose reflux as well. A simple antacid and some dietary changes will often help.

Syncope

Syncope, or passing out, is scary when it does happen. If this happens when you are exercising, as mentioned earlier, this needs to be looked at further. Luckily, most times syncope is due to common causes like not eating or not drinking enough. When the body is low on fluids or sugar, it can react poorly, in this case by passing out. This usually happens when one suddenly gets up from bed or stands from a sitting position. Most of us have had the sensation of getting up too fast, getting a little lightheaded, and needing to take a second or two to gather ourselves. When one is hungry or mildly dehydrated, we can pass out from this before our body can compensate and adjust. It can even happen when you have a strong emotional reaction or distress. We have all heard of people passing out at the sight of blood or a sudden surprise. This doesn't just happen on TV but in real life as well. Overall, these syncopal episodes are attributed to what we call vasovagal reactions, and all that is usually needed is reassurance that this is a normal reaction.

Long QT Syndrome

In Chap. 15, hereditary conditions such as long QT syndrome are discussed. In this condition, there typically is an inherited/genetic component that causes prolongation of the QT interval on the ECG. The condition may cause syncope or even sudden death from a fast heart rhythm called ventricular tachycardia or ventricular fibrillation. It is often picked up on an ECG and can be made worse with certain medications or external stimuli (depending on what type of long QT syndrome one has). Chapter 15 also discusses some of the medications to be avoided with this condition. Most patients can be treated with medications, such as beta-blockers, but some do require an implantable defibrillator to prevent sudden death.

Kawasaki Disease

Kawasaki disease has been historically well known to pediatricians due to its interesting constellation of findings, its mysterious origins, and its serious consequences (especially with regard to the heart). Recently, it has become known to the general public because of its seemingly similar relation to the new condition, COVID-19-related Multisystem Pediatric Inflammatory Syndrome, which we will discuss later. To this day, no one knows how or why Kawasaki disease develops nor is there a specific test for it. What we do know is that there is a specific constellation of findings that help to make the diagnosis (see Table 44.3). These findings include conjunctivitis, rashes, fever of more than five days duration, cracked lips, swollen hands and feet that peel, strawberry tongue, and lymph node enlargement (especially on one side of the neck). Interestingly, all the symptoms may eventually go away, but the negative effects on the heart can last a lifetime.

This disease attacks the heart's coronary vessels and can cause coronary aneurysms (dilation of the coronary arteries) and in turn change the heart's dynamics, which can lead to heart attacks. Luckily, intravenous immunoglobulin and aspirin, when given early, are both effective in preventing future heart attacks. Multisystemic

Table 44.3 Kawasaki disease signs and symptoms

Conjunctivitis
Rash
Fever—prolonged more than 5 days
Cracked lips
Swollen hands and feet that progress to peeling
Strawberry tongue
Lymph node enlargement, especially on one side of the neck

inflammatory syndrome is a condition similar to Kawasaki disease and toxic shock-like syndrome that has been identified in children who have COVID-19. These patients develop very similar symptoms as in Table 44.3 and may have failure to thrive, tachycardia, altered color, chest pain, lethargy, and confusion. As of July 2025, 963 children in New York State have been identified with this condition, and they are typically treated with anti-inflammatory medications and supportive care in the pediatric ICU.

Rheumatic Fever

Rheumatic fever typically affects children from age 5 to 15 years. It is an autoimmune disorder that is caused by a streptococcal infection (a common bacterial infection that causes a sore throat, though rheumatic fever itself is uncommon). The best way to prevent it is prompt treatment of a strep throat infection with antibiotics. Symptoms include a rash (and nodules under the skin), fever, joint and chest pains, and palpitations. People who have had rheumatic fever are at risk of developing severe valve dysfunction later on in life that may need treatment.

Commotio Cordis

Commotio cordis is a condition that is typically caused by an object hitting the chest wall and compressing the heart during the vulnerable cycle of the heart. It can be triggered by being hit by a projectile object like a baseball, lacrosse ball, or hockey puck and can trigger ventricular fibrillation and potentially cause sudden cardiac arrest and sudden death. The only treatment for commotio cordis is CPR and early defibrillation. It is important to have automatic external defibrillators (AEDs) at sporting events for athletes of all ages in order to treat this deadly disease. Recently, in 2023, professional football player Damar Hamlin of the Buffalo Bills was struck directly in the chest by a tackle from an opposing team player, and immediately collapsed on the field, unresponsive with no pulse. The nation froze in collective shock as medical personnel immediately rushed to the scene. They began performing cardiopulmonary resuscitation and used an AED to restore his pulse, ultimately bringing him back to life. This was a real-life example of commotio cordis that demonstrated the lifesaving effects of AEDs.

Children and Atherosclerosis

My mom would always tell me, "Don't worry about eating that, you are young," as she would encourage me to not trim off the fat on the steak or some other fatty piece of meat. In the end, she was right and also wrong. She is right in that fats are much more complex than we thought back then, and some fats are not all bad or artery-clogging. She was wrong in that eating the wrong kinds of fats during your lifetime can lead to heart disease, and kids can start showing evidence of negative cardiovascular changes to their blood vessels (the early stages of atherosclerosis). In the end, moderation is the key even at a young age. Good habits started at a young age will help to keep the body, its organs, and blood vessels in optimal shape.

Connective Tissue Disorders and Autoimmune Diseases

45

Bernadette Riley

Heart disease affects special populations in different ways. Some examples are those who have connective tissue disorders and autoimmune diseases. Connective tissue is made up of two proteins, collagen and elastin, and they are responsible for holding the structures of the body together- including blood vessels and structures like heart valves. Connective tissue disorders are autoimmune rheumatic disorders that can affect the elasticity in the joints and cause pain. They can fall into two different categories: those that are genetic (inherited) and those that are acquired. The genetic variety is believed to include conditions such as Marfan syndrome, Ehlers-Danlos syndrome (EDS), and Hypermobility Spectrum Disorder (HSD). Acquired varieties may be related to vitamin deficiencies such as scurvy, and rheumatologic disorders such as systemic lupus erythematosus, rheumatoid arthritis, mixed connective tissue disorder, and Sjögren's syndrome, to name a few (see Table 45.1).

The first category consists of inherited conditions. Marfan syndrome is a connective tissue disorder involving a genetic mutation in the gene responsible for making fibrillin-1, an important component of elastic tissue. Abraham Lincoln was believed to have this condition. These patients are typically slender, with tall arms, legs, and fingers; flat feet; curved spine (scoliosis); and carved-out chest (pectus carinatum) or carved-in chest (pectus excavatum), a tall, arched palate; nearsighted; and a weakened aorta (prone to a leaky aortic valve and aortic aneurysms). Hypermobility of the joints is also a feature of Marfan syndrome.

B. Riley (✉)
Department of Family Medicine, New York Institute of Technology College of Osteopathic Medicine, Old Westbury, NY, USA
e-mail: briley@nyit.edu

© The Author(s), under exclusive license to Springer Nature Switzerland AG 2025
T. J. Cohen, R. S. Blumenthal (eds.), *Surviving and Thriving With Heart Disease*,
Contemporary Cardiology, https://doi.org/10.1007/978-3-032-00579-3_45

275

Table 45.1 Connective tissue disorders and their cardiac manifestations

Genetic

  Marfan's syndrome: Aortic aneurysm, aortic regurgitation, valvular disease, coronary artery disease, mitral valve prolapse, POTS, tachyarrhythmia

  Ehlers-Danlos syndrome (EDS): Mitral valve prolapse, aortic root dilation, POTS, tachyarrhythmia

  Hypermobility Spectrum Disorder (HSD): POTS, tachyarrhythmia

Acquired

  Scurvy: Blood vessel fragility, anemia, hypotension, cardiac enlargement

  Systemic Lupus Erythematosus: Accelerated atherosclerosis, dilated cardiomyopathy, myocardial fibrosis, heart failure

  Rheumatoid Arthritis: Heart failure, dilated cardiomyopathy, mitral valve regurgitation, conduction disease, pericarditis

  Mixed Connective Tissue Disorder: Pericarditis, mitral valve regurgitation, conduction disease, accelerated atherosclerosis

  Sjogren's Syndrome: Accelerated atherosclerosis, pulmonary hypertension, valvular regurgitation, pericarditis

These patients are often detected during a history and physical examination which identifies the characteristic body habitus (legs, arms, toes, and fingers disproportionately longer than the rest of the body; arm span divided by height of 1.03 or more; spider-like fingers called arachnodactyly; chest wall that caves in (pectus excavatum); high arched palate; and joint laxity) and/or picks up a cardiac murmur on auscultation consistent with mitral valve prolapse (a midsystolic click), mitral regurgitation (a holosystolic murmur), and/or aortic regurgitation (a diastolic decrescendo murmur). If any of the latter murmurs are present, an echocardiogram can be useful for identifying valve and aorta abnormalities.

If mild aortic valve disease or aortic root abnormalities are identified, they can be followed and managed with echocardiographic surveillance (echocardiogram every six months) and medications such as beta blockers. If more severe disease is identified or develops, heart surgery may be required (aortic valve replacement, aortic arch repair/replacement, potentially with a graft, and possibly reimplantation of their coronary arteries; also called the Bentall Procedure, which includes graft, valve replacement, and coronary artery reimplantation).

EDS is another inherited connective tissue disorder in which there is extreme skin and joint laxity and hypermobility, which is a common patient complaint. The skin may be very thin and bruise easily. Out of the 13 subtypes, hypermobile EDS (hEDS) currently does not have a genetic mutation associated with it, but is based on a strict clinical criteria checklist. Hypermobile joints are seen in most of the other EDS subtypes, as well as Marfan syndrome, and are required for a diagnosis of hEDS. Figure 45.1 shows a patient with increased hypermobility. Both EDS and Marfan syndrome can have mitral valve prolapse and aortic root weakening. The latter may place these patients at risk for aortic root dilatation and rupture. Patients who do not meet the strict clinical criteria for hEDS but have signs or comorbid conditions that affect them may have HSD.

These conditions can have cardiac manifestations, including palpitations, lightheadedness and dizziness (presyncope), and passing out (syncope). One common abnormality found in those with EDS and HSD is postural tachycardia syndrome

Fig. 45.1 A hypermobile patient demonstrating increased laxity of the joints

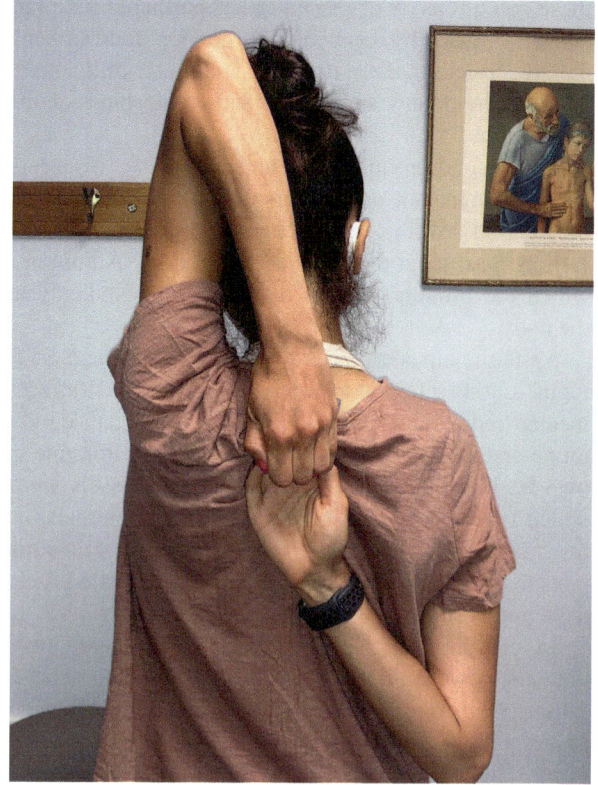

(POTS). POTS is defined as a heart rate increase of at least 30 beats per minute (bpm) or an increase to a rate higher than 120 bpm within the first 10 minutes of standing, in the absence of orthostatic hypotension. Sometimes these patients might also drop their blood pressure and present with lightheadedness and dizziness (presyncope) or even lose consciousness (syncope; see Chap. 10).

When EDS and HSD patients experience palpitations and syncope that are not postural in nature, or the mechanism of their presyncope and/or syncope remains unclear, they may benefit from short- and/or long-term ECG monitoring (sometimes with an implantable loop recorder). The latter is particularly useful for infrequent bouts of recurrent, unexplained syncope and can be implanted for over four years. Based on their clinical presentation, as well as the results of cardiac monitoring, a small percentage may benefit from electrophysiology testing (see Chap. 21), and catheter ablation if a focal arrhythmia source or extra pathway is identified (see Chap. 29).

Two cardiac conditions that could be seen in EDS are aortic root dilatation and mitral valve prolapse, both of which are diagnosed with echocardiograms. Some subtypes of EDS and Marfan syndrome are at greater risk for aortic root dilatation and rupture. Those types, such as vascular EDS, should be monitored closely by cardiac specialists.

It is important for specialized connective tissue treatment centers (such as the EDS/Hypermobility Treatment Center at NYIT) to partner with a local expert on these conditions. NYIT's center has partnered with the Long Island Heart Rhythm Center (directed by this book's author, Dr. Todd Cohen) in order to provide state-of-the-art services to these patients. The center utilizes a multidisciplinary approach to address the many symptoms and comorbid conditions seen in these special populations.

The second grouping of connective tissue disorders consists of acquired disorders, which include autoimmune diseases such as systemic lupus erythematosus and rheumatoid arthritis, mixed connective tissue disorder, and Sjögren's syndrome, as well as nutritional deficiencies like scurvy. Autoimmune disease is a condition in which the immune system of the body mistakenly attacks, rather than protects, the body.

Systemic lupus erythematosus, or SLE, is the most frequently diagnosed form of lupus. Lupus refers to a variety of diseases that affect the skin, and erythematosus means "reddening," because the disease can cause red skin lesions. It is an autoimmune disease, which means that the body's immune system mistakenly attacks its own healthy tissue. The heart and blood vessels are commonly involved in SLE, which may manifest as accelerated atherosclerosis, myocardial fibrosis, and even heart failure. Atherosclerosis (fat and plaque deposition within arterial walls) happens faster in patients with SLE and is associated with an increased risk of cardiac ischemic events.

Myocardial fibrosis, or scarring of the heart, may also be observed in these patients; however, it doesn't reflect the duration or severity of the disease. The heart muscle walls may become stiff and unable to fill or pump effectively. In advanced cases, patients may develop dilated cardiomyopathy, and heart failure may also occur. The cardiac pathology in SLE may be the result of the systemic inflammation of the disease plus the synergistic effects of traditional risk factors such as diabetes, hypertension, or hyperlipidemia.

Rheumatoid arthritis (RA) is similar to SLE in that it is an autoimmune disease, but the former primarily affects the joints. It is characterized by morning stiffness, arthralgias, and arthritis. It is believed that inflammatory and prothrombotic (clot-forming) processes contribute to cardiovascular disease, which is the third leading cause of death in RA patients. Heart disease may include dilated cardiomyopathy, mitral regurgitation, heart failure, conduction disease, and pericarditis. This autoimmune disease can also cause vasculitis (inflammation of blood vessels) with the deposition of granulomas on the pericardium, myocardium (muscle wall), heart valves, coronary arteries, aorta, and/or the conduction system (which are distinct to RA). Atrial fibrillation and other conduction disturbances and arrhythmias may result.

Patients with mixed connective tissue disease have coexisting features of SLE, RA, scleroderma (hardening of the skin and connective tissues), and/or polymyositis (chronic inflammation of the muscles). This hybrid disorder can have cardiac manifestations similar to the previously mentioned autoimmune disorders, but the incidence of primary cardiac involvement is less. In this condition, high pressures can occur on the right side of the heart (the result of pulmonary hypertension caused by pulmonary fibrosis), which can eventually lead to cor pulmonale (right-sided heart failure) if left untreated. Occasionally, mitral valve prolapse is reported.

In addition, inflammation involving the sac around the heart can occur (pericarditis), often associated with fluid buildup inside the sac (pericardial effusion), and pericardial thickening is common. Rarely, fluid can build up inside the pericardium such that blood flow out of the heart is impaired. This is called cardiac tamponade and may be associated with a drop in blood pressure and hemodynamic collapse. When this occurs, fluid needs to be drained from the pericardium immediately, either with a needle (pericardiocentesis) or a surgical procedure (pericardial window).

Sjögren's syndrome is an autoimmune disorder of unknown etiology characterized primarily by dysfunction of white blood cells, causing them to target the salivary and lacrimal glands. It is believed to be precipitated by genetic susceptibility paired with a bacterial or viral infection. Extraglandular disease could involve the heart when this syndrome is associated with SLE or RA, though the mechanism is not well understood. Sjögren's patients (without overt heart disease) experience valvular regurgitation, pericardial effusion, pulmonary hypertension, and increased left ventricular mass index at a higher frequency when compared to age-matched controls.

Finally, scurvy is unique from the previous conditions in that it is characterized as a nutritional deficiency of vitamin C. Vitamin C, or ascorbic acid, is a water-soluble vitamin critical for normal collagen synthesis. The blood vessels become fragile when levels are insufficient, leading to the clinical presentation of cutaneous lesions and rashes. Signs of deficiency typically appear after one to three months and may overlap with the previously mentioned rheumatologic and autoimmune diseases. Anemia is present in 75 percent of cases and can cause heart failure due to the high-output state. Hypotension may also occur because the vessels are unable to vasoconstrict due to their fragility. Other cardiac complications include enlargement, hemopericardium, and sudden death.

It is evident that these connective tissue disorders and autoimmune diseases are related to a wide spectrum of cardiac manifestations. Although the etiology and pathogenesis of many of these diseases aren't completely understood, it is important for patients to be managed by both a rheumatologist and a cardiologist to receive comprehensive care and optimize symptom management.

Part VII
Being Proactive

Being proactive is being in the driver's seat of your own heart health. It means a heart-healthy diet, regular exercise, and stress reduction. It also means knowing your numbers: heart rate, blood pressure, cholesterol (LDL, HDL, and triglycerides), weight/BMI, blood glucose and A1C, and your ejection fraction (EF). The "Surviving and Thriving" card provided in Appendix J gives you a mechanism to "Know Your Numbers" and have a "Plan B." On the "Plan B" side, you should write your essential medical information such as medications, allergies, implantable devices, healthcare proxy, etc. (remember to attach a copy of your most recent ECG; also see Chap. 52: Defensive Patienting). The "Know Your Numbers" side is for you to track your heart rate, blood pressure, weight/BMI, fasting blood glucose, HbA1c, and ejection fraction.

Keep your "Surviving and Thriving" card in your wallet with your other important cards—your driver's license, credit cards, and health insurance card. This is an important personal medical information document that is also used as a tracking and reminder tool, and it can be photographed with your smartphone and stored there for easy access (with privacy protection, of course). Either cut out the card from the book, photocopy or scan it, or download and print out the card from www.liheart-rhythmcenter.com (click the "Create Your Surviving and Thriving Card"). And then fill in both sides! You can update it as many times as you want. The trick is not only *knowing* your numbers but *using* them as targets toward your ideal blood pressure, cholesterol, weight/BMI, blood glucose/HbA1c, and ejection fraction.

In this final part of the book, my goal is to get you to be proactive about your heart health. These chapters contain ideas and strategies to help you take charge of your own heart health. We also talk about robotics, learning CPR (cardiopulmonary resuscitation), support groups, defensive patienting, supplements, and racial and ethnic disparities in health care. We all need to be aware of all the factors that come into play in managing our own heart health. So just do it!

Preventing Heart Disease

46

Todd J. Cohen

An old adage says, "An ounce of prevention is worth a pound of cure." That means, it is best to head off heart disease by "good clean living." But what is meant by the term —*good clean living*? It entails eating a well-balanced diet rich in fruits and vegetables, limiting excess fatty or fried foods, reducing red meat and alcohol consumption, not smoking, avoiding substance abuse, and staying well-hydrated. Following these lifestyle pillars can help you lead a healthy life. Combine that balanced diet with regular exercise, relaxation, and a good night's sleep, and you have charted a good course.

Of course, it is best to prevent heart disease before it even happens. It is important to realize that the buildup of plaque within the coronary arteries begins in childhood and is a lifelong process. If you have a family history of heart disease (especially heart disease before the age of 50 years), it is especially important that you do whatever you can to keep your heart healthy. If your mother or father had a heart attack before age 50, you should definitely check your cardiac risk factors (blood pressure, cholesterol, glucose, weight or BMI, and smoking history), and if they are abnormal, you and your healthcare provider will need to intervene to get those risk factors under control.

The pillars of eating right, exercising regularly, and minimizing your stress cannot be overstated. This book provides a means for you to understand heart disease, the tests necessary to diagnose it, monitor it, and the treatments necessary to get it under control. But even more importantly, the book gives you some unique tools to help you relax (yoga, meditation, and other forms of mindfulness) and exposes you to smartphone Apps that may be useful to track your progress and fitness, and even

T. J. Cohen (✉)
NYIT College of Osteopathic Medicine, New York, NY, USA
e-mail: tcohen03@nyit.edu

© The Author(s), under exclusive license to Springer Nature Switzerland AG 2025
T. J. Cohen, R. S. Blumenthal (eds.), *Surviving and Thriving With Heart Disease*,
Contemporary Cardiology, https://doi.org/10.1007/978-3-032-00579-3_46

Table 46.1 Preventing heart disease

Remember the old adage: "An ounce of prevention is worth a pound of cure!"
Remember the three pillars: eat right, exercise regularly, and minimize stress!
Use every tool in this book, including all the information contained in the lifestyle modification chapters, mindfulness, yoga, and use Apps to maximize heart disease prevention.

explores wearable as well as implantable technology. Written in the post-pandemic era, the book gives heart disease patients and their families every tool to make their lives more meaningful to thrive with their disorder. For more information, see Chaps. 38, 39, 40, 41, and 42, or the entire book for that matter. Table 46.1 provides some takeaway points from this brief chapter.

Cardiopulmonary Resuscitation and the Automatic External Defibrillator

47

Todd J. Cohen

Cardiopulmonary resuscitation (CPR) is a method of resuscitating an unconscious person who has no significant blood pressure or who has inadequate circulation by providing chest compressions and ventilation (breaths delivered to the person's airway). It is important to understand that to learn CPR, especially for a layperson, it is essential to take a course in Basic Life Support from a certified instructor (typically offered by the American Red Cross or the American Heart Association). By definition, a person who does not have a palpable pulse has inadequate circulation. When someone collapses from any cause and is not breathing and has no palpable pulse, CPR must be initiated *immediately* and *effectively* if the person is going to have any chance for survival. By alternately compressing the chest over the lower part of the person's chest bone (called the *sternum*) and then allowing it to relax, it is possible to help circulate blood throughout the body. In addition, by providing mouth-to-mouth ventilation to the person, you support the breathing, or pulmonary, component of *cardiopulmonary* resuscitation. In general, 30 chest compressions are given, followed by two breaths, and this sequence is repeated until a defibrillator arrives at the scene.

Most cases of sudden cardiac arrest are caused by ventricular tachycardia or ventricular fibrillation, which almost always require prompt defibrillation to achieve a good outcome and a successful resuscitation. CPR courses are available through local hospitals, support groups such as the Sudden Cardiac Arrest Association, and organizations such as the American Heart Association and the American Red Cross (see Chap. 51). These courses now teach the "C-A-B" of CPR. The C stands for *C*hest compression first, followed by opening the *A*irway, and last but not least *B*reathing. A CPR certification card is given to participants when they complete the course.

T. J. Cohen (✉)
NYIT College of Osteopathic Medicine, New York, NY, USA
e-mail: tcohen03@nyit.edu

© The Author(s), under exclusive license to Springer Nature Switzerland AG 2025
T. J. Cohen, R. S. Blumenthal (eds.), *Surviving and Thriving With Heart Disease*,
Contemporary Cardiology, https://doi.org/10.1007/978-3-032-00579-3_47

The first step in performing CPR is to determine whether the person is unconscious (does not respond to shouting or tapping and is not breathing) as detailed in Fig. 47.1. If so, this is an emergency, and it is imperative to call for help (911). CPR should be initiated on a flat surface (*CIRCULATION*) as follows. The operator should kneel on the side of the unconscious person, and their hands should be positioned over the center of the chest bone with elbows locked. The compressions are performed with the heel of one hand on the chest, and the other hand on top of that one. Strong and effective chest compressions are essential to help provide oxygen and blood flow throughout the body. Each compression should be to a depth of at least 2 inches; after compression, the chest should passively relax and expand back to baseline, and the process should be repeated for a total of 30 compressions, at a rate of 100 to 120 beats per minute.

Performing chest compressions to the rhythm of the refrain of the Bee Gees' song "Stayin' Alive" (from the movie *Saturday Night Fever*) is useful for approximating this rate. Remember: "Ah, ha, ha, ha, stayin' alive, stayin' alive" (repeat, repeat, repeat). Note: circulation can be assessed by checking the unconscious

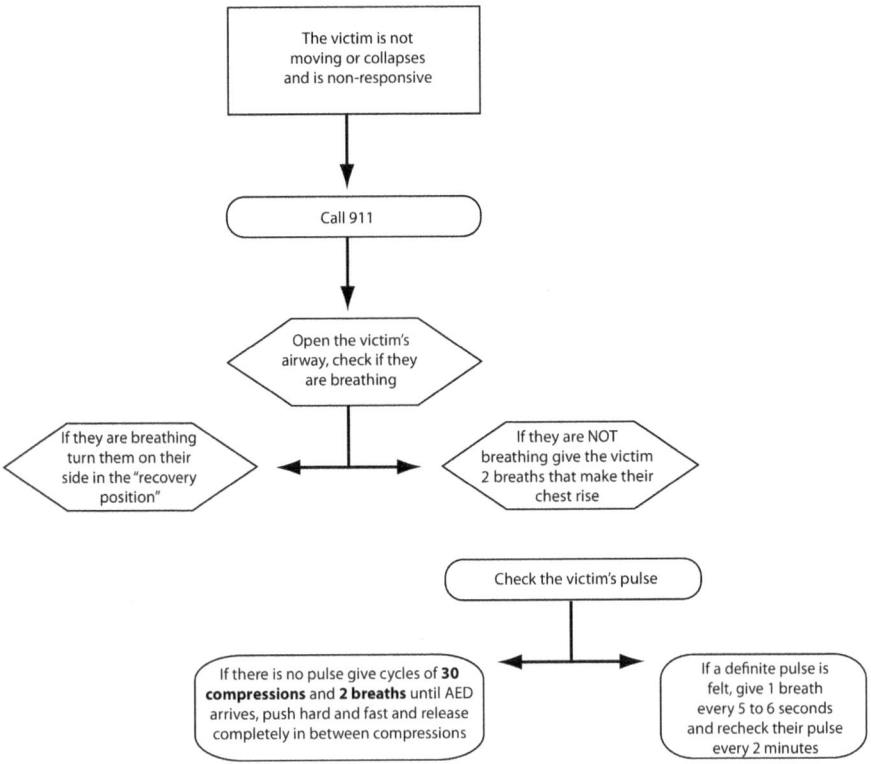

Fig. 47.1 The proper protocol when dealing with an unconscious person and the initiation of CPR. (Adapted from T.J. Cohen, *A Patient's Guide to Heart Rhythm Problems* (Baltimore, MD: The Johns Hopkins University Press, 2010), p. 157)

person's pulse, either at the neck level, where the carotid pulsation can be felt, or at the wrist, where the radial pulse may be felt. Note that checking for a pulse can be unreliable.

The *AIRWAY* should be open and not obstructed (CPR teaches the operator to open up an obstructed airway using a head tilt-chin lift method; i.e., the head is tilted backward and the chin is lifted upward). The *airway* can be assessed immediately by listening and feeling for breathing from the person's nose and mouth. Also, look to see if the chest is rising and falling from respiration. After 30 chest compressions, if the person is not breathing, two breaths should be given *(BREATHING)*. Each breath should be given in pairs of two, each lasting 2 seconds in duration. Periodically, a breathing check should be performed to determine whether the person has recovered and has started to breathe again. This check should be performed quickly and for no more than 10 seconds. The 30–2 chest compression-breathing sequence should be repeated until an automatic external defibrillator arrives. If the pulse recovers and the person is still not breathing, give one breath every 5 to 6 seconds.

It is important to practice the techniques of CPR periodically to retain the appropriate skills. Recertification in CPR (Basic Life Support) is required every 2 years to maintain certification. Important information about performing CPR on adults, children, and infants is provided in Table 47.1.

How to perform appropriate CPR is demonstrated in Figs. 47.2 and 47.3. During chest compression (Fig. 47.2), air is pressed out of the lungs, and blood is expelled

Table 47.1 How CPR should be performed on adults, children, and infants

First, call 911.			
Maneuver	Adult (older than 8 years)	Child (1 to 8 years)	Infant (under 1 year)
How to open airway	Head tilt, chin lift	Head tilt, chin lift	Head tilt, chin lift
How often to breathe mouth to mouth	2 breaths at 2 seconds	2 breaths at 2 seconds (make chest rise)	Two breaths at 2 seconds (make chest rise)
Where to check pulse	Carotid (neck) or radial (wrist)	Brachial (arm) or femoral (groin)	Brachial (arm) or femoral (groin)
Where to do compressions	Lower half of sternum, between nipples	Lower half of sternum, between nipples	Just below nipple line
How to do compressions	Push hard and fast with heel of one hand, with other hand on top	Push hard and fast with heel of one hand, possibly with second hand on top	Push hard and fast with two fingers
How deeply to compress	1.5 to 2 inches	Approx. 1/3 to 1/2 the depth of the chest	Approx. 1/3 to 1/2 the depth of the chest
How fast to compress	Approx. 100 compressions per minute	Approx. 100 compressions per minute	Approx. 100 compressions per minute

Source: Derived from 2020 American Heart Association. Guidelines for Cardiopulmonary Resuscitation and Emergency Cardiovascular Care. Circulation. 2020;142(supplement 2): S337–S357

Fig. 47.2 The compression phase, or active phase, of CPR. Compressions are administered over the chest bone. (Adapted from T.J. Cohen, *A Patient's Guide to Heart Rhythm Problems* (Baltimore, MD: The Johns Hopkins University Press, 2010), p. 158)

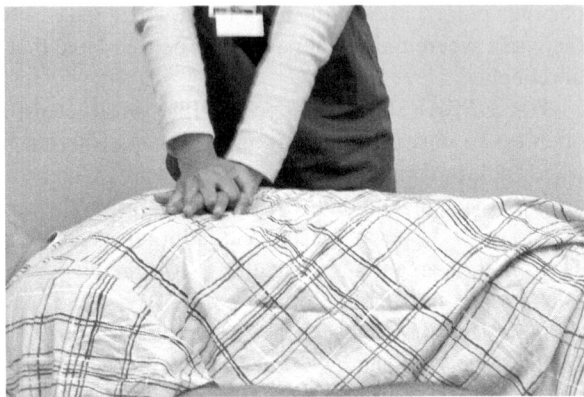

Fig. 47.3 The passive relaxation phase of CPR, which follows an active compression administered to the chest. (Adapted from T.J. Cohen, *A Patient's Guide to Heart Rhythm Problems* (Baltimore, MD: The Johns Hopkins University Press, 2010), p. 159)

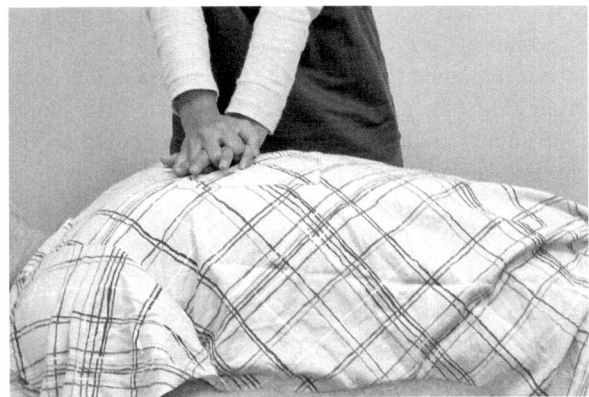

from the heart to the rest of the body. The passive relaxation phase of CPR (Fig. 47.3) follows the compression phase. During the passive relaxation phase, the chest passively expands, which helps the lungs to fill with air and the heart to fill with blood.

Automatic External Defibrillator (AED)

An automatic external defibrillator (AED) is a self-guided electronic device, usually the size of a lunch box, that is used to shock a person out of ventricular tachycardia or ventricular fibrillation. Skin patches are connected to the chest and hooked into the AED. An illustration is typically provided in the AED kit to demonstrate where the patches should be placed on the chest. The AED aurally guides you through the usage of the system, telling you how to detect the heart rhythm abnormality and how to deliver a shock.

AEDs are often successful in treating life-threatening arrhythmias like ventricular tachycardia and ventricular fibrillation. AEDs are available in many public areas, such as airports, schools, supermarkets, and sports arenas.

Mechanical Devices that Help with CPR (Alternatives to Standard CPR)

If you see a mechanical or handheld device resembling a toilet plunger, you should note that this device (coinvented by the author of this book) actively expands the chest and assists with blood returning to the heart as well as the breathing process (a technique called active compression-decompression CPR). The device took many years to develop and is currently approved for use in the United States and abroad. Figure 47.4 shows one version of a handheld CPR device, called the ResQPUMP, which is approved together with the ResQ Pod, in order to help resuscitate patients (manufactured by Zoll Medical Corp., Chelmsford, MA). A mechanical version of this device, the Lukas 3 CPR device, can automatically provide this enhanced CPR (manufactured by Physio-Control, Redmond, WA; a Division of Stryker Corporation, Kalamazoo, MI).

Fig. 47.4   The ResQ Pump ACD CPR device coinvented by the author of this book. The device, used together with the ResQ Pod, can augment CPR and is approved by the FDA and used clinically. (Reproduced with permission from HMP Communications LLC from Practical Electrophysiology, Third Edition)

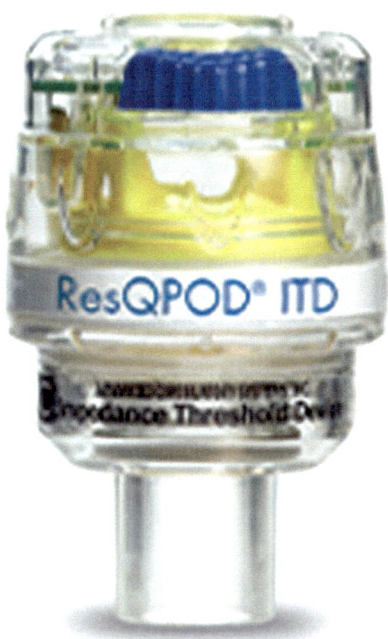

Who Should Learn CPR and Learn How to Use an AED?

Everyone! Particularly, anyone who is at risk for heart rhythm problems or sudden cardiac arrest, or who knows someone who is at risk for any of these problems, should learn CPR and how to use an AED. People overseeing large areas where people congregate, such as shopping malls, supermarkets, government centers, large businesses, arenas and stadiums, churches, temples, bus and train stations, airports, and any other means of mass transportation, as well as at competitive sporting events at any level, should learn CPR and how to use an AED. A person surviving a sudden cardiac arrest in the community relies on the willingness and ability of a bystander to effectively perform CPR and properly use a defibrillator. Time is of the essence when performing these life-saving measures.

Patient Follow-Up: Remote Monitoring and Telemedicine

48

Terri Seppala and Todd J. Cohen

This book emphasizes how important it is for you to establish an open and honest dialogue with your physician. Let your doctor know how you are feeling, and tell your doctor about any symptoms you may be experiencing. If it is your first visit to your heart doctor's office, he or she will complete a history, perform a physical examination, and do an ECG. That is, of course, if you are able to see your doctor in person. During the 2020 COVID-19 pandemic, emergency provisions were put in place to provide for new and old patient visits via the computer or smartphone (i.e., virtually) in order to provide safe and uninterrupted medical care. This is called telehealth and will be discussed by our expert, Terri Seppala, below.

Following an in-person or telehealth visit, routine blood work and other diagnostic tests may be ordered, depending on your symptoms. Your physician will also review any current medications that you are taking, including over-the-counter drugs and supplements. Keep a current list of all your medications and the dosages you take in your wallet at all times. You might also carry a copy of a recent ECG wherever you go, because this document may help guide medical care should you develop cardiac symptoms. The "Surviving and Thriving" card included with this book provides you with a good means to record important medical information and track your important health-related numbers. You can learn more about this card throughout this book (see Chap. 52), and get your card in Appendix J or create your

---

Terri Seppala has died before the publication of this book.

T. Seppala
CEO and President of Telehealth Associates, East Setauket, NY, USA

T. J. Cohen (✉)
NYIT College of Osteopathic Medicine, New York, NY, USA
e-mail: tcohen03@nyit.edu

© The Author(s), under exclusive license to Springer Nature Switzerland AG 2025
T. J. Cohen, R. S. Blumenthal (eds.), *Surviving and Thriving With Heart Disease*,
Contemporary Cardiology, https://doi.org/10.1007/978-3-032-00579-3_48

card using the "Create My Surviving and Thriving Card" button at https://www.liheartrhythmcenter.com.

Medical follow-up with your doctor is essential. If you have a heart condition or are at risk of a heart problem, getting good care and advice is essential. A referral from a local and trusted doctor is often useful. Search the Web and see what information is available about doctors you are considering (including whether they provide telehealth services). Investigate their background, education, and professional experiences. Doing a good background check can help determine which provider is a good choice for you. Once you meet the doctor (in person or virtually), think about whether he or she satisfies your objectives regarding your health, respects your healthcare decisions, and takes the time to answer your questions. Answering your questions is important, but if he or she is busy, don't be turned off.

A busy doctor and practice may be a sign of the physician's success. You should also engage the nursing staff in conversation and get to know them because nurses are often the first point of contact for patients. Some busy practices employ allied professionals such as nurse practitioners and physician assistants who may also be useful in providing your care, relaying information to your physician, and renewing prescriptions.

Doctors follow up with patients with heart rhythm disease in several ways. If you are taking medications, you will need to see your physician routinely. As discussed in Chap. 25, many drugs have side effects that can be serious, and many drugs can potentially interact adversely with other medications. Tell your doctor whether the medication is improving your symptoms or making them worse. Discuss with your doctor any supplements you add to your diet, such as fish oil, vitamins, garlic, red yeast rice, and herbal supplements.

Remote Monitoring of Implantable Devices

Patients with implantable devices previously needed to be seen in person in their doctor's office. Now, however, advances in technology make it possible for patients to have their devices checked remotely, by means of a cellular service (or some other type of communication). The communication may interface with your smartphone or some other means of wireless communication. If you have a device, it is possible to follow up through a remote monitoring service available through the device manufacturer, a third party, or your doctor's office. Web-based systems that provide home-based remote monitoring include Biotronik's Home Monitoring, Boston Scientific's Latitude, Medtronic's CareLink, and Abbott's Merlin. These systems will still need to be overseen by one of the services listed above.

To take advantage of the flexibility of this system, you must know how to set up your monitor and how to send a transmission. Some devices and systems have a bedside monitor that will allow you to send information when you feel or detect something is not right. This monitor might regularly sweep information from your implantable device, but you must be near it (bedside or in close proximity to this device) for this to occur. The monitoring system may include a wand that is placed over your device, which transmits the reading to your doctor, or it might communicate wirelessly using a technology such as Bluetooth, in order to collect the information from the device and send it to a smartphone which then transmits information through a cellular service to a cloud based remote monitoring system. This permits almost real-time detection of heart rhythm problems and allows you, as the patient, to send alerts to your doctor. For heart failure patients, almost all implantable defibrillators and heart failure treatment devices (biventricular devices) have an impedance-based measuring system built into the device in order to detect fluid accumulation. The basis of these systems was developed by the author of this book, and the first iteration appeared in the Medtronic defibrillator line of products and is called Optivol™. Other devices, such as Abbott's pacemaker/defibrillators, have implemented similar systems with a different name called CorVue™.

Boston Scientific uses a system called HeartLogic™ that incorporates transthoracic impedance sensing with other variables (such as heart sounds, activity, respiration, and nighttime heart rate). Remote monitoring of heart failure may employ a scale (Boston Scientific's Latitude™ NXT Remote Patient Monitoring System includes this), pulse oximeter, and blood pressure cuff. This information can be collected wirelessly, and the information can be sent to a cloud-based monitoring system. The Center for Medicare Systems provides for the reimbursement of remote physiologic monitoring of fluid accumulation every 31 days. The doctor, of course, can examine these values more frequently, if he or she wishes, based on the clinical circumstances (however, the latter may not be reimbursed, depending on your particular insurance plan).

Figure 48.1 shows a remote transmission received from a patient with atrial fibrillation. This patient had been using a novel method of preventing atrial fibrillation by taking a beta-blocker thirty minutes before having an alcoholic beverage. The method worked consistently until he forgot to take this medication. The remote strip demonstrates the absence of atrial fibrillation and its presence shortly after forgetting his prophylactic protection.

The process of sending the data from your device, either directly or indirectly, to your doctor's office may or may not be a regularly scheduled event. If you have a device that is not connected via Bluetooth to your cell phone and are going to send an unscheduled transmission, please let your doctor know about your intention to do so. A remote transmission that occurs without the knowledge of the healthcare team is a prescription for a problem, since the strip you transmit may not be reviewed immediately. It is recommended that you call after making a transmission to verify that they received the information. If you feel any seemingly non-life-threatening symptoms, *call the doctor's office.* He or she will determine whether more frequent transmissions are indicated or whether you need to be seen in person.

Remember, the remote transmission service is not a substitute for calling 911. If you are experiencing potentially life-threatening symptoms (such as chest pain, loss of consciousness, recurrent lightheadedness and dizziness, or acute shortness of breath), call 911. You can send an unscheduled transmission of data, but please remember to notify your doctor so that they are aware of the transmission and can act upon this information.

Alarms and alerts that are programmed by your doctor may trigger an alert on the monitoring system (CareLink, Merlin, etc.). Remember, these are not emergency

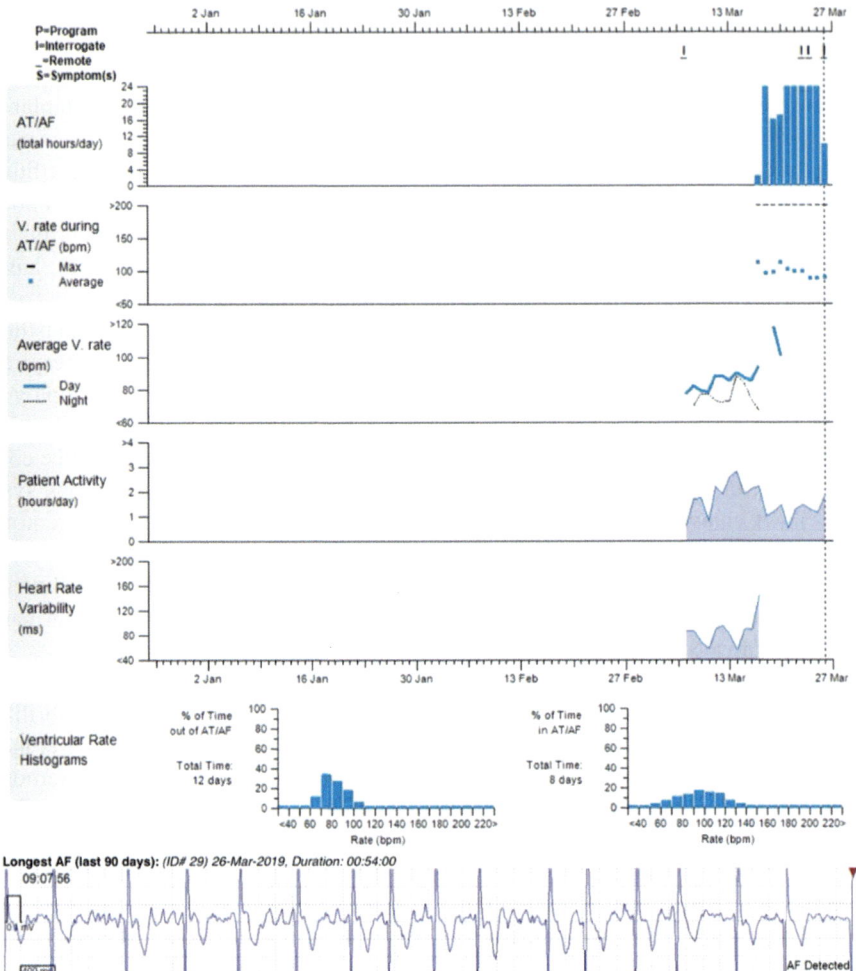

Fig. 48.1 A recording of atrial fibrillation from an implantable loop recorder, the result of not taking beta-blockers immediately before consuming alcohol. This patient had previously induced alcohol-induced defibrillation which was prevented by taking a beta-blocker 30 minutes prior to consumption. For more information, see Meshoyeorer DI and colleagues in EP digest, mentioned in the bibliography

services and should not be regarded as such. Occasionally, because of some communication issue between the device and the phone/monitor, information may be delayed in getting to the system. Therefore, these systems should not be regarded as life-essential, and any serious problems should prompt a call to your doctor or a visit to the emergency room. Not every remote monitoring program is set up in the same manner, so please check with your healthcare provider regarding their system and method.

Also, note there is another means for monitoring heart failure besides implantable heart rhythm devices. One example is the CardioMEMS™ HF system manufactured by Abbott Cardiovascular. This system employs a sensor device that is implanted in the distal pulmonary artery and can transmit heart rate and pulmonary artery pressures in order to remotely manage heart failure and has been demonstrated to reduce heart failure admissions.

How Often Do You Need to See the Doctor If You Are Being Monitored Remotely?

A patient should be seen at least once or twice yearly by their heart disease specialist. This could be via telehealth or in person. Without this kind of contact, it is easy for the patient to lose touch with their doctor and forget that the doctor has any oversight on their care. Do not hesitate to call your healthcare provider's office or make an appointment if you have any questions or concerns that you would like to address. If you are about to change physicians, call your current doctor's office to let them know. The office staff at the new doctor's office can help you set up your remote monitoring system for their office.

What Should You Tell Your Doctor?

Patients should never feel that their doctor does not have the time to listen to their concerns. If you feel this way consistently (rather than only occasionally, on a doctor's busy day), you may want to consider switching to a different doctor. Carry a list of current medications in your wallet at all times, including the name of each drug, the frequency and route of administration, and dosage. Alternatively, you should be able to access this information remotely through the portal of your electronic health record.

If you have not received an invite to your portal, please remind your healthcare provider to send you an invite, so that this information is readily available. The portal itself can provide an easy, safe, and secure means to communicate with your healthcare provider. If you are unsure why you are taking a specific medication, send a message or ask your physician. Tell him or her about any change in medications, change in medical condition, or change in address. Most importantly, tell your doctor how you are feeling. Remember to use your "Surviving and Thriving" card. It is your "Plan B," especially if you need to access important health information and you cannot get to your portal or contact your healthcare provider.

For people who have implantable heart rhythm devices such as defibrillators, call your physician's office if you have received a shock or shocking sensations related to the device. If you get more than two shocks from a defibrillator, call 911 for transport and go to the emergency room as soon as possible. Remember to carry your device identification card at all times. This information may also be written on your "Surviving and Thriving" card as well.

If you have any side effects from any medication, do not hesitate to call your doctor. If you have any recurrence of symptoms following a heart procedure or if you develop side effects from medications or think that you are experiencing a complication, notify your doctor immediately and arrange follow-up.

Bring the Clinic to the Home with Telehealth Visits (Terri Seppala)

Today, we use digital solutions in all aspects of our lives, from banking to retail, and healthcare is no different. Telehealth brings the clinic to where you are, giving you the ability to see the right provider when you need to. Telehealth is no longer an innovative fad—for most physicians, it's a necessity to meet patient demands for control over their time, flexibility, scheduling, privacy, and access to care. Whether you call it telehealth, telemedicine, virtual care, or connected care, it is the way medicine is being practiced now and in the future. Similar to remote monitoring, telehealth allows the doctor or healthcare provider to observe you, diagnose, and treat you with video and health monitoring devices. The healthcare provider can communicate back and forth with you in real-time on a video call using your tablet, laptop, computer, or smartphone. The provider can see and examine you through the microphone and camera on your device.

During the video call, the healthcare provider can remotely retrieve vital signs like your weight, temperature, blood pressure, and pulse from devices sent to your home, or you can provide your weight and temperature on the call. Telehealth visits can be very useful for disabled patients who have difficulty traveling to the doctor's office or for people living in remote areas who have to travel long distances for a routine visit. Even in urban, congested areas, on a snowy day if you need to see the doctor, taking a taxi, driving yourself, or calling an ambulance may create lengthy delays in getting to your appointment or to the emergency room.

With telehealth, you can pick up the phone and get a video visit without the constraints of physically getting to the clinic and waiting to see the doctor. Telemedicine is not just "medical facetime." If a video visit is not enough, there are telemedicine kits brought to your home for diagnostic assessments. Some are equipped with video tablets, stethoscopes, dermatology and ENT cameras, EKG leads, and ultrasound. These kits may be physically carried to your residence by a certified technician who "telepresents" you to a remote doctor or nurse practitioner.

The technician may serve as the "eyes and ears" of the doctor who is guiding their use of the diagnostic tools from the kit. One such kit is manufactured by MedPod™ and distributed by Henry Schein Inc. and called MobileDoc (Fig. 48.2). This is essentially a computer with a number of monitoring tools in a roller suitcase. The MobileDoc is intended to allow the patient to send the standard information to the healthcare provider, who may be seen via a virtual chat on the computer. In a recent study of 2000 patients, using these diagnostic kits reduced visits to the ER/Urgent Care clinic by 86% (see my company's website: https://www.telehealthassociates.com, under the "Case Study" tab under "Evaluation Report," for a

Fig. 48.2 MobileDoc by MedPodTM and distributed by Henry Schein Inc. MobileDoc is a telemedicine kit with diagnostic tools used in telemedicine visits

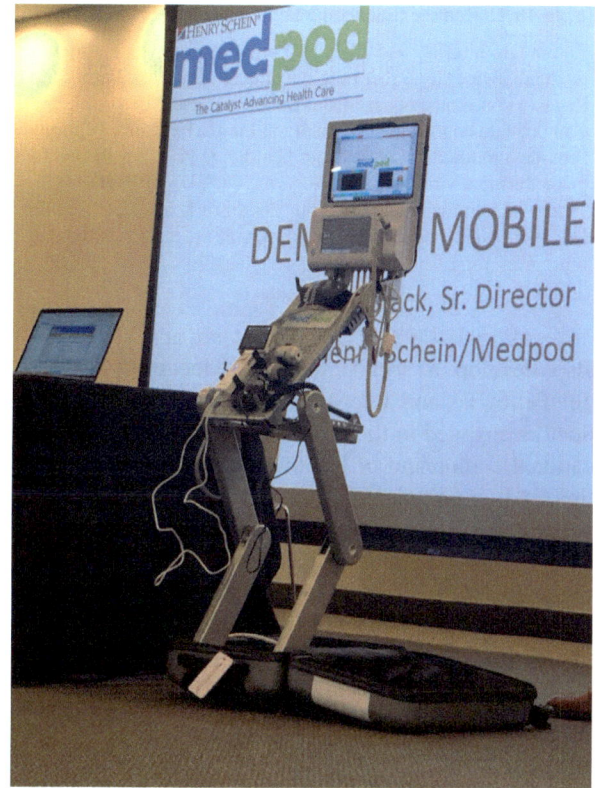

summary of this New York State Department of Health study). Also, the study showed that the doctor could treat the patient 50% faster than in an emergency room or Urgent Care clinic. Further, the doctor gets reimbursed the same amount for a telehealth visit as for an in-person clinic visit.

If telemedicine had been adopted by more doctors before the COVID-19 crisis, just imagine how the virus could have been lessened right away using telehealth-enabled devices. This includes video for medical and mental health appointments, remote patient monitoring to track COVID symptoms and other chronic diseases, and telemedicine diagnostic kits for symptom diagnosis. Additional information may be found at my company's website listed above.

Some doctors, such as the author of this book (Dr. Todd Cohen), had to rapidly adopt telehealth into their clinics during the COVID-19 pandemic, and make the transition immediately in order to provide immediate and consistent care to patients with heart disease. Dr. Cohen's journey in telehealth has been well cataloged by EP Lab Digest and video interviews as the emergency pandemic began. His methods have also been described in the journal itself, and he was able to incorporate a cloud-based telehealth solution as part of his electronic fax, which was directly connected to his electronic health record. His practice's system is entirely HIPAA compliant and versatile since it is accessible wirelessly and is cloud-based.

Table 48.1 Remote monitoring and telehealth versus in-person clinic visits

Remote monitoring and telehealth provide a convenient method to follow-up a patient's medical device (loop recorder, pacemaker, or defibrillator) and medical care.
Receive continuity of care from the convenience of your home.
Can provide continuous feedback on the performance of implantable devices.
Provide a method of seeing your healthcare provider from a far distance, or while sheltering in place during a viral outbreak (e.g., the COVID-19 pandemic).
Time efficient method to see your doctor or healthcare provider in follow-up.
In-person visits and device checks permit the ability to have hands-on care and permit device reprogramming.

In addition, Dr. Cohen and his team at NYITCOM in Old Westbury were able to also develop a secure medical education platform called TeleMedstudent™, TeleFellow™, and TeleMedEd™ in order to keep the medical students and student doctors engaged in their clinical rotations remotely during the pandemic. The educational component of his site provides a centralized source for updates, lectures, tips, and communication on telehealth at NYITCOM. You can get a flavor of this system through his practice's website at https://www.liheartrhythmcenter.com. Dr. Cohen's medical student Innovation Team won first place with TeleMedstudent™ in the 2020 OMED SOMA student research competition.

Many questions about the long-term adoption of telehealth were answered during the pandemic. Telehealth was a big success and proved extremely useful during a highly infectious period of time. After the return to a more normal clinic environment, one should not forget the importance of in-person visits, touching and palpating the patient, and listening to their carotid arteries, lungs, and heart. That being said, telehealth still provides a useful means to evaluate patients and their cardiac conditions, especially when they are at a distance. Table 48.1 reviews the advantages and disadvantages of remote monitoring and telehealth.

Smartphone and Wearable Technology and Heart Health

49

Nicole Hunzeker and Todd J. Cohen

Smartphones and technology can be valuable tools for promoting and maintaining heart health. There is an incredible variety of free, easily downloadable iPhone and Android applications for fitness, nutrition, yoga, and meditation that can help you develop and maintain healthy habits. The emergence of wearable technology, such as the Apple Watch (Fig. 49.1) and Fitbit, has made it even easier to promote healthy habits. The ease and accessibility of these resources make them incredible tools for taking control of your heart health and well-being.

N. Hunzeker
Department of Internal Medicine, NYU Langone Hospital, Brooklyn, Brooklyn, NY, USA

T. J. Cohen (✉)
NYIT College of Osteopathic Medicine, New York, NY, USA
e-mail: tcohen03@nyit.edu

Fig. 49.1 An Apple Watch being used to monitor patient heart health

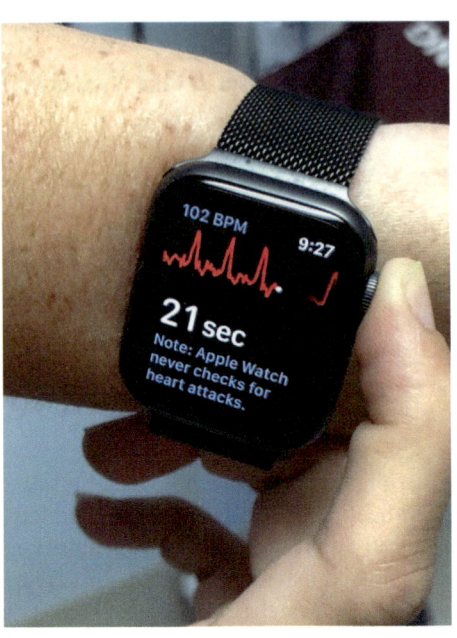

Smartphone Health Applications

The four main categories of smartphone health applications that will be discussed are fitness, nutrition, yoga, and meditation and can all be found in Table 49.1: Smartphone Health Applications. These can all be downloaded for free or for a nominal cost and accessed through the Apple App Store and the Google Play Store, for iPhone and Android users, respectively.

Smartphone applications can be incredibly useful in establishing and maintaining workout routines to promote heart health. Whether you're looking to work out in a gym, at home, or outside, there are smartphone applications that can support your goals. Applications such as *Jefit* provide weight-lifting routines to follow in the gym, but if you would rather work out at home, the application *You Are Your Own Gym* provides effective bodyweight exercise routines. For those who enjoy running or want to give it a try, *Nike+ Run Club* is an easy-to-use application that records the distance and time of your runs to track your progress and keep you motivated.

Another important component of cardiovascular health, nutrition, can be easily monitored via smartphone applications, which can increase the effectiveness of diets and promote healthy lifestyle maintenance. *MyFitnessPal* is an application that tracks the calories and macronutrients of the foods that you input into the application and calculates a daily total that can be very useful when attempting to maintain a caloric deficit for weight loss. For healthy cooking ideas, the application *Mealime* provides a robust catalog of healthy recipes with corresponding downloadable grocery lists. Another aspect of nutrition that is often overlooked is hydration. Unless

Table 49.1 Smartphone health applications

Name	iPhone/ Android	Cost	Description
Fitness			
Jefit	Both	Free	Weight-lifting gym exercise plans and built-in progress tracker
You Are Your Own Gym	Both	Free	At-home exercises using body weight only
Nike+ Run Club	Both	Free	Run tracking and activity log for all fitness levels
Nutrition			
MyFitnessPal	Both	Free	Quick and easy calorie counter and diet tracker
Mealime	Both	Free	Healthy recipes with premade grocery lists
Waterlogged	Both	Free	Hydration reminders throughout the day
Yoga			
Daily Yoga	Both	Free	Step-by-step guide for all yoga levels
Pocket Yoga	Both	$2.99	Detailed voice and visual instructions from various yoga instructors for all skill levels
Simply Yoga	Both	Free	20-, 40-, and 60-minute session options available
Meditation			
Headspace	Both	Free	Guided meditations to teach the user the fundamentals of meditation
The Mindfulness App	Both	Free	Guided meditations, mindfulness reminders, and a meditation journal
Buddhify	Both	$4.99	200+ unique meditations and calming exercises

your doctor has specifically advised you to limit your fluids, the application *Waterlogged* can help keep you hydrated by setting goals and sending reminders to drink water.

Yoga and meditation are incredibly beneficial practices for both physical and mental health (see Chap. 42 for information on their benefits). There are a multitude of smartphone applications that make practicing yoga and meditation accessible and convenient. *Daily Yoga* is a straightforward app, for example, that provides clear step-by-step images of hundreds of yoga poses. If you would rather have an instructor guide you through the poses, then *Pocket Yoga* is a perfect choice. To access premade yoga routines of 20, 40, or 60 minutes in length, download the application *Simply Yoga*.

For those looking to practice more mindfulness, there are plenty of smartphone applications from which to choose. For those just starting out with meditation, the application *Headspace* provides elegant guided meditations, teaching users the fundamentals of meditation. Similarly, *The Mindfulness App* provides users guided meditations, while also incorporating mindfulness reminders and a meditation journal. Sometimes, finding time to fit meditation into your schedule can be difficult. If that's the case, *Buddhify* provides both traditional meditation options as well as meditations on the go, or whenever you have a couple free minutes.

Smartphone applications geared toward promoting healthy habits are fantastic resources to help keep you on track with your fitness, nutrition, and mindfulness goals.

Wearable Health Technology

The two most popular wearable health technology products on the market are the Fitbit and the Apple Watch. Both are great options for reaching your health goals. Exploring the key features of each may provide insight into which may be a better fit for your particular goals.

The Fitbit is worn around the wrist like a watch, and it includes features such as health coaching, guided breathing, calorie tracking, sleep insights, reminders to move, heart rate tracking, and goal setting. The Fitbit allows users to record their steps, distance traveled, and calories burned. This data can be used to track the user's progress over time and keep them on target with their cardiovascular fitness goals. Using pulse readings during rest and exercise, Fitbit can also assign a "Cardio Fitness Level," which can range from "Poor, Fair, Average, Good, Very Good, or Excellent." These features allow users to have tangible measures to monitor their activity and fitness levels and therefore make Fitbit an excellent wearable health technology option.

The Apple Watch is another very attractive option for people looking to track and be in control of their movement and overall fitness. All versions of the Apple Watch include features such as step tracking, workout tracking, reminders to stand, and heart rate monitoring. Perhaps most importantly, the Apple Watch Series 4 version and above have an ECG application that can generate an ECG similar to a single-lead electrocardiogram. The device can detect arrhythmias and allow you to share this data with your doctor, which makes it a valuable tool that can identify underlying pathologies that often go undetected. In addition, the Apple Watch Series 6 or later versions can measure oxygen saturation, which can be very helpful in assessing the status of congestive heart failure (as well as any potential impact of COVID-19 on the cardiopulmonary system).

A key similarity shared by both the Fitbit and Apple Watch is the social motivation component of the technology. Users of both products can connect with their friends and family, share their fitness progress, and even compete with each other. This social component makes wearable technology more engaging for the user and can be very motivational for many people, which in turn can expedite their progress. Whether it be smartphone applications or wearable health technology, there are countless digital resources to help promote and maintain healthy behaviors. Finally, advances in artificial intelligence (AI) can empower both patients and physicians, while also helping to monitor and treat the entire gamut of cardiovascular diseases. In addition, AI may be able to help robotic medical devices (see Chap. 53) perform faster, safer, and more precisely.

Racial Disparities and Gender Differences in Heart Disease

50

Marilyn Chengot and Brittany Cohen

Racial disparities and gender differences are important factors in managing patients with cardiovascular disease (CVD). The gender and racial background of the patient influence the outcome of those who are being treated for CVD. Black patients have the highest rate of CVD (47%), and that rate is projected to rise to 50% by 2035 (according to an October 19, 2018 cover story in Cardiology Magazine, from the American College of Cardiology, entitled "One Size Does Not Fit All: The Role of Sex, Gender, Race and Ethnicity in Cardiovascular Medicine," https://www.acc.org/latest-in-cardiology/articles/2018/10/14/12/42/cover-story-one-size-does-not-fit-all-sex-gender-race-and-ethnicity-in-cardiovascular-medicine). A similar upward trend is predicted for the Hispanic population and women as a whole. *Bias is another important factor.* For example, women and minorities experiencing chest pain are much less likely to be referred for cardiac catheterization than a white man. Recognition of gender and racial differences regarding cardiovascular risks, prevention, and treatment is essential for improving the outcomes amongst minorities and women.

M. Chengot (✉)
Department of Cardiology, Amityville Heart Center, Amityville, NY, USA
e-mail: marilyn.chengot@gmail.com

B. Cohen
Electrical Engineer at ARC by ChargeItSpot, Philadelphia, PA, USA

T. J. Cohen, R. S. Blumenthal (eds.), *Surviving and Thriving With Heart Disease*,
Contemporary Cardiology, https://doi.org/10.1007/978-3-032-00579-3_50

Minorities face more barriers to CVD diagnosis than their white counterparts, resulting in suboptimal healthcare. These barriers stem from factors such as income inequality (resulting in a lack of healthcare coverage) as well as educational and environmental background, limited access to healthcare, and communication barriers. In a 2007 study, more than half of people of color weren't covered by health insurance, according to "FACTS: Bridging the Gap—CVD Health Disparities" from the American Heart Association (https://www.heart.org/idc/groups/heart-public/@wcm/@hcm/@ml/documents/downloadable/ucm_429240.pdf). High blood pressure, diabetes, and obesity (all key risk factors for CVD) are more prevalent in minorities.

Racial disparities have shown that a Black person is 42% less likely to receive an implantable defibrillator post a myocardial infarction than those who are Caucasian (also from the 2018 Cardiology Magazine cover story mentioned above). Black and Hispanic individuals are less likely than white individuals to have their heart-related symptoms taken seriously in clinical settings. Black and other minority populations face a higher risk of heart failure compared to White individuals. Among Black individuals, this increased risk is more often attributed to hypertension rather than coronary artery disease. Additionally, both Black and Hispanic individuals tend to have poorer glycemic control in comparison to their white counterparts.

Black individuals tend to have a higher sensitivity to salt, which, if left unmonitored, could lead to hypertension. In the United States, Black individuals also have the highest risk of hypertension, 41%, as opposed to anywhere else. This is in comparison with the white population at 28% (again from the 2018 Cardiology Magazine cover story). According to the above referenced, American Heart Association FACTS, it is important to note that most United States studies centered around race have focused on Black individuals (91%), as opposed to their other minority counterparts, Hispanic (26%), Asian (14%), and Native American individuals (5%).

Some minorities also face language barriers when communicating health issues to their doctors, which can result in inadequate care. In 2001, only 2% of cardiologists self-identified as Black, and 3.8% as Hispanic. Thus, it is no surprise that racial barriers exist. When surveyed about racial disparities in patient treatment (according to the above American Heart Association FACTS reference), only 35% of cardiologists acknowledged the importance of knowing about racial diversity while treating patients. When it comes to treating minorities, cardiologists need to be more aware of these racial differences and cognizant of racial bias.

Table 50.1 shows some heart disease-related issues found in both Hispanic and Black populations. Both have a sensitivity to salt; are prone to high blood pressure, diabetes, and obesity; have a tendency toward poor glycemic control; and have a

Table 50.1 Cardiac risk factors in Black and Hispanic individuals	High blood pressure, diabetes, obesity
	Salt sensitivity
	Poor glycemic control
	Higher risk of heart failure
	Higher risk of high blood pressure

Table 50.2 Cardiac risk factors related to the female gender

High testosterone levels before menopause
Increase in hypertension during menopause
Autoimmune diseases such as rheumatoid arthritis
Stress and depression

higher risk of high blood pressure and heart failure. These disparities are not a result of individual hospitals and clinics but as a systemic problem within the healthcare community.

Gender differences also play a crucial role in CVD treatment. A significant barrier related to women being treated for CVD is a result of a lack of knowledge in the cardiology community. Many CVD studies have been centered around men, and have not focused on gender; because of this, the cardiologist may be missing CVD signs due to symptoms not as easily characterized as "traditional." Women, in general, have been underrepresented in cardiovascular trials, including all areas of CVD (such as stenting and implantable defibrillators). Women tend to experience more subtle symptoms regarding heart attacks than men, which can be difficult to detect if the cardiologist isn't well-versed in gender differences.

Symptoms usually used to diagnose a heart attack include indigestion, shortness of breath, and back pain, but these symptoms are much less common in women, according to Dr. Lili Barouch, from Johns Hopkins School of Medicine, in her article entitled "Heart Disease: Differences in Men and Women," https://www.hopkinsmedicine.org/heart_vascular_institute/centers_excellence/women_cardiovascular_health_center/patient_information/health_topics/heart_disease_gender_differences.html. The specific risk factors regarding women who experience CVD are seen in Table 50.2 and include (1) higher levels of testosterone before menopause, (2) an increase in hypertension during menopause, (3) autoimmune diseases like rheumatoid arthritis, (4) stress and depression, and (5) unawareness that these issues could be risk factors for heart disease. The lack of gender-focused studies to understand differences in women's experiences with CVD compared to men has contributed to undiagnosed and untreated cases.

One example is that women may experience chest pain before menopause. Young adult women who complain of chest pain may not receive stress testing to the same degree as their age-matched male counterparts. Even though their incidence may be less, and their presentation might be different, it is important to be aware of this general bias, since coronary artery disease can still occur in women under the age of fifty.

With respect to bias, we have to accept the fact that there has been racial discrimination in the past. Table 50.3 reviews areas of bias in CVD, and in particular, there has been a lack of studies of minorities besides the Black population. Women have been underrepresented in many of the large clinical cardiovascular trials as well. Language barriers do exist, and we, as healthcare workers, have to make sure that we use all our tools to help improve this issue. Many diverse populations lack health insurance, yet they deserve humane treatment and guideline-driven therapy

Table 50.3 Areas of bias

Racial discrimination
Lack of studies on minorities beside black individuals
Lack of studies on female patients
Language barriers that hinder effective communication with their doctor
Lack of health insurance
Lower-income economic background
Lack of female and minority cardiologists

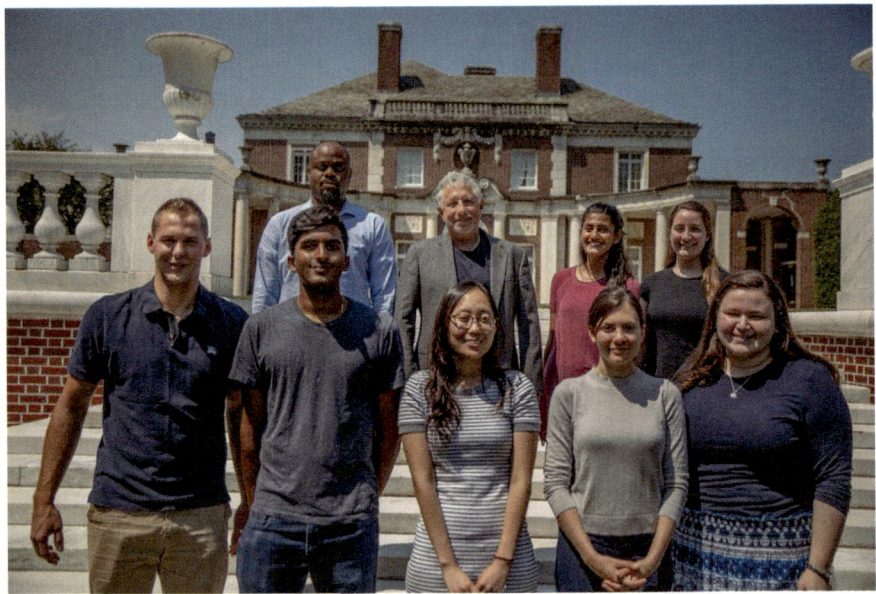

Fig. 50.1 Dr. Cohen and members of his first research team at NYITCOM pose for a picture in front of the de Seversky Mansion in Old Westbury, NY

just as much as those with coverage. This includes those who come from a poor economic background. Finally, healthcare workers must include all races, creeds, colors, and a more diverse gender mix in order to present a more understanding and empowered healthcare workforce that can better understand those being treated. Figure 50.1 shows Dr. Cohen's diverse research team at NYITCOM.

In closing, both gender and race have played vital roles in disparity when it comes to identifying CVD. Whether it is caused by racial discrimination or unawareness of female symptoms, these two groups have resulted in undetected signs and a lack of proper treatment. Because most cardiologists consist of white men, it is very important for them to be more aware of racial disparities and gender differences when handling their patients in order to provide the best care. More studies need to include greater representation of women and diverse groups (in addition to Black individuals) in order to truly understand the impact of heart disease on each unique population. In addition, awareness of ethnic differences and gender bias is essential for improving equitable access to cardiac testing and treatments across diverse populations.

Support Groups, Counseling, and Other Resources

51

Sarah Jane Muder and Todd J. Cohen

Information and support are available for patients and their families through organizations such as the Sudden Cardiac Arrest Association (www.suddencardiacarrest. org), American College of Cardiology (www.acc.org), the American Red Cross (www.redcross.org), and the Heart Rhythm Society (www.hrsonline.org). Support groups are beneficial for both individuals with heart disease, as well as family members and friends. These support groups provide education to keep patients and their loved ones up to date on current therapies, and offer a space for individuals to express their feelings about their disease. Talking with individuals who have had heart disease for many years is helpful in identifying realistic goals for the years following the diagnosis.

A diagnosis of a new cardiac disease can be just as emotionally taxing on family and loved ones as it can be on the individual. In addition, support groups can prove very helpful to those close to someone with cardiac disease. They allow families to explore and understand the impact of the disease process on loved ones. For more information about some heart-related support groups (including those related to hypertrophic cardiomyopathy), see Table 51.1.

Individuals should not ignore the benefits of seeking counseling upon diagnosis of a new cardiac illness. Counseling can help patients view their new diagnosis in a

S. J. Muder
Department of Obstetrics and Gynecology, St. Luke's University Health Network, Bethlehem, PA, USA
e-mail: sarah.muder@sluhn.org

T. J. Cohen (✉)
NYIT College of Osteopathic Medicine, New York, NY, USA
e-mail: tcohen03@nyit.edu

© The Author(s), under exclusive license to Springer Nature Switzerland AG 2025
T. J. Cohen, R. S. Blumenthal (eds.), *Surviving and Thriving With Heart Disease*,
Contemporary Cardiology, https://doi.org/10.1007/978-3-032-00579-3_51

Table 51.1 Heart-related support groups

American Heart Association (www.heart.org): Helps support and advance the diagnosis and treatment of cardiovascular disease and stroke.

American College of Cardiology (www.acc.org): A large society for cardiologists that supports their research, training, and maintenance of board certification. Also helps patients and families with education related to heart disease prevention and management.

American Red Cross (www.redcross.org): A global network of volunteers geared toward helping in emergencies and disasters. Also involved in donating blood, CPR, and resuscitation training.

Cardiac Arrhythmias Research and Education Foundation (www.longqt.org): Helps advocate for research and education in preventing sudden cardiac death.

Heart Rhythm Society (www.hrsonline.org): A large international society for heart rhythm specialists (electrophysiologists), ancillary professionals, and related personnel that supports all aspects of heart rhythm disorder understanding and advancement, including education, research, training, certification, treatment, and patient care.

Hypertrophic Cardiomyopathy Association (www.4hcm.org): Helps support patients with hypertrophic cardiomyopathy and their families.

Sudden Cardiac Arrest Association (www.suddencardiacarrest.org): Supports patients (and their families and friends) who have experienced or may be at risk for sudden cardiac arrest, with a focus on education in the prevention, resuscitation, and treatment of those at risk for sudden cardiac arrest.

Sudden Arrhythmia Death Syndromes Foundation (www.sads.org): Offers support for inherited heart rhythm conditions such as long QT Syndrome.

different light and develop coping strategies to survive and thrive with heart disease. Counseling services are becoming more and more widely used as scientific evidence illustrates the benefits that it can have on both physical and mental well-being. It is not uncommon for patients to become depressed or have anxiety after receiving a new medical diagnosis. Cardiac disease can bring with it many changes. Patients may not be able to enjoy the same activities that they once loved, which may cause substantial mental distress.

Finding a counselor or psychologist can be achieved by looking for in-network providers, using the help of your insurance company's website. You can also ask your primary care provider for a referral to a counseling service. Resources like Talk Space (talkspace.com) and BetterHelp (betterhelp.com) allow you to access a counselor on your own time and at affordable rates for those who do not have insurance.

The American Heart Association (AHA) makes a number of publications available to patients and their families to help with their care and the management of their health. AHA family resources include guidance on diet and weight management, as well as community-based CPR classes. Inviting family members and friends to become trained in CPR can help them feel like they are being proactive and involved in the health journey of their loved ones. The AHA can be easily accessed at www.heart.org.

Device companies have vast resources online. These resources include information regarding heart disease and arrhythmias, medications, catheter ablation, and devices. Access the manufacturers' websites at BIOTRONIK (www.biotronik.com),

Table 51.2 Contact numbers of some common device manufacturers	Abbott: 1-800-PACEICD Biotronik: 1-800-547-0394 Boston Scientific: 1-800-CARDIAC Johnson & Johnson: 1-800-652-6227 Medtronic: 1-800-MEDTRON

Boston Scientific (www.bostonscientific.com), Johnson and Johnson (www.jnj.com), Medtronic (www.medtronic.com), and Abbott (www.abbott.com). Technical support telephone numbers for each of these device manufacturers are listed in Table 51.2.

Books are a helpful resource in understanding a disease process, as well as reading about the experiences of others going through a hard time. This book is a fantastic start in the journey to understanding and accepting your condition, or the condition of a loved one. For more book recommendations, consult your local library. Many books have been written by doctors and patients (and even doctors who have unexpectedly become patients) on the subject of adapting to a new life after a medical diagnosis. You can also ask your librarian for book recommendations about thriving with a chronic disease.

Defensive Patienting: A Primer on Patient Safety

52

Todd J. Cohen

Patient safety is the foremost concern of healthcare providers when they diagnose and treat heart rhythm patients. When receiving their degree from medical school, doctors take the Hippocratic oath, by which, among other provisions, they vow to do no harm. Even so, doctors and other healthcare workers are human, and unfortunately, humans make mistakes. Hospitals and medical clinics have protocols (checks and balances) to help ensure a patient's privacy and safety. But patients also need to have a system in place, much like defensive driving. This is what I call *defensive patienting*. Defensive patienting adds protection for you and helps you to ensure your own safety. The following safety tips may help you in any number of healthcare situations.

First, you should be familiar with your own medical information and should have immediate access to it through your patient portal to your electronic medical record. If you don't have access to your portal, ask your healthcare provider for access. They will typically send you an email, and you will need to set up a username and password to gain access to your portal. This should allow you to securely access your medical information, schedule appointments, ask for prescription renewals, and communicate with your healthcare provider. However, there are times you might not be able to access your portal, whether you are traveling, experiencing technical issues, or simply forget how to log in. This is why I recommend a backup plan (Plan B). If you don't already have one, you should put one in place right now. All your medical information should be included on your "Surviving and Thriving" card found in this book in Appendix J and can serve as a backup plan if you cannot access your portal. The card puts two key principles of this book to work for you.

T. J. Cohen (✉)
NYIT College of Osteopathic Medicine, New York, NY, USA
e-mail: tcohen03@nyit.edu

Throughout this book, I have emphasized "knowing your numbers" so you can know where you are with respect to your cardiac risk factors. These include blood pressure, cholesterol (LDL, HDL, and triglycerides), obesity (weight and BMI), and diabetes (fasting blood glucose and A1C level). I also have emphasized the importance of having a Plan B. Like the song written by John Seppala, every heart disease patient needs a fallback plan to get on with their life. Each book contains your own personal "Surviving and Thriving" card, which you can fill out and carry with you. It has two sides: one side is "Know Your Numbers," and the other side is "Plan B" (see Fig. 52.1a, b).

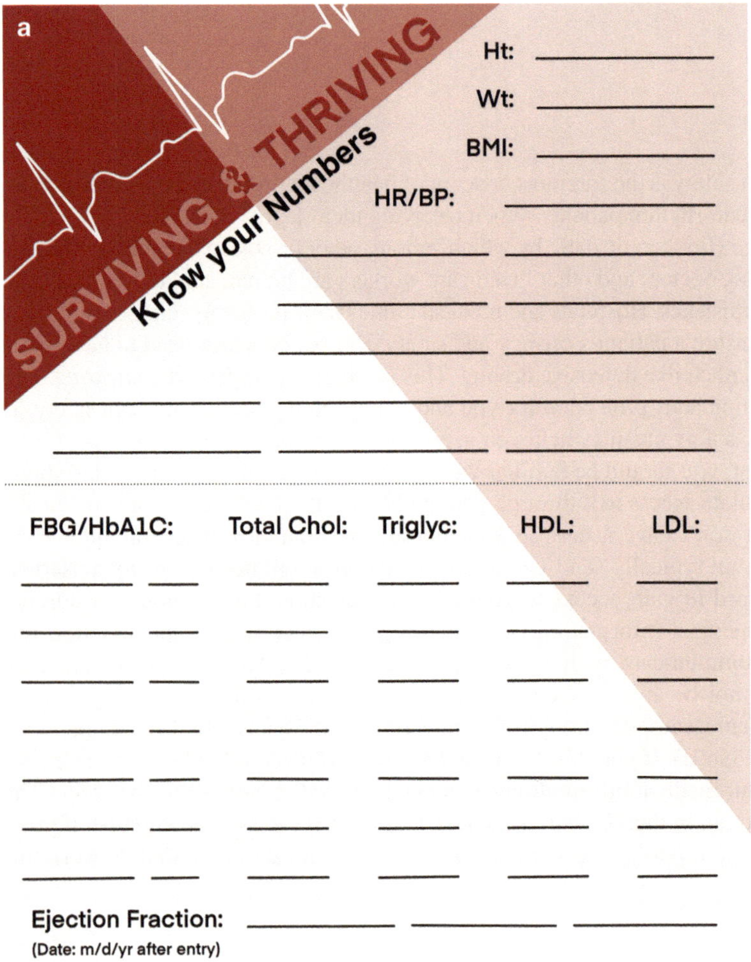

a

SURVIVING & THRIVING

Know your Numbers

Ht: _____

Wt: _____

BMI: _____

HR/BP: _____

FBG/HbA1C:	Total Chol:	Triglyc:	HDL:	LDL:

Ejection Fraction: _____ _____ _____
(Date: m/d/yr after entry)

Fig. 52.1 (a, b) This figure shows an image of your "Surviving and Thriving" Card. The card has two sides and contains your essential medical information ("Plan B" side), and a mechanism to track your numbers ("Know Your Numbers" side). Appendix J is your actual card, which you should cut out, fill out, and keep with you, along with a copy of your ECG. Keep them in your wallet, purse, glove compartment, or any other easily available place. You can also make copies by accessing my practice's website at https://www.liheartrhythmcenter.com. (Note: this is the same as the figure of Appendix J (but I intend to show both of these figures on one page here; one under the other))

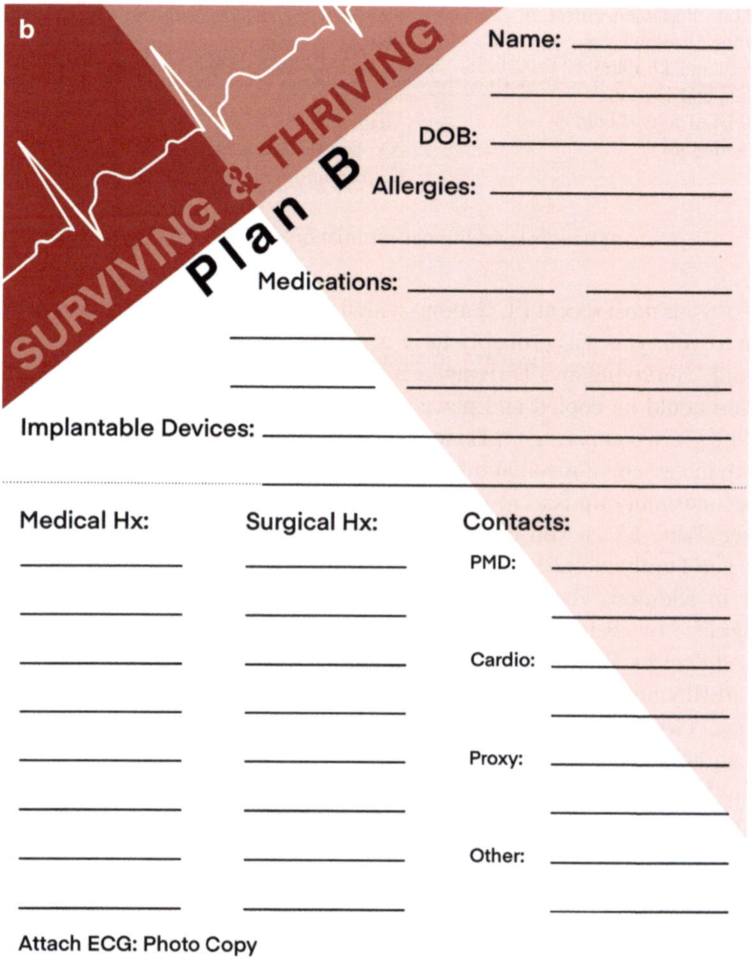

b

SURVIVING & THRIVING Plan B

Name: _____
_____

DOB: _____

Allergies: _____
_____

Medications: _____ _____
_____ _____ _____
_____ _____ _____

Implantable Devices: _____
_____

Medical Hx:	Surgical Hx:	Contacts:
_____	_____	PMD: _____
_____	_____	_____
_____	_____	Cardio: _____
_____	_____	_____
_____	_____	Proxy: _____
_____	_____	_____
_____	_____	Other: _____
_____	_____	_____

Attach ECG: Photo Copy

Fig. 52.1 (continued)

You can cut or punch out the card from this book, and write your own personal information on it, or you can go to my website, https://www.liheartrhythmcenter. com, and hit the "Create Your Surviving and Thriving Card" button, fill out the card, and then print it out. You can update the card as often as you would like and print it out, ensuring to put the most recent date to make sure you have your most recent information.

Table 52.1 shows the essential information that you should carry as a backup when you can't access your portal. The Plan B side includes your name and birth date to provide double identification. You can list your main medical conditions, including implanted devices, allergies, and medications. In addition, carry contact information, including the name of your healthcare proxy (the person who will make medical decisions for you if you become incapacitated). You should also carry

Table 52.1 Portable medical information (available via your portal and a backup "Surviving and Thriving" card and ECG copy should be carried with you)

Full name and date of birth
Medical conditions
Implantable devices and materials
Allergies
Medications
A copy of a recent ECG
Contact information, including a healthcare proxy

a copy of your most recent ECG along with the card. Should something unexpected happen to you, you will probably have access to your portal, but just in case, you have your "Surviving and Thriving" card with your essential medical information. This card could be copied and placed in your smartphone, wallet, purse, or even your car's glove compartment. This will provide any healthcare provider who assists you with the essential medical information needed to expedite your treatment.

A second safety tip is to research hospitals, medical clinics, and doctors in your area (see Table 52.2). You can gather information from doctors, as well as from friends and family members who have received care from those institutions or providers. In addition, you can search the Internet and employ a service such as Healthgrades (www.healthgrades.com), which supplies ratings of medical institutions and doctors along with other information about them. Organizations such as the Heart Rhythm Society (www.hrsonline.org) and the American Board of Internal Medicine (www.abim.org) provide useful information regarding the board-certification status of heart rhythm specialists and other physicians.

A third safety tip is to do what's necessary to prepare for a test or procedure. For a summary of how you can protect your rights and help avoid medical errors, see Table 52.3. You must be aware of what is going on. You should make sure you are getting the right procedure on the correct part of the body by confirming this information with each new healthcare provider who approaches you. You need to be on your toes. Make sure you know and understand your condition and any tests that are ordered. What is involved in the tests? What are the risks, benefits, and alternatives? Did the doctor take time to explain these to you, and do you have any questions? If you do not understand something, it is your responsibility to stop and ask questions. Question, question, question! And keep asking until your questions are answered to your satisfaction. Except in an emergency, do not go forward with any tests or procedures until you are satisfied that you understand the what, why, how, and by whom.

The fourth tip to keep in mind is that patients are entitled to privacy based on the Health Insurance Portability and Accountability Act (HIPAA). Doctors cannot disclose a patient's medical information to anyone, including family members and friends, without the patient's permission. A patient's medical information, including the medical record, is private, and rules exist regarding with whom this information can be shared. For more information about HIPAA privacy rules, see https://www.hhs.gov/ocr/privacy/hipaa/understanding/index.html.

Table 52.2 Research the hospital and the doctor	Look into the experience of doctors and the experiences of other patients. Make use of services such as HealthGrades (www.healthgrades.com). Review information from the Heart Rhythm Society (www.hrsonline.org). Consult the American Board of Internal Medicine (www.abim.org).

Table 52.3 Preparing for a test or procedure

1. Be aware.
2. Know and understand what tests have been ordered.
3. Do not just go with the flow.
4. Prevent "wrong patient, wrong procedure, wrong site" errors by actively participating in the safety procedures:
   Double identification: Staff will check your first name and last name and date of birth to confirm your identity. Make sure they get the spelling and the dates right!
   Time out: Prior to any invasive procedure, a time out is required to confirm that the right patient, the right procedure, and the right site will be operated on (or will undergo a test or procedure). This must be performed with the entire medical team before proceeding.
5. Understand the risks, benefits, and alternatives before consenting to any test, procedure, or surgery.
6. Question, question, question.

Finally, a patient who is not independently competent requires the input of a healthcare proxy to help make medical decisions. Ideally, a healthcare proxy is appointed by the patient in a legal document prepared *before* the patient is incompetent or has any need for the proxy. The proxy and all paperwork confirming that person's role as proxy needs to be readily available and accessible. The proxy's contact information should be in the patient's medical chart (and should be on your "Surviving and Thriving" card). The contact information of important family members should also be readily available.

"Defensive patienting" is a primer for protecting the patient in the complex medical network. Heart problems and procedures are intrinsically complicated. This book is intended to empower all patients and their families and friends to get the best care from their healthcare providers. I hope this book will help with your "Defensive patienting" by increasing your understanding of your heart, any possible heart conditions that you may have, as well as what you can do to optimize your treatment.

Robotics and Heart Disease

53

Zachary Coopee, Robert Hubley, and Todd J. Cohen

Part of being a proactive patient is questioning the tools and methods your physician recommends or uses for treatment. If your doctor discusses using an advanced surgical robot to perform a heart procedure, such as cardiac catheterization, ablation, or open-heart surgery, you and your doctor need to be comfortable with these procedures before agreeing. Surgeons typically must perform hundreds of procedures before becoming proficient in using an advanced surgical robot. You should be concerned if your doctor does not have adequate experience.

Robotic surgery began in 1985, and there are already certain procedures, such as open-heart surgery, that are often performed with an advanced surgical robot. As of 2019, the da Vinci® Surgical System (dVSS), shown in Fig. 53.1, has been used in over five million surgical procedures worldwide, as of 2020, according to Intuitive Surgical Corporation, located in Sunnyvale, CA. However, it is still important to ask your doctor about the advantages and disadvantages of robotic surgery. According to recent research completed in 2016, robotic surgery has been shown to be at least

Z. Coopee
Department of Anesthesiology, Yale School of Medicine, New Haven, CT, USA
e-mail: zachary.coopee@yale.edu

R. Hubley
Department of Internal Medicine, Walter Reed National Military Medical Center, Bethesda, MD, USA
e-mail: roh2wf@virginia.edu

T. J. Cohen (✉)
NYIT College of Osteopathic Medicine, New York, NY, USA
e-mail: tcohen03@nyit.edu

© The Author(s), under exclusive license to Springer Nature Switzerland AG 2025
T. J. Cohen, R. S. Blumenthal (eds.), *Surviving and Thriving With Heart Disease*,
Contemporary Cardiology, https://doi.org/10.1007/978-3-032-00579-3_53

Fig. 53.1 The use of the DaVinci Surgical System in procedures involving the heart. (Image courtesy of Intuitive Surgical, Inc.)

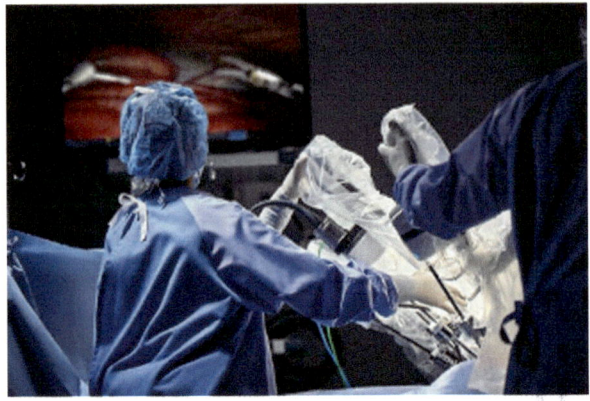

Fig. 53.2 Dr. Cohen operating during an electrophysiology study using the Amigo Remote Catheter System

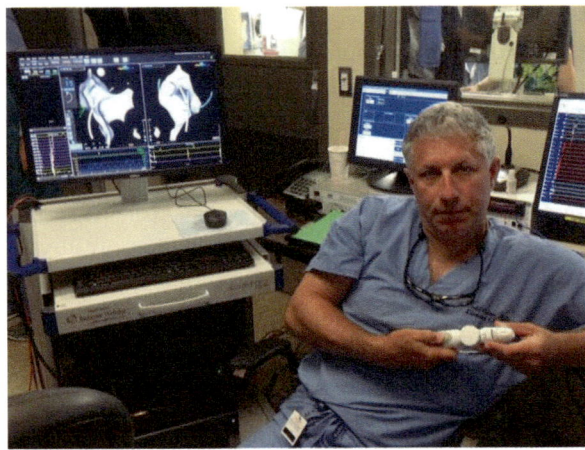

as effective as conventional surgical approaches, but more quality evidence is needed to make further conclusions.

Dr. Todd Cohen, one of this book's authors and editors, developed a robotic system for performing heart rhythm procedures, such as electrophysiology studies, mapping, and catheter ablation, called the Amigo™ Remote Catheter System (Fig. 53.2). This system allows operators to remotely manipulate standard catheters from outside the fluoroscopy field. The Amigo™ (Fig. 53.3) has been successfully used in a variety of electrophysiology and mapping procedures, and it appears to be at least equivalent to manually performed procedures. One major advantage of the Amigo™ is that it helps minimize operator fatigue by eliminating the need to wear lead, since the doctors are located in a separate control room outside of the fluoroscopy field. Dr. Cohen's experience with developing and using this system is well chronicled in "The Amigo ™ Remote Catheter System: From Concept to Bedside," published in the Journal of Innovations in Cardiac Rhythm Management (see Bibliography under Shaikh ZA et. al).

Fig. 53.3 The Amigo remote Catheter System, which was developed for procedures including electrophysiology studies, mapping, and cardiac ablations

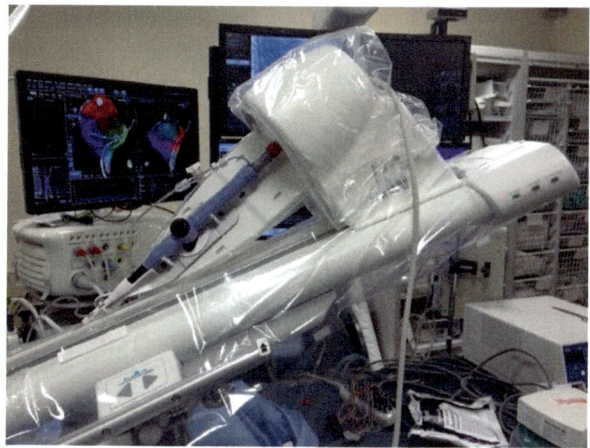

Table 53.1 Questions to ask your doctor about robotic surgery

1. Why do I need robotic surgery? Why will it help with this procedure?
2. What are the benefits of this specific robotic procedure?
3. What is your experience performing this surgery?
4. What were the outcomes of your previous robotic procedures? Any complications?
5. If I elect not to have a robotic surgery, what are my other options?
6. Will robotic surgery take longer than conventional surgical approaches?
7. How will my recovery time be affected compared to other surgical options?
8. Is this procedure covered by my insurance? Will it cost me more out of pocket?

Other robotic systems have been developed for interventional cardiology and may assist in the performance of a cardiac catheterization procedure and/or stent deployment. One such system, Corindus Vascular Robotics, acquired by Siemens Medical Solutions, uses a remote coronary wire/catheter manipulation platform, analogous to the electrophysiology platform employed by the Amigo™, to assist in percutaneous vascular and coronary artery procedures, such as stent deployment (robotic-assisted percutaneous coronary intervention). Table 53.1 lists some questions to ask your doctor before you undergo a robotic procedure. Specifically, you should ask them about their experience with these systems before undergoing any robotic procedure.

In summary, advanced surgical robots are frequently used in heart procedures. However, robotic surgery is rarely the only surgical option and you should not feel compelled to agree to robotic surgery. You should understand the associated risks and benefits, as well as the surgeon's experience with the particular robotic system, before agreeing to undergo any robotic cardiac procedure.

Supplements

54

Nicole Hunzeker and Todd J. Cohen

With so many supplements on the market, navigating which ones are right for you can be a challenging task. Many claim a benefit to heart health, but are any of these claims substantiated? It is important to understand that supplements in general can vary according to their preparation and that any claims may not be scientifically based. Also, remember to talk to your physician about what supplements you are taking or considering. Some information on supplements can be found in Chaps. 37 and 38. This chapter elaborates on some of the principles already discussed and presents additional advice to those interested in preventing and treating heart disease.

The American Heart Association (AHA) recommends getting your needed nutrients, vitamins, and antioxidants from food intake rather than supplements. However, while the benefits and risks of supplements are still being studied, this chapter will review some of the data related to supplements and cardiovascular health. *Specifically, my team will review garlic, green tea, Coenzyme Q10, omega-3 fish oil, and multivitamins. And after each discussion, I (Dr. Todd Cohen) will give my recommendation in italics. I will also review the AHA's stance on coffee and alcohol consumption and give my advice on these beverages.*

First, garlic may have some beneficial effects on heart disease risk factors. Varshney and Budoff published an article entitled "Garlic and Heart Disease" in the Journal of Nutrition in 2016 (see Bibliography). They reviewed all double-blind randomized human studies, including meta-analyses through May 2013. They concluded that a definite benefit of garlic intake on cardiovascular disease has not yet

N. Hunzeker
Department of Internal Medicine, NYU Langone Hospital, Brooklyn, Brooklyn, NY, USA

T. J. Cohen (✉)
NYIT College of Osteopathic Medicine, New York, NY, USA
e-mail: tcohen03@nyit.edu

been proven. They did find evidence that garlic supplementation can modestly decrease blood pressure and total cholesterol, and may help reduce the risk of cardiovascular events. The most consistent effects were identified in aged garlic extract, which was also beneficial in reducing the inflammatory marker C-reactive protein (CRP). The problem was the inconsistency of the various garlic preparations. *My overall recommendation is that you should consider adding fresh garlic to your food in order to enhance the taste, rather than add salt.*

Green tea consumption has been suggested as possibly being beneficial to the heart and possibly even lowering LDL levels. Some studies have suggested a benefit to those with atrial fibrillation, and studies have even suggested that green tea may prevent heart attacks or strokes. *There is no conclusive scientific proof of these facts in any controlled, randomized, blinded study, and I am concerned about coming to any conclusion with a wide variety of tea preparations. Additionally, green tea can contain oxalates, and heavy consumption might contribute to kidney stone formation. My best recommendation is if you enjoy green tea, drink it in moderation.*

Coenzyme Q10 (CoQ10) is a naturally occurring molecule involved in harvesting cellular energy and is an antioxidant found in the human body and in some foods that we eat. Studies on the benefits of CoQ10 have been inconclusive, particularly regarding its effects on improving cardiac events and outcomes. *In general, I do not routinely recommend that my patients add CoQ10 to their diet.*

Lastly, omega-3 fatty acids (typically found in fish oils) have been purported to have a beneficial effect on your heart. The various preparations of omega-3 fatty acids make it difficult to decide which one to buy (and which specific preparation). Previously, omega-3 fatty acids have been shown to help reduce triglycerides in those with high levels. Recently, the REDUCE-IT trial, published by Deepak Bhatt and colleagues in 2020 in Circulation (see Bibliography), demonstrated that icosapent ethyl (a specific omega-3 formulation) reduced cardiovascular events by 25% in those patients with elevated triglycerides and on statins who had heart disease (or were at risk of developing heart disease). *At present, adding fish consumption (specifically oily fish like salmon) and flax seeds to a heart-healthy diet is probably more prudent than over-the-counter omega-3 fatty acid supplementation.*

The AHA does not recommend taking mineral or vitamin supplements but rather recommends getting these nutrients by eating a well-balanced diet. This is probably the best way to think about heart health. Remember to eat plenty of fruits and vegetables and aim for a moderate intake of saturated fat, salt, and sugar. Try to eat tree nuts and whole, unprocessed grains. In the long run, you will be better off. The US Preventive Services Task Force also found that there was not sufficient evidence to support taking multivitamins to prevent cardiovascular events (International Journal of Preventive Medicine 2018).

With respect to diet, nutrient supplements, minerals, or vitamins, a large analysis of 277 clinical trials conducted by researchers from Johns Hopkins Medicine (see Khan SU et al. in the Bibliography) found little evidence supporting their benefits for improving heart disease or longevity. *So, unless you are identified by a physician as having a vitamin or mineral deficiency, specific vitamin supplementation is unnecessary, especially if you eat a well-balanced diet.*

   This information and any information regarding claims surrounding the usage of supplements must all be considered with a critical mind. There is a substantial lack of randomized controlled research studies about these topics, and many limitations and confounding variables exist across studies in the field. For example, people who go out of their way to take supplements to improve their health often may prioritize and care about their health to a higher degree than the average person. A person who cares about his or her health enough to seek out supplements also likely routinely exercises, eats healthy, and regularly engages in other healthy habits. This information suggests that these types of health-conscious people are going to have more favorable health outcomes regardless of the supplement's effect. In addition, it is important to keep in mind the potential risks of dietary supplements. The long-term usage of any nutrient in high enough quantities can become toxic, and also, drug interactions can occur between prescribed medication and supplements. Furthermore, the efficacy, purity, and safety of supplements do not have to be tested before marketing the products, unlike prescription medications.

   Finally, coffee and alcohol might not be considered a supplement, but many people with heart disease can still enjoy these foods in moderation. Over the years, modest coffee consumption and even a glass of red wine a day have been deemed safe and even potentially beneficial to those who want to prevent heart disease (and even those who might have heart disease). According to the AHA, coffee can help your energy level and focus and is associated with a lower risk of type 2 diabetes and Parkinson's disease (they highlight one study lowering the risk of Alzheimer's disease). They even note that regular consumption could lower one's mortality from heart disease, suicide, and nervous system disorders.

   One study noted that drinking up to six cups of coffee per day modestly reduces one's risk of coronary artery disease, heart failure, and even stroke. A concern may not be the coffee itself but what one adds to it (cream and sugar). *Many of you have heard about the health benefits of drinking a glass of red wine each day. There have been no conclusive health studies (randomized double-blinded trials) that have proven this point. Therefore, alcohol consumption is not recommended by the AHA for any health benefits. But my personal recommendation is that it is okay in moderation (one four-ounce glass per day; and probably best not every day). If you have any palpitations or other symptoms, please talk to your doctor.*

   In conclusion, it is important to understand which supplements have evidence for being beneficial to your cardiovascular health. The current stance of the AHA is not to rely on supplementation but rather to obtain appropriate nutrients by consuming a wide variety of foods from each food group, as explained above. Coffee may be beneficial, but alcohol consumption should be in moderation, if at all.

Infections of the Heart

Emily Dries and Todd J. Cohen

Infections of the heart are rare but serious complications caused by microbes such as bacteria and viruses. These infections are classified by where the infection occurs: the endocardium (innermost layer of your heart), myocardium (your heart muscle), or the pericardium (the outer covering of your heart).

Endocarditis

An infection of the endocardium is called infective endocarditis. The endocardium lines the heart chambers and valves to provide protection. Infective endocarditis occurs when an infection travels through the blood to the heart, causing an infected heart valve. The infection can originate from another area of the body, or enter the body through the mouth or skin. It can also be a rare complication (less than 1% incidence) from an implanted heart rhythm device, such as a pacemaker or defibrillator, with wires that were inserted through a vein into the heart.

There are many risk factors for endocarditis. Older patients (over 60 years old) are at greater risk for endocarditis due to the increased likelihood of comorbid heart or valve conditions. Men are more likely than women to get infective endocarditis. Intravenous drug use is another risk factor, as it can introduce pathogens (like bacteria) into your bloodstream, where they can then travel to the heart.

E. Dries
Department of Pediatrics, The Children's Hospital at Montefiore, Bronx, NY, USA

T. J. Cohen (✉)
NYIT College of Osteopathic Medicine, New York, NY, USA
e-mail: tcohen03@nyit.edu

Bacteria present in the oral cavity can also seed infection, and, as such, preventive antibiotics may be given to patients undergoing invasive dental procedures. Other procedures, including insertion of wired pacemakers and defibrillator devices, also pose a risk, and patients may receive an antibiotic pouch that is placed in the device pocket before closure to help lessen the risk of infection. Other risk factors include structural heart disease, valvular heart disease (Chap. 12), congenital heart disease (Chap. 15), prosthetic heart valves, or the presence of intravascular or implantable heart rhythm devices (pacemakers and defibrillators).

Infective endocarditis is most commonly caused by bacteria. The three most common bacteria are staphylococci (such as *Staph. aureus),* streptococci (such as viridans group strep), and enterococci. The most common pathogens will vary based on geographic region and individual patient risk factors. Fungi are a much rarer cause of infective endocarditis.

Endocarditis can lead to complications such as heart damage and septic emboli from the infected valve (little collections of infection that break off and enter the bloodstream). The symptoms of endocarditis include fever and chills from the infection. Other symptoms can result from endocarditis complications, such as septic emboli, which may result in organ damage.

If your doctor suspects infective endocarditis, they will order tests such as a blood culture, a chest x-ray, an ECG, and an echocardiogram. Infective endocarditis can be treated with antibiotics, although surgery may be warranted if the infection is severe. If a leaded pacemaker or defibrillator becomes infected, all the hardware will need to be removed, and the patient will be treated for at least 6 weeks with antibiotics. A temporary pacemaker and/or wearable defibrillator may be required to tide the patient over until the infection is resolved.

Removal of pacemaker or defibrillator leads is performed via a procedure called a *laser lead extraction.* This procedure should be performed at a specialized center by a doctor with extensive extraction experience and with open heart surgery backup immediately available, since a complication such as the tear of the heart or blood vessel can be fatal unless immediate surgical treatment is available. If you need this procedure, ask your doctor about their personal experience with this procedure, including the risk of complications.

Myocarditis

Myocarditis is inflammation of the muscular tissue of the heart (or myocardium). Myocarditis can be caused by an autoimmune disease (such as systemic lupus erythematosus, see Chap. 45), bacteria, viruses, a parasite, or even some medications.

Infectious myocarditis is most commonly caused by viruses but can also be caused by bacteria and fungi. Some common viruses involved include coxsackievirus (the virus responsible for hand-foot-mouth disease, seen most commonly in children), adenovirus, hepatitis C, and cytomegalovirus. Chagas disease (more common in Mexico, Central America, and South America) is caused by the parasite *Trypanosoma cruzi* (usually through a bite from the blood-sucking triatomine bug) and is an important cause of ventricular tachycardia and sudden death.

Symptoms of myocarditis vary based on the part of the heart involved, the extent of involvement, and the cause of the inflammation. Some symptoms can include fatigue, muscle aches, chest pain, heart failure, and heartbeat changes. If your doctor suspects myocarditis, they will run some tests that might include blood work, ECG, chest x-ray, echocardiogram, or an MRI. A definitive diagnosis can be made by an endomyocardial biopsy, but a diagnosis can also be made based on clinical criteria.

Treatment for myocarditis depends on the cause and severity of the inflammation. Treatment targets both the cause and the effects of myocarditis on the heart and body (i.e., heart failure and arrhythmia symptoms). If severe, surgical interventions can be necessary. Chagas disease, for example, may require antiparasitic medications, heart failure medications, and even an implantable defibrillator.

Pericarditis

Pericarditis refers to inflammation of the pericardium, which is the membrane surrounding the heart. There are many causes of pericarditis, including infection, metabolic disorders, cancers, rheumatic diseases, and gastrointestinal diseases. Infectious causes of pericarditis occur when a pathogen (most commonly a virus) infects the pericardium. If symptoms can be controlled, the exact cause of pericarditis does not often need to be identified.

Symptoms of pericarditis can include fever and chest pain. The chest pain may be sharp or dull, and it may worsen with deep breaths and improve with leaning forward. When your doctor listens to your heart, they may hear a friction rub, which is an abnormal heart sound (that sounds like the rubbing from sandpaper). The testing for pericarditis includes blood tests, ECG, chest x-ray, and echocardiogram.

Treatment for pericarditis aims to control symptoms and reduce inflammation. Pain control can include aspirin, nonsteroidal anti-inflammatory medications (such as ibuprofen), or colchicine, which is also used to treat gout. If the cause of pericarditis is identified, treatment can be tailored to the underlying cause. Rarely, the amount of fluid inside the pericardium can build up and put extensive pressure on the heart, causing the walls of the right atrium and/or right ventricle to collapse, which prevents blood from filling into the heart. This is called *cardiac tamponade*. It can be the result of an underlying disease (such as cancer or an infection), a tear in a blood vessel, or perforation of the heart (cardiac perforation). The latter may be a rare complication from a heart procedure (such as an electrophysiology study, pacemaker or defibrillator implant, cardiac catheterization/stenting/TAVR procedure, or cardiac catheter ablation), or the result of trauma such as a fall, fight, or car accident.

When this occurs, it requires immediate treatment with intravenous fluids, supportive care with medications, and an emergent procedure either performed with a needle (*pericardiocentesis*) or the creation of a surgical window (*pericardial window*) to drain the fluid out of the pericardium. Often, a tube is left in the pericardium for a few days to permit further drainage and prevent fluid buildup. This tube is eventually removed.

Heart Disease and Infections (Including COVID-19)

Heart disease can limit your body's ability to fight off infections. For example, research has shown that the common influenza affects patients with heart disease more severely than those without heart disease. For this reason, patients with heart disease should stay up to date with vaccinations and be cautious with their exposures.

A recent example of this increased vulnerability is the COVID-19 pandemic caused by the SARS-CoV-2 virus. Between March and June 2020, the Long Island Heart Rhythm Center (Dr. Cohen's clinic) had seven patients test positive for COVID-19 or be diagnosed clinically with the disease. The Centers for Disease Control and Prevention reports that patients with heart conditions, such as heart failure, coronary artery disease, cardiomyopathy, or hypertension, are at a higher risk of severe illness from COVID-19. This respiratory virus can place severe strain on the cardiovascular system and may cause the following: heart failure (either indirectly from the stress of the infection on the cardiovascular system, or directly by infecting the heart muscle and causing myocarditis), heart rhythm problems (cardiac arrhythmias), and result in a heart damage (a heart attack), to name a few.

Current treatment for these conditions includes supportive measures (such as oxygen, pressor support, placing the patient prone, and treating the cardiac condition) and may include drugs such as dexamethasone and remdesivir when indicated. Additional medical treatments are needed to help improve the prognosis of those severely affected by this illness. These treatments are evolving, so please check with your healthcare professional to determine the best way to treat cardiac COVID-19 effects. Figure 55.1 shows Dr. Cohen wearing an N-95 mask during COVID-19 pandemic while operating in the hospital. Table 55.1 reviews some facts about infections of the heart.

Fig. 55.1 Dr. Todd Cohen
wearing an N-95 mask
while operating in the
hospital during the
COVID-19 pandemic

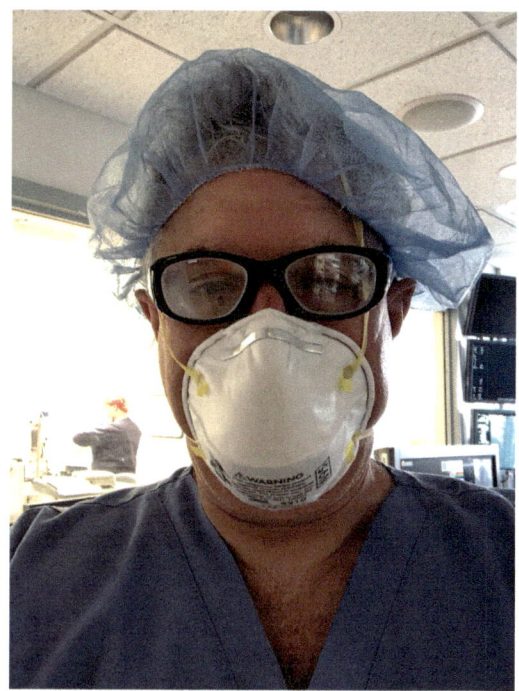

Table 55.1   Facts about infections of the heart

Infections of the heart are rare but potentially serious.
Endocarditis is an infection of the endocardium, the lining of the heart valves and chambers.
Myocarditis is an infection of the myocardium, the muscular tissue of the heart.
Pericarditis is inflammation of the pericardium, the surrounding membrane of the heart.
Underlying heart disease can limit your body's immune response to fight off other infections.
Symptoms of these infections vary but can include fever, chills, muscle aches, or chest pain.
Chagas disease is caused by a parasite, more common in Mexico, Central America, and South
America, and can result in heart failure and ventricular tachycardia. An implantable defibrillator
may help prevent sudden death.
COVID-19 can affect the heart either directly or indirectly and can cause heart attacks and
myocarditis.

Correction to: Surviving and Thriving With Heart Disease

Todd J. Cohen and Roger S. Blumenthal

Correction to:
T. J. Cohen, R. S. Blumenthal (eds.), *Surviving and Thriving*
With Heart Disease, **Contemporary Cardiology,**
https://doi.org/10.1007/978-3-032-00579-3

This book was inadvertently published with incorrect author details for all the chapters in the FM and chapter opening pages. In addition, the city and author information was missing in the Preface content. The caption for Figure 42.1 was incorrectly captured with courtesy information "Figure drawn by Aidan Conway". This has been updated in this corrected version.

The updated version of this book can be found at
https://doi.org/10.1007/978-3-032-00579-3

Appendix A: When an Electrophysiology Study Is Appropriate

1. To evaluate specific heart rhythm abnormalities (arrhythmias) such as slow heart rhythms (bradycardias) and fast heart rhythms (tachycardias).
2. To treat heart rhythm abnormalities and assess therapies including heart rhythm drugs, for catheter ablation therapy, to assess heart rhythm surgery, and to determine the need for a pacemaker or defibrillator.
3. To evaluate events or symptoms suggesting heart rhythm abnormalities, including cardiac arrest, loss of consciousness (syncope) of unknown etiology with data pointing towards a heart-related cardiac diagnosis, and unexplained palpitations.
4. To evaluate risk of rapid heart rhythms from the lower chambers of the heart (ventricular tachycardia or ventricular fibrillation).

Note: Be sure to talk with your doctor about any terms you do not completely understand.

Source: Homoud, M. K. (2020). Invasive diagnostic cardiac electrophysiology studies. In B. C. Downey (Ed.), *UpToDate*. Retrieved from http://www.uptodate.com//home

T. J. Cohen, R. S. Blumenthal (eds.), *Surviving and Thriving With Heart Disease*, Contemporary Cardiology, https://doi.org/10.1007/978-3-032-00579-3

Appendix B: When an Implantable Permanent Pacemaker Is Appropriate

1. In general, irreversible slow heart rhythm abnormalities that correlate with significant symptoms. This includes sinus node dysfunction, acquired high-grade heart block (see book for details). Talk with your doctor about the necessity of a pacemaker for the following additional conditions, since they may recommend it:
2. Symptomatic Mobitz type I (Wenckebach) second-degree atrioventricular block, Mobitz type II second-degree atrioventricular block, or third-degree atrioventricular block/complete heart block; physicians may still recommend a pacemaker even without symptoms in those instances.
3. Chronic bifascicular block with syncope of unknown etiology and severe conduction disease on an EP study.
4. Hypersensitive carotid sinus syndrome and neurocardiogenic syncope.
5. Prevention and termination of atrial arrhythmias (when other therapies fail).

Note: It is important for your doctor to correlate your symptoms with your slow heart rate, and that the doctor makes sure the problem is irreversible. If it is not clear that you need a pacemaker, long-term monitoring (either with an external or implantable cardiac monitor) can help with correlating your symptoms to the heart rhythm problem and determine whether a pacemaker will be helpful. Be sure to talk with your doctor about any terms you do not completely understand.

Source: Link, M. S. (2020). Permanent cardiac pacing: Overview of devices and indications. In B. C. Downey (Ed.), *UpToDate*. Retrieved from http://www.uptodate.com/contents/permanent-cardiac-pacing-overview-of-devices-and-indications

T. J. Cohen, R. S. Blumenthal (eds.), *Surviving and Thriving With Heart Disease*, Contemporary Cardiology, https://doi.org/10.1007/978-3-032-00579-3

Appendix C: When an Implantable Cardioverter Defibrillator Is Appropriate

1. Secondary prevention (after an event such as cardiac arrest from ventricular tachycardia or ventricular fibrillation) or in a patient with risk factors such as nonsustained ventricular tachycardia and a prior heart attack who has inducible sustained ventricular tachycardia.
2. Primary prevention (prior to an event, also called *prophylactic*) in those who have high risk conditions such as a prior heart attack (at least 40 days ago) and ejection fraction of 30% or less, moderate to severe heart failure, familial sudden death syndromes such as Brugada syndrome and arrhythmogenic right ventricular cardiomyopathy/dysplasia (ARVC/D), noncompaction of the left ventricle, hypertrophic cardiomyopathy, long QT syndrome, cardiac sarcoidosis, catecholaminergic polymorphic ventricular tachycardia, and in high risk patients with advanced heart failure as a bridge to cardiac transplantation.

Note: Be sure to talk with your doctor about any terms you do not completely understand.

Source: Ganz, L. I. (2019). Implantable cardioverter-defibrillators: Overview of indications, components, and functions. In B. C. Downey (Ed.), *UpToDate*. Retrieved from http://www.uptodate.com/contents/implantable-cardioverter-defibrillators-overview-of-indications-components-and-functions

Appendix D: When Biventricular Therapy Is Appropriate

1. A combination of reasons, including each of the following: Moderate to severe heart failure despite treatment with optimal medical therapy, unless the patient cannot tolerate these medications, a left ventricular ejection fraction of 35% or less, and a wide QRS complex on ECG (bundle branch block pattern).
2. A combination including each of the following: asymptomatic or mild heart failure on optimal medical therapy, a left ventricular ejection fraction of 30% or less, and a wide QRS complex on ECG.
3. If standard right ventricular pacing occurs all the time (pacer dependent) in order to prevent or treat heart failure/symptoms and improve the ejection fraction, or following ablation of the AV junction in which right ventricular pacing occurs all the time (pacemaker dependent)

Note: Be sure to talk with your doctor about any terms you do not completely understand.

Sources: Adelstein, E., Saba, S. (2019). Cardiac resynchronization therapy in heart failure: Indications. In S. B. Yeon (Ed.), *UpToDate*. Retrieved from http://www.uptodate.com//home

T. J. Cohen, R. S. Blumenthal (eds.), *Surviving and Thriving With Heart Disease*, Contemporary Cardiology, https://doi.org/10.1007/978-3-032-00579-3

Appendix E: When a Stent Is Appropriate

1. Symptomatic blockage in a coronary (heart) artery that is amenable to the placement of stent(s) in order to open up the artery and maintain coronary artery flow.
2. The above indication involving single or two-vessel coronary artery disease. Occasionally, an experienced operator may tackle more complicated anatomy (more blockages) with the availability of cardiac surgery backup.

Talk to your doctor about the risks, benefits, and alternatives of stenting, coronary artery bypass surgery, and/or medical therapy. Remember to ask questions.

Sources: Cutlip, D., Levin, T. (2020). Revascularization in patients with stable coronary artery disease: Coronary artery bypass graft surgery versus percutaneous coronary intervention. G. M. Saperia (Ed.), *UpToDate*. Retrieved from http://www.uptodate.com//home

T. J. Cohen, R. S. Blumenthal (eds.), *Surviving and Thriving With Heart Disease*, Contemporary Cardiology, https://doi.org/10.1007/978-3-032-00579-3

Appendix F: When a TAVR or Valve Replacement Is Appropriate

1. Valve repair or replacement is appropriate when the patient has severe and/or critical aortic stenosis with symptoms (chest pain, shortness of breath and fatigue), lightheadedness or dizziness, and/or syncope and is not high-risk for open heart surgery. 2. TAVR may be beneficial in symptomatic and severe aortic stenosis with a significant surgical risk. The FDA has approved TAVR for patients who have a low surgical risk as well. Please talk to your doctor, regarding the risks, benefits, and alternatives of this procedure.

Shared decision-making is needed between the treating physician and implanting physician.

Sources: Gaasch, W. H. (2020). Indications for valve replacement in aortic stenosis in adults. S. B. Yeon (Ed.), *UpToDate*. Retrieved from http://www.uptodate.com//home

https://www.onlinejacc.org/content/75/10/1208 (FDA approval)

T. J. Cohen, R. S. Blumenthal (eds.), *Surviving and Thriving With Heart Disease*, Contemporary Cardiology, https://doi.org/10.1007/978-3-032-00579-3

Appendix G: When a Watchman-Type Device Is Appropriate

1. Atrial fibrillation and high risk of stroke (are above the age 65, have diabetes, high blood pressure or heart failure).
   AND
2. (at least one of the following):
   (a) Recurrent bleeding from anywhere precluding long-term safe use of blood thinners.
       (bleeding from the gastrointestinal tract, intracranial being the most common).
   (b) Persistent fall risk (such as old age, neurological condition)
   (c) Lifestyle that increases the risk of trauma and bleeding

Shared decision-making is needed between the treating physician and implanting physician.
Sources: Hijazi, Z. M., Saw, J., (2020). Atrial fibrillation: Left atrial appendage occlusion. G. M. Saperia (Ed.), *UpToDate*. Retrieved from http://www.uptodate.com//home

T. J. Cohen, R. S. Blumenthal (eds.), *Surviving and Thriving With Heart Disease*, Contemporary Cardiology, https://doi.org/10.1007/978-3-032-00579-3

Appendix H: When a Heart Transplant Is Appropriate

1. A patient with persistent New York Heart Association (NYHA) functional class IV heart failure symptoms despite treatment with medications and/or cardiac resynchronization therapy (CRT). Patients with life-threatening arrhythmias that do not respond to medications, procedures to correct the rhythm, surgery, and/or implantable devices can also be considered.
   AND
2. Age less than 65 years of age with no terminal or other life-threatening illness or infection.

This is complex decision made with your heart failure physician, surgeon, and transplant team. Factors include your mental and physical condition, comorbid conditions, and the availability of a suitable donor.

Sources: Mancini, D. (2020). Heart transplantation in adults: Indications and contraindications. S. B. Yeon (Ed.), *UpToDate*. Retrieved from http://www.uptodate.com//home

T. J. Cohen, R. S. Blumenthal (eds.), *Surviving and Thriving With Heart Disease*, Contemporary Cardiology, https://doi.org/10.1007/978-3-032-00579-3

Appendix I: Know Your Numbers

Use this page as a comprehensive means to track your heart health metrics. Maintaining thorough documentation of your numbers compared to normal ranges can be very helpful for identifying changes over time.

T. J. Cohen, R. S. Blumenthal (eds.), *Surviving and Thriving With Heart Disease*, Contemporary Cardiology, https://doi.org/10.1007/978-3-032-00579-3

	BP	Weight	BMI	HR	Fasting Blood Glucose	HbA1C	Total Cholesterol	HDL	LDL	Triglycerides	EF
Normal Values	Less than 120/80 mmHg		18.5–24.9	60–100 bpm	Less than 100 mg/dL	Less than 5.7%	Less than 200 mg/dl	60 mg/dl or higher	100 mg/dl or lower	Less than 150 mg/dl	50–70%
Date:											
Date:											
Date:											
Date:											
Date:											
Date:											
Date:											
Date:											

Appendix J: Surviving and Thriving Card

Below is your Surviving and Thriving Card. This gift to you provides a means for keeping your essential medical information in one place (the "Plan B" side) as well as tracking your progress ("Knowing Your Numbers" side). Cut it out and then fill it out! You can also access copies from my practice's website at: www.liheart-rhythmcenter.com, where you can create as many Surviving and Thriving Cards as you like! Keep them in an easily available spot such as your wallet, purse, or glove compartment. You can also have a copy on your smartphone (just keep it private and secure—i.e., password protected. This card can serve as a backup when you cannot access your electronic medical record through your portal (Fig. A1).

T. J. Cohen, R. S. Blumenthal (eds.), *Surviving and Thriving With Heart Disease*, Contemporary Cardiology, https://doi.org/10.1007/978-3-032-00579-3

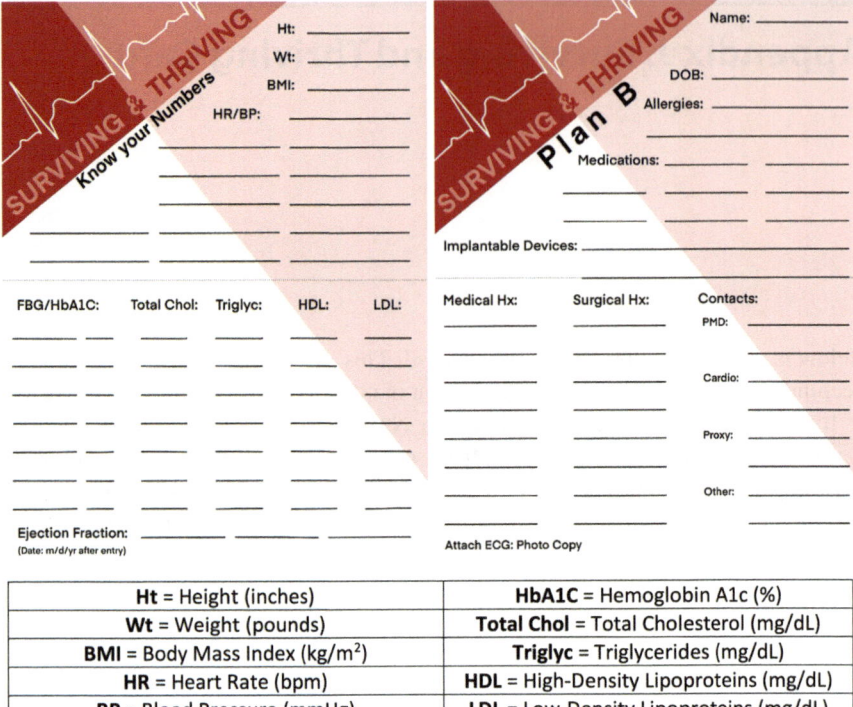

Ht = Height (inches)	HbA1C = Hemoglobin A1c (%)
Wt = Weight (pounds)	Total Chol = Total Cholesterol (mg/dL)
BMI = Body Mass Index (kg/m^2)	Triglyc = Triglycerides (mg/dL)
HR = Heart Rate (bpm)	HDL = High-Density Lipoproteins (mg/dL)
BP = Blood Pressure (mmHg)	LDL = Low-Density Lipoproteins (mg/dL)
FBG = Fasting Blood Glucose (mg/dL)	Ejection Fraction (%)

Fig. A1 Reduced image of your "Surviving and Thriving" Card. The card has two sides and contains your essential medical information ("Plan B" side), and a mechanism to track your numbers ("Know Your Numbers" side). Appendix J is your actual card that you should cut out, fill out, and keep with you, together with a copy of your ECG. Keep them in your wallet, purse, glove compartment, or any other easily available place. You can also make copies by accessing my practice's website at www.liheartrhythmcenter.com

Appendix K: Additional Information on Diets Discussed in Chapter 39

Adapting a new diet can be an intimidating undertaking, but these sample meal suggestions can get you started off on the right foot.

Diet	Breakfast	Lunch	Dinner	Snack
DASH	Oatmeal with fruit	Tuna salad	Whole wheat spaghetti, Caesar salad	Nuts, fat free Greek yogurt
Mediterranean	Greek yogurt with fruit	Vegetable soup with a whole grain roll	Roasted chicken & sautéed vegetables	Apple slices with almond butter
Ornish	Scrambled egg whites with side of berries	Vegetarian chili & corn bread	Salmon & quinoa salad	Hummus & sliced vegetables
Weight Watchers	Yogurt with granola & honey	Tomato, hummus & chicken sandwich	Vegetable stir fry	Banana with peanut butter
Sugar Busters	Vegetable omelet	Baked salmon with brown rice and broccoli	Southwest salad with grilled chicken	Assorted nuts
American Heart Association Diet	Avocado whole grain toast	Turkey burger with a side salad	Baked fish with brown rice and roasted asparagus	Fruit smoothie

Food Journal

Tracking your progress with your heart-healthy diet can help sustain these positive changes long term. Use the chart below to record your food intake and stay on track with eating healthy.

T. J. Cohen, R. S. Blumenthal (eds.), *Surviving and Thriving With Heart Disease*, Contemporary Cardiology, https://doi.org/10.1007/978-3-032-00579-3

Week 1

	Monday	Tuesday	Wednesday	Thursday	Friday	Saturday	Sunday
Breakfast							
Lunch							
Dinner							
Snacks							

Week 2

	Monday	Tuesday	Wednesday	Thursday	Friday	Saturday	Sunday
Breakfast							
Lunch							
Dinner							
Snacks							

Week 3

	Monday	Tuesday	Wednesday	Thursday	Friday	Saturday	Sunday
Breakfast							
Lunch							
Dinner							
Snacks							

Week 4

	Monday	Tuesday	Wednesday	Thursday	Friday	Saturday	Sunday
Breakfast							
Lunch							
Dinner							
Snacks							

Appendix L: Additional Information on Exercises Discussed in Chapter 39

If you're looking to begin an exercise regimen and are not sure where to start, use the following information as a starting point for ideas on ways to be active and how to track your progress. The American Heart Association recommends getting at least 150 minutes of moderate-intensity aerobic activity or 75 minutes of vigorous aerobic activity per week. This could mean exercising for 30 minutes of moderate-intensity exercise, 5 times a week, or 25 minutes of vigorous aerobic activity, 3 times a week.

Exercise type	Moderate vs. Vigorous intensity	Special notes
Brisk Walking	Moderate	Brisk pace is considered at least 2.5 mph
Biking	Moderate	Moderate intensity is considered biking under 10 mph
General Gardening	Moderate	Considered raking, trimming shrubs, etc.
Water Aerobics	Moderate	Great option for anyone with joint issues
Running	Vigorous	Be sure to properly stretch before and after to avoid muscle strain
Swimming	Vigorous	Great option for anyone with joint issues
Biking	Vigorous	To be considered vigorous exercise, needs to be at a pace over 10 mph
Aerobic Dancing	Vigorous	Examples include Zumba, Jazzercise, Masala Bhangra, and ballroom dancing
Jumping Rope	Vigorous	Great way to quickly burn calories

My Weekly Exercise Tracker:

Week 1

	Monday	Tuesday	Wednesday	Thursday	Friday	Saturday	Sunday
Exercise Type:							
Minutes:							
Total			Total Weekly Minutes of Exercise: _____				

T. J. Cohen, R. S. Blumenthal (eds.), *Surviving and Thriving With Heart Disease*, Contemporary Cardiology, https://doi.org/10.1007/978-3-032-00579-3

Week 2

	Monday	Tuesday	Wednesday	Thursday	Friday	Saturday	Sunday
Exercise Type:							
Minutes:							
Total		Total Weekly Minutes of Exercise: _____					

Week 3

	Monday	Tuesday	Wednesday	Thursday	Friday	Saturday	Sunday
Exercise Type:							
Minutes:							
Total		Total Weekly Minutes of Exercise: _____					

Week 4

	Monday	Tuesday	Wednesday	Thursday	Friday	Saturday	Sunday
Exercise Type:							
Minutes:							
Total		Total Weekly Minutes of Exercise: _____					

Glossary

Ablation A procedure performed to get rid of, treat, and potentially cure a heart rhythm problem. See also *catheter ablation*.

Accessory pathway An extra electrical connection between the atrium and ventricle, in addition to the AV node.

Acetylsalicylic acid (aspirin) An antiplatelet medication useful in preventing and treating a heart attack (myocardial infarction). Also, part of a regimen used after stent placement.

Active compression-decompression CPR A technique of CPR that uses a suction cup-type device to compress and decompress the chest and is approved as an alternative to standard CPR. The technique was coinvented by Dr. Todd Cohen.

Alcohol A direct and indirect toxin to the heart that can in excess cause atrial fibrillation, cardiomyopathy, and holiday heart (ventricular tachycardia and fibrillation with binge drinking). Beverages such as beer, liquor, and wine are best consumed in moderation.

Alcohol septal ablation A catheterization procedure in which alcohol is infused in a septal coronary artery branch to relieve the outflow tract obstruction seen in some forms of hypertrophic cardiomyopathy. See also *hypertrophic cardiomyopathy*.

Aldosterone A hormone produced by the adrenal glands that plays a critical role in regulating the levels of salt and water in the body and, therefore, influences blood pressure.

Alpha-blocker A type of medication that blocks the alpha-adrenergic receptor. This medication may be used to treat high blood pressure, Raynaud disease, and benign prostatic hypertrophy (BPH). Medications may have both alpha- and beta-blocker properties and may be used to treat heart failure as well as high blood pressure.

Alpha-glucosidase inhibitors A class of antidiabetic drugs used in the treatment of type 2 diabetes that act by stopping enzymes that breakdown carbohydrates in the small intestine. This slows down the breakdown of carbohydrate and allows the carbohydrates to enter the blood more slowly from the digestive tract thus preventing high blood sugar. Examples include acarbose (Precose) and miglitol (Glyset).

© The Editor(s) (if applicable) and The Author(s), under exclusive license to Springer Nature Switzerland AG 2025
T. J. Cohen, R. S. Blumenthal (eds.), *Surviving and Thriving With Heart Disease*, Contemporary Cardiology, https://doi.org/10.1007/978-3-032-00579-3

American College of Cardiology Support group for cardiology-related individuals and their patients. www.acc.org

American Heart Association Support group for patients and families related to heart disease. www.heart.org

American Red Cross Global support group for disaster relief and learning CPR. www.redcross.org

Amigo™ A robotic system invented by Dr. Todd Cohen used for cardiac catheter ablation.

Amiodarone A drug used to treat heart rhythm problems such as atrial fibrillation, atrial flutter, ventricular tachycardia, and ventricular fibrillation. Usually viewed as the strongest and most effective medication with the most side effects (can affect the eyes, skin, lungs, liver, and thyroid).

Amyloidosis A disease in which a protein called amyloid builds up in the heart and other organs. It can cause restrictive cardiomyopathy. See also *cardiomyopathy, restrictive cardiomyopathy*.

Anesthesia A state of controlled, temporary loss of sensation or awareness that is induced by certain medications for medical purposes.

Angioplasty A procedure in which a balloon catheter is placed into a coronary artery to open up a blocked blood vessel. See also *percutaneous coronary intervention*.

Angiotensin-converting enzyme inhibitor (ACE inhibitor) A medication used to treat high blood pressure and treat or prevent heart failure.

Angiotensin II receptor blocker (ARB) A medication used to treat high blood pressure and treat or prevent heart failure.

Angiotensin receptor-neprilysin inhibitor (ARNI) A class of medication used to treat heart failure. May be preferable to either an ACE inhibitor or an ARB in the treatment of mild to moderate heart failure.

Angina A condition in which the heart is deprived of oxygen and may be manifested by chest, arm, throat, back, and/or abdominal pain or discomfort and shortness of breath.

Annuloplasty A procedure to tighten or reinforce the ring (annulus) around a valve in the heart.

Antiarrhythmic drugs or medications A type of drug or medication that may affect special channels within the cells (often sodium or potassium channels). These medications may be quite potent and often have the side effect of proarrhythmia, in which a worse heart rhythm problem, such as ventricular tachycardia, may occur.

Anticoagulant Blood thinner used to prevent clot formation and stroke. This medication includes the oral version called warfarin (Coumadin) and the intravenous or subcutaneous injectable heparin (low-molecular-weight heparin).

Antiplatelet drugs A class of drugs that interfere with the aggregation of platelets (i.e., make your blood cells less "sticky") to prevent the formation of cholesterol plaques (atherosclerosis), blood clots, heart attacks, and strokes. See also *acetylsalicylic acid, clopidogrel, platelets*.

Antitachycardia pacing Pacing stimulation techniques for termination of tachyarrhythmias. May be automatically applied by an ICD and has the ability to painlessly terminate ventricular tachycardia. See also *defibrillator, tachycardia, ventricular tachycardia.*

Aortogram A minimally invasive procedure that uses a catheter to inject contrast medium into the aorta to visualize the aortic root, coronary artery origins, and other blood vessels, such as the left common carotid artery, left subclavian artery, and brachiocephalic artery.

Aortic aneurysm A weakness in the wall of the aorta which dilates and balloons out. Can be a precursor to aortic dissection.

Aortic dissection A rip or tear in the wall of the aorta that can result in a life-threatening bleed.

Aortic regurgitation A leaky aortic valve, which can put increased stress on the left ventricle. Significant aortic regurgitation can result in heart failure symptoms.

Aortic stenosis Narrowing of the aortic valve that results in a decrease in cardiac output from the heart. Symptoms include syncope (loss of consciousness), heart failure, and angina.

Aortic valve The valve that directs blood flow from the left lower chamber of the heart (left ventricle) to the rest of your body.

Apolipoproteins A particle that carries cholesterol particles in the blood and influences how cholesterol particles are cleared from tissues and blood. May be associated with the development of vascular disease (and eventually heart disease).

Apple Watch A form of wearable technology capable of recording an ECG and more recently oxygen saturation. May be useful in detecting atrial fibrillation and guiding fitness. Series 4 or greater can record your ECG, and Series 6 or greater can also record your oxygen saturation.

Arrhythmia A condition in which the heart beats in an irregular or abnormal rhythm.

Arrhythmogenic right ventricular dysplasia (also called arrhythmogenic right ventricular cardiomyopathy, arrhythmogenic right ventricular cardiomyopathy/dysplasia, arrhythmogenic right ventricular dysplasia/cardiomyopathy, ARVD, ARVC, ARVC/D, or ARVD/C) A hereditary condition in which fat is deposited in the heart, typically in the right ventricle. Patients with this condition are predisposed to ventricular tachycardia.

Asystole A markedly slow heart rhythm (bradycardia) in which the heartbeat pauses for a prolonged period, usually much longer than 6 seconds.

Assist devices Also known as mechanical circulatory support; pumps which can be installed in the heart and aid the patient in properly pumping blood from the heart. May be used for both short-term and long-term use. Also, may be left, right, and biventricular assist devices.

Asthma A chronic inflammatory disease of the airway in which there is reversible airway hyperreactivity causing the airway to narrow. A form of chronic obstructive pulmonary disease (COPD).

Atherosclerosis Fat and calcium deposits inside blood vessel walls that lead to plaques and coronary artery disease. Diabetes, high blood pressure, smoking, and high cholesterol all contribute to blood vessel wall damage and subsequent plaque formation. Disruption or erosion of these plaques may lead to a heart attack (myocardial infarction). See also *myocardial infarction*.

Atria The upper chambers of the heart. There is a right and a left atrium.

Atrial fibrillation A very fast and irregular abnormal heart rhythm coming from the upper chambers of the heart (atria). Atrial fibrillation is often caused by triggers from within the pulmonary veins.

Atrial flutter An organized or regular fast heart rhythm coming from the upper chambers of the heart (atria).

Atrial septal defect (ASD) A hole in the interatrial septum in the upper chambers of the heart between the right and left atria. If significant in size, may require closure either surgically or percutaneously with a medical device.

Autoimmune disorder A disorder in which a person's immune system labels its own body cells as foreign and attacks them, causing inflammation. May affect any organ or organ system, and to date, there are over 80 types of classified autoimmune diseases. See also *connective tissue disorder*.

Automatic external defibrillator (AED) An external device, about the size of a lunch box, that is used to treat sudden cardiac arrest by shocking ventricular tachycardia or ventricular fibrillation. Patches are placed on the patient's chest, and the device provides audible prompts guiding the operator through a number of steps resulting in a shock (defibrillation) if necessary. These devices should be readily available in public places, such as planes, stadiums, churches, temples, museums, and schools. See also *defibrillator, ventricular fibrillation, ventricular tachycardia*.

Autonomic nervous system A part of the human nervous system that acts unconsciously and is responsible for respiratory rate, heart rate, digestion, sexual arousal, pupillary response, and urination. This system is responsible for the fight-or-flight response. See also *dysautonomia*.

AV node A part of the heart's wiring system, which creates a delay for the electrical signal as it leaves the atria and conducts to the ventricles.

AV node reentry A rapid rhythm involving an extra connection in the middle of the heart (the AV node).

Bariatric surgery Surgeries that involve making changes to your digestive system to aid in weight loss, especially when lifestyle modifications (e.g., diet and exercise) have proven to be unsuccessful.

Bempedoic acid An alternative or synergistic acting drug to statins that act to reduce cholesterol levels in the bloodstream by blocking cholesterol synthesis.

Beta-blocker A type of medication used to lower blood pressure, slow down a rapid heart rhythm, and prevent and treat heart failure and ischemia (the lack of blood flow to the heart). This medication blocks the beta-adrenergic receptor.

Bias An overt or covert influence on how one reacts to patient differences. Important for healthcare providers to be aware of, in order to optimize medical care to all groups of patients.

Bifascicular block A condition in which two of the three major fascicles of the heart's conduction system are blocked. These fascicles include the left anterior and posterior fascicles of the left bundle branch, and the right bundle branch, which is considered a single fascicle.

Biguanides An antidiabetic drug used to manage type 2 diabetes by helping control blood sugar by decreasing the absorption of sugar from the intestines, decreasing the liver production of glucose, and improving the cell's sensitivity to insulin. May also help with weight loss. Example includes metformin.

Bile acid High cholesterol fats produced in the body that help with absorbing fat from food.

Bile acid resins A class of drugs that bind to fats specifically bile acids thus facilitating their removal from the body. This allows for a lower level of cholesterol in the body, and thus, more cholesterol is used for essential cell function and slower development of atherosclerosis. May result in vitamin deficiencies. Examples include cholestyramine and colesevelam.

Bioprosthetic valve A replacement valve made from animal structures such as cows (bovine) or pigs (porcine).

Biventricular device A device that paces (stimulates) both ventricles of the heart to improve its performance. This is also called cardiac resynchronization therapy (CRT) or biventricular pacing. See also *cardiac resynchronization therapy*.

Blalock-Taussig shunt A surgical procedure, invented at Johns Hopkins Hospital by Helen Taussig, Alfred Blalock, and Vivian Thomas, in order to treat tetralogy of Fallot. Also called the blue baby operation.

BNP (brain natriuretic peptide or B-type natriuretic peptide) Blood level is useful in determining the presence of heart failure.

Body mass index (BMI) This index can be used as an indicator of body fat. It is derived by one of the following formulas:

Using the metric system

BMI (kg/m^2) = weight in kilograms $\div$ (height in meters)^2

Using the English system

BMI (kg/m^2) = weight in pounds $\times$ 703 $\div$ (height in inches)^2

Bradycardia A slow heart rhythm, typically fewer than 60 beats per minute. Bradycardias may be significant when the heart rate is lower than 40 beats per minute, especially if the patient is symptomatic.

Brugada syndrome A hereditary condition in which there are specific electrocardiographic findings and patients are at risk for sudden cardiac arrest. These high-risk patients can benefit from an implantable defibrillator.

Buddhify App that helps with mindfulness; see www.buddhify.com.

Bundle branch block A condition diagnosed by an abnormal finding on the ECG, in which there is disease in at least one of the electrical branches that send electricity to the lower chambers of the heart. Typically, there is a right and a left bundle branch, and when a block or a delay occurs in either electrical structure, significant conduction disease may be present. An EP study may be useful in elucidating the amount of conduction disease.

Bupropion An antidepressant that is also effective at smoking cessation by decreasing nicotine cravings.

Calcification The accumulation of calcium salts into body tissue which can cause the tissue to harden.

Calcium channel blockers A type of medication that blocks the calcium channel and can cause a slow heart rate and a drop in blood pressure. It can be used to control rapid rhythms from the upper chambers (supraventricular tachycardia). See also *verapamil, diltiazem.*

Cardiac catheterization A procedure in which a catheter (tube) is placed within the heart for diagnostic and/or therapeutic purposes. See also *coronary angiography, percutaneous coronary intervention, stent.*

Cardiac magnetic resonance imaging (MRI) A noninvasive procedure that may be used to visualize the heart and its surrounding structures.

Cardiac output The amount of blood pumped out of the heart in liters per minute. An indication of the strength of the heart along with the ejection fraction. See also *ejection fraction.*

Cardiac resynchronization therapy (CRT) The therapy provided by a biventricular pacing device. The timing of right and left ventricular pacing is performed to provide a more uniform (synchronous) ventricular contraction. See also *biventricular device.*

Cardiac tamponade A compression that results when fluid builds up in the sac around the heart to the point that blood flow is impeded; the patient may have a potentially life-threatening drop in blood pressure, requiring abrupt removal of the fluid either by a needle or creation of a surgical pericardial window to relieve the tension. Cardiac tamponade may be the result of a perforation either from a needle, device wire or lead, or a heart catheter. In any case, emergency care is necessary to promptly treat this problem. See also *pericardial effusion, pericardiocentesis, pericardial window.*

Cardiac transplantation (heart transplantation) A complicated surgical procedure in which a diseased heart is replaced by a healthy heart from a recently deceased patient.

Cardiologist A doctor who specializes in the heart.

CardioMEMS™ HF System A remote monitoring system for treating heart failure, which remotely monitors pulmonary artery pressures. The system is manufactured by Abbott Cardiovascular and has been shown to decrease heart failure admissions.

Cardiomyopathy A weak heart muscle. This might be caused by various conditions, including but not limited to coronary artery disease (possibly including a heart attack), high blood pressure, valve disease, chemotherapy / radiation treatment, pregnancy, alcohol, hereditary conditions, infections, infiltrative conditions, and otherwise unknown causes.

Cardiopulmonary resuscitation (CPR) A method of chest compressions and mouth-to-mouth ventilation to help resuscitate an unconscious patient in cardiac arrest.

Cardioversion A procedure performed to convert an abnormal heart rhythm back to a more normal rhythm. This can be performed with drugs (also called pharmacological cardioversion) or with electricity (electric shock, also called electrical cardioversion).

CareLink™ A remote device monitoring service provided by Medtronic Corp.

Catecholamine polymorphic ventricular tachycardia (CPVT) A hereditary condition in which exercise brings out polymorphic ventricular tachycardia and is associated with sudden death.

Catheter ablation A procedure in which a catheter is placed through a vein or artery to map, treat, and potentially cure a heart rhythm abnormality (arrhythmia). See also *ablation*.

CHA2DS2-VASc score A stroke risk score advocated by the American Heart Association, American College of Cardiology, and Heart Rhythm Society. The score gives similar points for the risks of CHADS2 with the following changes: one point for age of 65 years or older, another two points for age of 75 years of older, one point for being female (sex category or Sc), and one point for vascular disease (such as heart attack, peripheral vascular disease, or aortic plaque). A score of 1 for men, or 2 for women, warrants anticoagulation therapy consideration in order to reduce the risk of stroke from atrial fibrillation.

Chagas disease A disease caused by the parasite Trypanosoma cruzi in which the heart can develop a myocarditis. The parasite is transmitted by Triatomine bugs (also called kissing bugs; a type of reduviid bug). It is more common in Mexico, Central America, and South America. It is associated with heart failure, ventricular tachycardia, and sudden death. Treatment includes antiparasitic medications and an implantable defibrillator.

Cholesterol A fatlike substance that is found in all the cells of the body. It is required to make hormones, vitamin D, and helps digest foods. Cholesterol may be further broken down into different types. When a certain type of cholesterol gets inside damaged blood vessels and becomes oxidized, it leads to atherosclerosis. See also *low-density lipoprotein, high-density lipoprotein, atherosclerosis.*

Cholestyramine A medication known as a bile acid sequestrant (also known as *bile acid resin*) used to treat high cholesterol.

Chronic obstructive pulmonary disease Also known as COPD, this is a lung disease that makes it hard to breathe. There are two forms: chronic bronchitis, which involves a long-term cough with mucus, and emphysema, which damages the lungs overtime. Most people have a combination of both. In COPD, the air becomes trapped in the lungs, and people with this condition are unable to fully exhale and experience shortness of breath.

Clopidogrel (Plavix) An antiplatelet medication used with acetylsalicylic acid (aspirin) following stent placement to prevent re-occlusion of the coronary artery.

Coenzyme Q10 A supplement often taken together with a statin, but not recommended by the author on a routine basis.

Coffee A supplement to a heart healthy diet that may be safe up to 5 cups per day. Be careful adding cream and sugar to your diet when enjoying this beverage.

Cognitive behavioral therapy A short-term mental therapy to help change your thought pattern. Useful for depression, anxiety, mental illness, and obsessive-compulsive disorder.

Commissurotomy An open-heart surgery that repairs narrowing of the mitral valve (mitral stenosis). During this surgery, the patient is placed on a heart-lung bypass machine, while the surgeon removes calcium deposits and other scar tissue from the valve leaflets.

Commotio cordis Ventricular tachycardia or fibrillation caused by a projectile hitting the chest during the vulnerable cycle of the heart. Can be treated with a rapid response using an automatic external defibrillator (AED). Can happen with projectile sports such as baseball, hockey, and lacrosse.

Complete heart block (complete AV block or third-degree heart block) A condition in which the electrical activity from the upper chamber cannot conduct down to the lower chamber. All electrical activity from the upper chambers to the lower chambers is completely blocked.

Computerized axial tomography (CT) angiogram A test in which a patient is given contrast dye intravenously and then receives radiation to help doctors visualize the heart, its blood vessels, and surrounding structures. This test is also useful prior to an atrial fibrillation ablation procedure in visualizing the number and configuration of pulmonary veins that attach to the left atrium.

Computer tomography angiography (CT angiography or CTA) A test in which contrast dye is administered to visualize the heart and its coronary arteries and determine whether blockages are present.

Congenital heart disease An inherited heart disorder due to a genetic defect that is present at birth and results in a distortion of cardiac anatomy.

Congestive heart failure (CHF or heart failure) A condition in which the heart fails to perform normally and fluid backs up into the lungs or other parts of the body. The patient may exhibit symptoms of fatigue, shortness of breath, leg swelling, and other forms of fluid accumulation.

Connective tissue A group of specialized cells made up of two proteins, collagen and elastin, that work together to hold the structures of the body together.

Connective tissue disorder Autoimmune disorders that affect elasticity of body tissues and cause pain. May be acquired or inherited and affect multiple body systems, including the heart and cardiovascular system. See also *connective tissue, autoimmunity, Ehlers-Danlos syndrome, Marfan syndrome, systemic lupus erythematosus, scleroderma, polymyositis, Sjogren's syndrome, scurvy.*

Corindus Vascular Robotics A robotic system for performing cardiac catheterization, PCI, and stenting. The system was acquired by Siemens Medical Solutions.

Cor pulmonale A change in right ventricular shape and function as lung (pulmonary) disease.

Coronary arteries Blood vessels to the heart that provide the heart with oxygen and nutrient rich blood.

Coronary artery bypass surgery Also known as coronary artery bypass grafting (CABG), this is an open-heart surgery that uses a healthy blood vessel from the leg, arm, or chest and redirects blood around a section of a blocked artery in the heart. This improves blood flow to the heart muscle.

Coronary artery disease (also known as CAD) When arteries that supply the heart become hardened from cholesterol deposits forming plaques (atherosclerosis).

As the plaque grows blood flow to the heart decreases, which can lead to chest pain (angina), myocardial infarction, heart rhythm abnormalities (arrhythmias), and/or weaken the heart muscle, resulting in heart failure.

Coronary artery dissection A tearing of the wall of a coronary artery which may result in the lack of blood flow to the heart and/or bleeding into the pericardial sac.

Coronary angiography (angiogram) A procedure in which a catheter is placed inside the heart and contrast dye is administered to visualize the coronary arteries.

Cortisol A hormone produced in the adrenal glands in response to low blood sugar and stress. This hormone increases blood sugar, suppresses the immune system, and aids in the metabolism of carbohydrates, fats, and proteins.

COVID-19 A condition caused by the coronavirus SARS-CoV-2, which caused a worldwide pandemic in 2020, associated with fever, cough, loss of smell, pneumonia, myocarditis, and even death.

CPR Cardiopulmonary resuscitation is a technique for providing respiration and circulation to the body during cardiac arrest.

Cyanosis A blue tint to the skin when there is diminished oxygenation of body cells.

Daily yoga A smartphone health application that provides step-by-step images of hundreds of yoga poses.

da Vinci Surgical System A robotic system for performing heart surgery manufactured by Intuitive Surgical Corp. in Sunnyvale, California.

DASH diet Dietary Approaches to Stop Hypertension (DASH) emphasizes foods that are lower in sodium and encourages foods that are rich in potassium, calcium, and magnesium. The diet advocates for plenty of vegetables, fruits, and low-fat dairy products as well as nuts, whole grains, fish, and poultry. Red meat, sweets, processed foods, and sugary beverages are discouraged. It is a low-saturated-fat diet with less than 2300 mg of sodium per day.

Deep venous thrombosis Also known as a DVT, this is a serious condition where a blood clot forms in a vein deep inside the body. DVTs typically form in the thigh or lower leg but can also develop in other areas of the body. Symptoms include leg pain often in the calf, similar to cramping or soreness, warmth to the touch in the affected area, and a swollen, red, or discolored leg on the affected side. It may occur without any noticeable symptoms. The blood clot may travel to the lungs and lead to a life-threatening condition called a pulmonary embolism. See also *pulmonary embolism*.

Defensive patienting The term used to describe how patients should protect their privacy and safety as they enter into medical care. It is analogous to defensive driving.

Defibrillation A procedure in which an electrical shock is delivered to the chest wall or internally to the heart to terminate an abnormally fast heart rhythm (tachycardia).

Defibrillator A device used to shock the patient's heart out of a very rapid rhythm (tachycardia) into a more normal rhythm.

Diabetes Persistently high blood sugar which damages blood vessels, kidneys, eyes, nerves, and extremities over time if not controlled by lifestyle and/or medication. May be diagnosed at a young age from autoimmune disease (Type 1 diabetes) or from the body's inability to respond to insulin (Type 2 diabetes). See also *insulin*.

Diabetic ketoacidosis A life-threatening condition in people with type 1 diabetes who cannot produce their own insulin. In the absence of insulin, glucose cannot enter the cells, and the body begins to produce ketones, products of fat breakdown for energy. It presents with deep labored breathing, excessive thirst, frequent urination, abdominal pain, nausea, vomiting, confusion, weakness, and fruity-scented breath. See also *diabetes*.

Diaphoresis Sweating, especially to a higher degree. It is a common symptom of heart attack (myocardial infarction), along with chest pain that may or may not radiate to the chest, jaw, arms, shoulder blades or back, although abdominal pain or even no pain may occur. Other symptoms include shortness of breath, dizziness, nausea, vomiting, fatigue, palpitations, and even collapse from a heart rhythm problem. Call 911 if you ever experience these symptoms. If an aspirin is available, it is helpful to chew as well. See also *myocardial infarction*.

Diastolic blood pressure Also known as the bottom number; the blood pressure after the heart is finished contracting and is relaxing.

Digitalis A medication that can help strengthen a weak heart in a patient with congestive heart failure. Can also be used to slow down heart rhythm problems such as rapidly conducting atrial fibrillation.

Dilated cardiomyopathy A weakening of the heart muscle in which part or all of the heart muscle dilates. See also *cardiomyopathy*.

Diltiazem A calcium channel blocker that works on both heart muscle and blood vessels. Works to slow down heart rate and rhythm as well as increase blood flow through arteries, thus lowering blood pressure. See also *calcium channel blocker, verapamil*.

DPP-4 inhibitors (dipeptidyl peptidase IV inhibitors) A class of antidiabetic agents used for the treatment of type 2 diabetes that works by preventing GLP-1 from being broken down by inhibiting DPP-4. This allows blood sugars to fall. Examples include sitagliptin (Januvia), saxagliptin (Onglyza), linagliptin (Tradjenta), and alogliptin (Nesina). See also *GLP-1 inhibitors*.

Diuretic (water pill) A medication used to remove excess fluid that builds up in congestive heart failure. These drugs may alter electrolyte levels, such as potassium, and therefore, blood needs to be periodically obtained to ensure that the electrolytes are within normal limits.

Dofetilide A heart rhythm drug that may be useful in treating atrial fibrillation and atrial flutter. This medication can worsen heart rhythm problems (such as by causing proarrhythmia). See also *proarrhythmia*.

Dronedarone A heart rhythm drug that may be used to treat atrial fibrillation and atrial flutter. May be less effective than amiodarone.

Dysautonomia An abnormality of the autonomic nervous system. May be acute or chronic and may be associated with other degenerative or autoimmune diseases. Proper functioning of the heart, bladder, intestines, sweat glands, pupils, and blood vessels may be affected. See also *autonomic nervous system, postural orthostatic tachycardia syndrome.*

Echocardiogram (echo) A test that uses sound waves (ultrasound) to visualize the heart, its structure, and its function. It is typically performed in two dimensions, showing cross-sections of the heart (called a two-dimensional echocardiogram). See also *transesophageal echocardiogram.*

Edward Sapien 3 transcatheter heart valve system A TAVR (transcatheter aortic valve replacement) system that is used to insert a TAVR valve that is balloon-expandable, low profile, stented, and comprised of bovine pericardium.

Ehlers-Danlos syndrome A group of inherited connective tissue disorders that are generally characterized by joint hypermobility, skin hyperextensibility, and tissue fragility. Musculoskeletal pain, arterial, intestinal, and uterine fragility or rupture, scoliosis, mitral valve prolapse, and aortic root dilatation are other common symptoms. There are 13 subtypes, and almost any organ system may be affected. See also *dysautonomia, postural orthostatic tachycardia syndrome, connective tissue disorder.*

Eicosapentaenoic acid (EPA) Also known as Vascepa, a fatty acid shown to lower cardiovascular events (heart attack and stroke) by about 25% when used with a statin in those with vascular disease.

Ejection fraction (EF) A measure of the function of the heart. EF can be determined by tests such as an echocardiogram, an angiogram, or a nuclear imaging study. In general, the ejection fraction is a measure of the fraction of blood ejected from the heart. An ejection fraction less than 50% is abnormal.

Electrocardiogram (ECG or EKG) A test in which electrodes attached to the limbs and/or chest record electrical activity that is related to the heart, its rhythm, and its functionality.

Electrophysiologist A doctor who diagnoses and treats heart rhythm abnormalities. This doctor must train first in internal medicine and cardiology and subspecialize in the field of electrophysiology. An electrophysiologist may perform an EP study, a catheter ablation, or a device implant if warranted.

Electrophysiology The study of the electrical activity of the heart.

Electrophysiology study (EP study) A procedure in which catheters are placed in veins (and occasionally in arteries) and threaded into the heart to study the electrical activity of the heart and to induce abnormal heart rhythms.

Embolism Obstruction of an artery, typically by a blood clot. May originate in one part of the body and migrate via the circulatory system to create a blockage in another part of the body. May also be caused by a fat globule, an air bubble, or other foreign substance.

Entresto A combination of an ARB (valsartan) and sacubitril that helps rid the body of excess fluid and helps alleviate symptoms of heart failure. This drug also helps lower blood pressure. This combination medication is approved for people with chronic heart failure and with a reduced ejection fraction.

Epinephrine A hormone produced in the adrenal glands that plays an important role in the fight-or-flight response. Also known as adrenaline.

Ethnic differences Differences exist based on one's ethnicity, and an awareness may help look for specific medical problems and assure appropriate medical care.

Event recorder A device used to record heart rhythm events in real time. Events are only recorded when the device is activated.

Ezetimibe A drug that works by preventing cholesterol absorption in the small intestine from food in order to produce cholesterol-lowering effects.

Femoral artery A large artery in the thigh and the main arterial supply in the thigh and leg.

Fibrates A class of oral medications that decrease triglycerides as well as some effect on lowering LDL and raising HDL. Examples include gemfibrozil and fenofibrate. They work by helping the body use fatty acids for energy instead of depositing them into atherosclerotic plaques.

First-degree AV block A form of heart block in which there is a delay in the conduction from the atrium to the ventricle. A specific ECG pattern is observed.

Fish oil A combination of docosahexaenoic acid (DHA) and eicosapentaenoic acid, is useful for decreasing triglyceride levels as well as reducing arthritic pain.

Fitbit A form of wearable technology capable of recording an ECG and may be useful in detecting guiding fitness.

Flecainide A heart rhythm medication useful in treating supraventricular tachycardias (including atrial fibrillation) in patients with structurally normal hearts.

Food and Drug Administration (FDA) A United States organization responsible for protecting the public health and security of human and veterinary drugs, biological products, and medical devices and ensuring the safety of the United States food, cosmetics, and products that emit radiation.

Functional tricuspid regurgitation A problem with the ring that surrounds the tricuspid valve (annulus) causing the tricuspid valve to not close tightly enough causing blood to flow backward into the right upper heart chamber (atrium) when the right lower heart chamber (ventricle) contracts.

Garlic A supplement that is best used to season your foods in a heart-healthy diet.

Gastric bypass surgery A form of bariatric surgery in which a sleeve is inserted around the stomach to make the patient feel full after eating certain food portions. Used when lifestyle modifications (e.g., diet and exercise) have proven to be unsuccessful. See also *bariatric surgery*.

Gemfibrozil A medication from a group known as fibrates that is used to treat high cholesterol and high triglycerides; currently, fenofibrate is prescribed much more commonly when a patient is also on a statin.

Gender differences Differences in heart disease exist depending on one's gender. Gender may affect whether an individual receives a particular therapy or access to a trial. It is important to be aware of, in order to provide equal and fair access to healthcare for all patients.

Glucagon A hormone produced in the pancreas that balances the effects of insulin by increasing blood sugar.

Glucagon-like peptide 1 receptor agonists (GLP-1 receptor agonists) An antidiabetic drug class used to manage type 2 diabetes that works by decreasing the release of glucagon and decreasing the stomach from emptying. May also help the pancreas make more insulin-producing cells (beta cells). Includes exena-tide (Byetta), dulaglutide (Trulicity), semaglutide (Ozempic), and liraglutide (Victoza). See also *glucagon*.

Glycemic index The measure of how quickly a substance can raise blood sugar. The higher the glycemic index, the faster the substance raises blood sugar and leads to a spike in insulin.

Green tea A supplement to a heart-healthy diet, best enjoyed in moderation.

Handoff The transfer of care from your primary care physician (PCP) to the specialist (such as the cardiologist), in which they will treat the patient and eventually "handoff" the patient back to the PCP.

HDL Good cholesterol component; see high-density lipoprotein for more information.

Headspace A smartphone health application that provides elegant guided meditations teaching users the fundamentals of meditation.

Health Insurance Portability and Accountability Act (HIPAA) Federal law that ensures the privacy of a patient's medical information.

Heartbeat The beating or pulsation of the heart; a single pulsation or beat of the heart.

Heart Rhythm Society A society for electrophysiologists, and other heart rhythm-related patients, staff, physicians, and manufacturers. www.hrsonline.org

Heart transplantation See *cardiac transplantation*.

Hemochromatosis A disorder in which iron deposits in the body and its organs. It can cause a form of restrictive cardiomyopathy. See also *cardiomyopathy, restrictive cardiomyopathy*.

Hemoglobin A1C (HbA1C) A blood test that indicates how your blood sugar has been over the past 3 months; used to diagnose and manage diabetes mellitus. Less than 5.7% is normal, 5.7–6.4% is prediabetic, and greater than 6.5% is considered to be diabetic. See also *diabetes*.

Heparin An anticoagulant medication useful in preventing the formation of blood clots and decreasing the growth of blood clots that have already formed. See also *anticoagulant*.

High-density lipoprotein Also known as HDL, it is a molecule which helps transport lipids throughout the body. HDL protects our blood vessels. HDL absorbs cholesterol from body cells and transports it back to the liver, slowing plaque formation and atherosclerosis. >60 mg/dL is a desirable level of HDL. Men are at risk if their HDL <40 mg/dl, and women are at risk if their HDL is <50 mg/dl. Also known as the "good" cholesterol. See also *low-density lipoprotein, atherosclerosis*.

High-grade AV block A form of heart block in which electrical activity from the upper chambers is not consistently conducted to the lower chambers. In particular, more than one consecutive atrial beat fails to conduct to the lower chamber.

His bundle Part of the wiring system of the heart that is below the AV node. If the His bundle is severely diseased, a patient may be at risk for heart block, and a pacemaker may be indicated.

HMG-CoA reductase inhibitors (statins) A class of medications useful in treating high cholesterol and, to a lesser degree, high triglycerides.

Holter monitor A device used to record continuous heart rhythm information typically over 1 to 2 days.

Homocysteine Common amino acid found in your blood; a high level may be linked to heart disease. Also associated with a deficiency in vitamins B6, B12, and folic acid.

Hydralazine Used to treat high blood pressure by relaxing blood vessels so blood can flow more easily through them.

Hyperosmolar hyperglycemic state A life-threatening complication of diabetes mellitus type 2, where older individuals are subject to physical or emotional stress, forget to drink water, and become dehydrated, leading to very high blood glucose levels. Symptoms include dehydration, excessive thirst and urination, weakness, leg cramps, vision problems, and altered levels of consciousness. See also *diabetes*.

Hypertension Persistently elevated high blood pressure, where the high force of blood against blood vessels damages them and leads to atherosclerosis. May be primary, where no cause can be identified, or may be secondary to another medical condition. See also *atherosclerosis*.

Hypertensive crisis Blood pressure that is greater than 180/120 mmHg. Further categorized as hypertensive urgency and hypertensive emergency.

Hypertensive emergency Blood pressure that is greater than 180/120 mmHg complicated by organ dysfunction (e.g., stroke, heart failure, renal failure, blindness).

Hypertrophic cardiomyopathy A condition in which the heart muscle is thickened and the heart's contraction may be very strong (hyperdynamic). A very thick heart muscle, significant family history of sudden death, the presence of ventricular tachycardia, or loss of consciousness (syncope) may all suggest the need for an implantable cardioverter defibrillator (ICD).

Hypoglycemia Low blood sugar that may be life-threatening and lead to presyncope, syncope, arrhythmia, pale skin, tremor, anxiety, sweating, hunger, and irritability. More severe symptoms include confusion, visual disturbances, seizures, and loss of consciousness. See also *presyncope, syncope, arrhythmia*.

Hypotension Low blood pressure which may be associated with symptoms of lightheadedness and passing out. See also *syncope, presyncope*.

Hypothyroidism An endocrine or glandular condition in which the thyroid gland fails to produce enough thyroid hormone. As a result, the heart may beat very slowly, and occasionally, atrial fibrillation may occur. Treatment of a slow rhythm problem (bradycardia) may require medications such as thyroid hormone replacement.

Ibutilide An intravenous heart rhythm medication useful in treating atrial fibrillation and atrial flutter. May also cause proarrhythmia. See also *proarrhythmia*.

Implantable cardiac monitor (implantable loop recorder) An implantable device that can record heart rhythm-related information. Other physiological information might also be recorded.

Implantable cardioverter defibrillator (ICD) A device that uses electrical energy to treat rapid and slow heart rhythms. High energy (DC energy) may be delivered to shock the patient out of a very fast rhythm (tachycardia).

Inflammation The body's immune response against harmful stimuli. Inflammation may be acute, such as a response to an infection, such as the flu, which helps eradicate the invader. However, inflammation may also be chronic, where the same immune response persists for months or even years and damages tissue. This is the underlying mechanism of atherosclerosis and heart disease, diabetes, asthma and many other medical conditions. Chronic inflammation is generally the product of both lifestyle and genetics.

Informed consent The process in which a doctor informs the patient of the risks, benefits, and alternatives to a given procedure. The patient should be given time to ask questions, and those questions should be answered to his or her satisfaction prior to consenting to a procedure.

INR (international normalized ratio) A blood test used to determine how thin the blood is as a result of a patient being on warfarin (Coumadin).

Isthmus Also known as the cavo-tricuspid isthmus, it is a body of fibrous tissue in the lower right atrium between the tricuspid valve and the inferior vena cava. It is a common target of treating atrial flutter via catheter ablation. See also *atrial flutter, catheter ablation.*

Insulin A hormone produced by the pancreas that enables body cells to take up carbohydrates and use them for energy. Without insulin production, or if the body cannot respond to the insulin secreted, blood sugar remains elevated and leads to chronic inflammation. See also *diabetes, inflammation.*

Interventionalist A doctor who performs interventions (i.e., invasive procedures). With respect to the heart, an interventionalist typically performs cardiac catheterization, in which catheters are inserted into the heart and its arteries and contrast dye is delivered to visualize its structures. The doctor may decide to deliver a stent (piece of mesh metal) to keep a blockage open.

Intra-aortic balloon pump A catheter-implanted device that is placed outside of the heart in a region of the major artery that carries blood away from the heart. This device inflates a balloon during heart relaxation (diastole) and deflates during contraction (systole) thus improving the pumping function of the heart as the hear can be more easily filled.

Intracardiac echocardiography (ICE) A procedure in which a catheter is inserted into the heart to visualize internal structures, guide a transseptal procedure, and monitor for pericardial effusion formation (a possible complication from catheter ablation in which blood leaks into the sac around the heart).

Ischemia The lack of blood flow to the heart muscle itself.

Ischemic cardiomyopathy A weak heart muscle caused by the lack of blood flow to the heart (ischemia) or damage to the heart as a result of a heart attack (myocardial infarction).

Isosorbide dinitrate Used to treat chest pain (angina) by relaxing the blood vessels of the heart so the heart does not need to work as hard and therefore does not need as much oxygen.

Iyengar yoga A form of yoga that has an emphasis on detail, precision, and alignment in the performance of yoga postures.

Jardiance (empagliflozin) A treatment for type 2 diabetes when diet and exercise do not provide sufficient blood sugar control. It is an SGLT2 inhibitor that inhibits the reabsorption of glucose by the kidneys. This class of medication is standard treatment for heart failure.

Jefit A smartphone health application that provides weight-lifting routines to follow in the gym.

Joint hypermobility syndrome A connective tissue disorder characterized by chronic musculoskeletal pain due to joint hyperextensibility. It shares many clinical features of Ehlers-Danlos syndrome, hypermobility type. See also *connective tissue disorder, Ehlers-Danlos syndrome.*

Kardia A mobile app that can be used to record an ECG rhythm strip using a smartphone. Accessible through https//www.alivecor.com/kardiamobile.

Kawasaki disease Is an inflammatory disease in children with over 5 days of fever, conjunctivitis (eye infection), and inflammation of blood vessels.

Kidney failure Also known as end-stage renal disease, this is the last stage of chronic kidney disease. The kidneys are responsible for clearing salt and waste from the body, and thus at this stage, salt, water, and waste begin to build up in the body. Dialysis or a kidney transplant is critical.

Know Your Numbers An important theme of this book in which you need to take responsibility for your own health and know important numbers such as your cholesterol (LDL/HDL/triglycerides), fasting blood sugar and A1C level, BMI and weight, and ejection fraction (EF).

Latitude A remote device monitoring service provided by Boston Scientific Corp.

LDL Bad cholesterol component; see low-density lipoprotein for more information.

Lead extraction A procedure to remove a pacemaker or defibrillator lead or leads from the heart. The procedure may involve special cutting tools that employ laser or radiofrequency energy.

Left atrial appendage A small muscular sac in the top of the left upper chamber of the heart (left atrium). A common site for clot formation.

Left ventriculogram A catheterization procedure in which a catheter is advanced into the left ventricle and contrast dye is injected to visualize the function of the left ventricle and calculate the ejection fraction. A similar procedure could be performed in the right ventricle, in which case it would be called a right ventriculogram. See also *ejection fraction.*

Leptin This is a hormone released from fat cells and is also known as the satiety hormone. This hormone helps lower appetite and allows the body to dip into stored fat for energy.

Lipoprotein a [LP(a)] Substances made of protein and fat that carry cholesterol through your bloodstream. Elevated levels have been linked to the development of vascular and some types of valvular disease.

Long QT syndrome A hereditary condition identified by abnormalities in the ECG and the patient's history, which may place the person at risk for ventricular tachycardia and sudden cardiac arrest.

Loop recorder A device used to record heart rhythm information. Once symptoms are identified and the device is activated, information that has been recorded is stored along with additional recorded data.

Low-density lipoprotein Also known as LDL, it is a molecule made up of both protein and lipid (fat) that transports lipids from the liver to the rest of the body. Ideally, LDL levels should be <100 mg/dL to minimize cholesterol buildup in blood vessel walls and subsequent plaque formation and atherosclerosis. In people with coronary artery disease, it should be <70 mg/dl and <55 mg/dl in those with diabetes and a history of acute coronary syndrome. Also known as the "bad" cholesterol. See *atherosclerosis, high-density lipoprotein*.

LUCAS 3 CPR Device A device manufactured by Physio-Control (Redmond, WA) that uses a suction cup for automatic mechanical active compression-decompression using Dr. Cohen's proprietary suction cup method.

Lyme disease A disease, following a tick bite, caused by a bacterium (*Borrelia burgdorferi*) found on a deer tick. This disease may result in slowing of the heart rate and a heart block. In severe cases, myocarditis might also occur. Disease in the wiring system of the heart is usually restricted to the sinus and AV nodes and is typically reversible following treatment with antibiotics. See also *myocarditis*.

MADIT-CRT study A study that demonstrated that biventricular defibrillators improve survival with fewer heart failure interventions, even in asymptomatic or mildly symptomatic heart failure patients (NYHA Class I or II) with an EF of 30% or less and a wide QRS complex.

Magnetic resonance imaging (MRI) A test that uses strong magnetic fields to image the body, heart, and other organs.

Marfan syndrome An inherited connective tissue disorder where patients are typically slender with tall arms, legs, and fingers. They also may have a curved spine and a caved-out chest or a carved-in chest. Hypermobility of the joints is also a feature. These patients may also have a weakened aorta and an echocardiogram is useful at identifying valve and aortic abnormalities. See also *echocardiogram, connective tissue disorder*.

Mealtime A smartphone health App that provides a robust catalogue of healthy recipes with corresponding downloadable grocery lists.

Mechanical valve A replacement valve made from nonorganic substances such as metals and plastics.

Meditation Technique to reduce stress through mental imagery.

Medtronic CoreValve™ A replacement valve that is a self-expanding, supra-annular, stented valve which is comprised of porcine pericardium.

Merlin Remote device monitoring system provided by Abbott/St. Jude Medical. Also called Merline.net™ and available at www.merlin.net.

Mexiletine A heart rhythm medication useful in treating ventricular tachycardia and ventricular fibrillation.

Mindfulness An awareness of the present and being in the moment.

MitraClip™ (device) A small clip that is attached to the mitral valve. It is placed using a minimally invasive procedure, guiding a catheter from the groin or chest to the heart. This device treats mitral regurgitation (MR) by helping the valve close more completely, helping restore proper blood flow through the heart and body. Also see *transcutaneous mitral valve repair or TMVr*.

Mitral regurgitation A leaky mitral valve that may result in an increased demand on the left side of the heart and symptoms of heart failure.

Mitral stenosis Narrowing of the mitral valve resulting in decreased blood flow into the left ventricle.

Mitral valve prolapse (also called MVP) A floppy redundant and sometimes leaky mitral valve that is often associated with palpitations. Severe mitral valve prolapse may lead to mitral regurgitation over time.

Mixed connective tissue disease An autoimmune disorder involving the joints and muscles with features of systemic lupus erythematosus, rheumatoid arthritis, polymyositis, and scleroderma. This disorder may also affect the heart.

MobileDoc A telehealth kit manufactured by MedPod™ for telehealth with contains multiple telehealth tools in a roller suitcase.

Mobitz type I second-degree heart block (Mobitz type I second-degree AV block or Wenckebach) A type of heart block that usually occurs in the AV node in which each atrial beat takes longer and longer to get to the ventricles until a beat is eventually blocked. If this rhythm is asymptomatic, it is not necessary to implant a pacemaker.

Mobitz type II second-degree heart block (Mobitz type II second-degree AV block) A type of heart block that may occur in the His bundle or below, in which each atrial beat is followed by a ventricular beat in a regular sequence, and then suddenly one atrial beat fails to conduct to the ventricle (a block occurs). The presence of this type of heart block often indicates the need for a permanent pacemaker.

Morphine An opiate (narcotic) analgesic drug used to treat moderate to severe pain that cannot be controlled by other pain medications. Works by controlling the nervous system (e.g., brain) response to pain. It is highly addictive.

Multisystem inflammatory disorder An inflammatory response in children similar to Kawasaki disease that occurs in COVID-19.

Multivitamins A supplement that may not be necessary unless one has a particular vitamin deficiency. Best to obtain through a balanced, heart-healthy diet.

My fitness pal A smartphone health application that tracks calories and macronutrients of foods that you can input into the application and calculates your daily total calorie intake.

Myocardial infarction (heart attack) Irreversible damage to the heart muscle as the result of a blockage in an artery to the heart. May be an indicator for an implantable cardioverter defibrillator (ICD), especially if the ejection fraction is less than or equal to 30%.

Myocarditis An inflammation of the heart muscle, which may be caused by an infection (such as bacteria or virus) or an autoimmune condition (such as systemic lupus erythematosus). Myocarditis might also be found in some patients with peripartum cardiomyopathy. See also *peripartum dilated cardiomyopathy, systemic lupus erythematosus.*

New York Heart Association (NYHA) Classification of Congestive Heart Failure A classification based on the presence of heart failure related to the amount of activity. Class I has no symptoms with exertion; Class II has mild symptoms with a great deal of physical exertion. Class III has symptoms with mild exertion, and Class IV has symptoms at rest. This classification is used to guide the implantation of defibrillators and heart failure devices (on optimal medical therapy).

Neurocardiogenic syncope See *vasovagal syncope*—a type of syncope in which a hyperactive vagus nerve response is triggered, typically while standing, that produces bradycardia and hypotension (drop in blood pressure).

Niacin (nicotinic acid) Also known as vitamin B3; a medication used to treat high cholesterol and high triglycerides.

Nike+Run Club A smartphone health app that tracks your runs by recording distances and times.

Nitroglycerin A drug that increases blood flow in arteries (vasodilator) so the heart does not need to work so hard and thus uses less oxygen; used primarily to treat chest pain (angina).

Nonfluoroscopic three-dimensional mapping A method used during an EP study to help identify the location of heart rhythm problems, along with the position of catheters within the heart.

Novel oral anticoagulants (NOACS) Includes apixaban (Eliquis), dabigatran (Pradaxa), and rivaroxaban (Xarelto) used to prevent the formation of blood clots. A superior alternative to warfarin for preventing strokes in patients with atrial fibrillation, since there is no need to avoid vitamin K-rich foods or routine monitoring of PT/INR.

NPO (nil per os) Means "nothing by mouth." Typically, patients must have nothing to eat or drink for at least 6 hours prior to any procedure. Medications with a sip of water may be permitted. Please ask your doctor for specific instructions.

NSAIDs Nonsteroidal anti-inflammatory drugs such as ibuprofen, which may interfere with certain medications. Please talk to your doctor prior to taking this type of treatment along with your heart medications.

Obesity Categorized as a BMI of 30 or more. Associated with increased risk of heart disease, stroke, type 2 diabetes, and certain cancers. See also *body mass index (BMI).*

Omega-3 fish oil A supplement to your diet, best to get through fish and flax seeds in your diet.

Optimizer Smart System A device that offers cardiac contractility modulation and may help those with NYHA Class III heart failure, with a left ventricular ejection fraction from 25% to 45%, who do not qualify for cardiac resynchronization therapy (a biventricular implant). It should not be used in patients with permanent or long-standing abnormal heart rhythm (atrial fibrillation) or flutter, in patients with a tricuspid valve from man-made materials, and in patients in whom vascular access to implant the electrodes is impossible.

OptivolTM A modified measurement obtained by measuring transthoracic impedance between the lead and the pulse generator (available in Medtronic defibrillators). Can indicate fluid accumulation in the lungs (and indicator of heart failure).
CorVue™ (Abbott) and HeartLogic™ (Boston Scientific) offer other similar systems to remotely monitor heart failure.

Oral glucose tolerance test A test that measures your blood sugar 2 hours after
drinking a sugary drink; used to diagnose and manage diabetes mellitus. A glucose level of less than 140 mg/dl is normal, 140–199 mg/dl is prediabetes, and
200 mg/dl or more is diabetic. See also *diabetes*.

Organic tricuspid regurgitation A problem with the tricuspid valve itself, causing it to not close tight enough and causing blood to flow backward into the right
upper heart chamber (atrium) when the right lower heart chamber (ventricle)
contracts.

Orthostatic hypotension A condition notable for a drop in blood pressure and an
increase in heart rate while going from supine to standing.

Orthostatic intolerance A condition notable for symptoms of tachycardia, lightheadedness and dizziness, and/or syncope associated with going from supine to
standing. *See POTS*.

Osteopathic manipulative medicine (OMM) A hands-on, manual medicine
approach and treatment provided by osteopathic medical physicians in the
United States. Involves the treatment of a patient's structural dysfunction of the
musculoskeletal system.

Over-the-counter medications (OTCs) Drugs you can purchase without a prescription from your doctor.

Overweight Categorized as a BMI of 25–30. See also *body mass index (BMI)*.

Oxygen saturation The fraction of oxygen-saturated hemoglobin (*hemoglobin—*
the protein in our blood that carries oxygen) relative to total hemoglobin (unsatu-
rated hemoglobin + oxygen-saturated hemoglobin). Normal arterial blood oxygen
saturation levels in humans are between 95% and 100%. Also called *Sp02*.

Ozempic (semaglutide) A diabetes medication that is also an anti-obesity medication used for long-term control of excess weight. It was developed by Novo
Nordisk and approved for use in the United States in 2017. Ozempic is an injectable medication, but the oral form is called Rybelsus.

Pacemaker A device that is implanted to treat slow heart rhythms (bradycardias).
It can also be used to treat heart failure. It is a component of an implantable cardioverter defibrillator (ICD).

Palpitations The noticeable feelings of having a fast-beating, pounding, or fluttering heart.

Patent foramen ovale A congenital heart defect present at birth where patients
have a flap that persists and covers the hole (foramen ovale) between the right
and left atrium that did not seal the way it should after birth. If associated with
recurrent strokes or ministrokes, despite anticoagulation, it may need to be closed
either surgically or interventionally with a medical device. See also *septal defect*.

PCP (primary care physician) Typically, the primary person responsible for your
medical care. Often an internist or family medicine doctor.

PCSK9 inhibitors (evolocumab) A cholesterol-lowering drug that acts by inhibiting the destruction of LDL receptors and thus increases the reuptake of LDL, which can help slow the atherosclerosis process. See also *LDL, low-density lipoprotein.*

Percutaneous coronary intervention (PCI) A procedure that is performed to open up a blocked coronary artery. A balloon catheter may be placed across the blocked vessel to open up the blockage (percutaneous transluminal coronary angioplasty). A stent (expandable piece of metal) may then be inserted to keep the coronary artery open. See also *angioplasty, stent, percutaneous transluminal coronary angioplasty.*

Percutaneous transluminal coronary angioplasty (PTCA) A procedure in which a balloon catheter is placed across a coronary artery blockage to open up the occlusion, and a metal stent is deployed at the site to keep the blood vessel open. See also *angioplasty, percutaneous coronary intervention, stent.*

Pericardial effusion The presence of blood or other fluid in the pericardial sac around the heart. This may be the result of a cardiac perforation, in which blood may flow into the sac. If blood continues to flow into the pericardial sac, it may put pressure on the heart muscle itself and potentially prevent blood from leaving the heart. If the latter occurs, the patient may have a life-threatening condition called cardiac tamponade, which requires immediate treatment. See also *pericardium, cardiac tamponade, pericardiocentesis, pericardial window.*

Pericardial window Surgical removal of a part of the pericardium, which allows doctors to drain excess fluid, treating pericardial effusion and cardiac tamponade. See also *pericardium, pericardial effusion, cardiac tamponade.*

Pericardiocentesis A procedure done to remove fluid that has built up in the pericardium and to treat pericardial effusion and cardiac tamponade. See also *pericardium, pericardial effusion, cardiac tamponade.*

Pericarditis Inflammation of the pericardium, the two thin layers of tissue that surround and protect the heart, help it pump, and hold it in place. May present as sharp, stabbing chest pain that worsens with deep breathing and is relieved by leaning forward, though presentations commonly vary from person to person. Must rule out heart attack. See also *myocardial infarction.*

Pericardium The membrane enclosing the heart, consisting of an outer layer and an inner double layer. See also *pericardial effusion, cardiac tamponade, pericardiocentesis, pericardial window.*

Peripartum dilated cardiomyopathy A cardiomyopathy of unknown etiology occurring around the time of pregnancy. Myocarditis may be seen in many patients with this disorder. See also *myocarditis.*

PET scan A positron emission tomography (PET) scan is useful in seeing how well the heart muscle itself is working. A nuclear tracer is injected through a vein, similar to what happens during a nuclear stress test, in order to identify differences in heart metabolism. This test may provide additional information above and beyond the normal nuclear stress test.

Plan B An important theme of this book, to always have a backup plan for life and whatever you do. Also, an important component of your Surviving and Thriving Card which includes a backup to your important medical information, which you should have easily available wherever you go.

Platelets A type of blood cell that helps form blood clots in order to slow or stop bleeding when there is an injury to a blood vessel to help wounds heal.

Pocket Yoga A smartphone health App to learn yoga at your own pace through step-by-step guidance with an instructor.

Polymyositis A chronic inflammatory disease that causes muscle weakness on both sides of the body. The most common muscles affected are closest to the trunk and are the hips, thighs, shoulders, neck, and upper arms. See also *connective tissue disorder*.

Postural orthostatic tachycardia syndrome (POTS) A specific group of symptoms, such as lightheadedness, dizziness, and presyncope, that frequently occur when standing upright (in contrast to laying horizontally) accompanied by a substantial increase in heart rate. Other symptoms include difficulty thinking and concentrating, fatigue, exercise intolerance, blurry vision, palpitations, and nausea. See also *dysautonomia, Ehlers-Danlos syndrome, autonomic nervous system, orthostatic intolerance, presyncope, connective tissue disorder*.

Prediabetes The presence of an elevated glucose level that is not high enough to qualify for diabetes. This often progresses to diabetes unless steps such as diet and exercise are taken prophylactically. See also *diabetes, insulin*.

Premature contractions Premature contractions are extra heartbeats that disrupt the regular heart rhythm. They may originate in the atria or in the ventricles.

Presyncope Lightheadedness and dizziness short of true loss of consciousness. The feeling that one is going to "black out" without actually blacking out.

Primary prevention The aim to prevent disease or injury before it ever occurs.

Proarrhythmia A side effect of a medication or device in which a rhythm problem is worsened or exacerbated. A drug such a procainamide may cause a form of ventricular tachycardia called *torsades de pointes*. Treatment is often to stop the trigger through other medications such as lidocaine; even pacing therapy may be necessary. See also *torsades de pointes*.

Procainamide A heart rhythm medication used occasionally in intravenous form to provoke ECG changes seen in Brugada syndrome. Infrequently used as a treatment of heart rhythm problems due to the presence of more efficacious medications with fewer side effects (including proarrhythmia). See also *proarrhythmia*.

Propafenone A medication used to treat atrial fibrillation and atrial flutter, especially in a patient with a structurally normal heart. Proarrhythmia may be a side effect. See also *proarrhythmia*.

Pseudoaneurysm Occurs when a blood vessel wall is injured, causing blood to leak from the vessel and surround the tissue. May be a complication of cardiac catheterization.

Psoriasis A skin disorder notable for increased scaly and flaky skin.

Pulmonary embolism A sudden blockage in a lung artery. May originate from a blood clot in the leg (deep venous thrombosis). This may be life-threatening, and symptoms include shortness of breath (sudden, worse with exertion), chest pain (sharp and more pronounced with deep breaths), and a blood-streaked cough. Other symptoms include arrhythmia, presyncope, diaphoresis, fever, leg pain, and clammy or discolored skin. Risk factors include heart disease, cancer, hereditary conditions that affect clotting, and prolonged immobilization (long car ride, bed rest after surgery). Smoking, high BMI, pregnancy, and supplemental estrogen are also risk factors. See also *deep venous thrombosis, arrhythmia, presyncope, diaphoresis.*

Pulmonary fibrosis Scarring and thickening of the lungs that can impair lung function and breathing. It is a rare side-effect of long-term amiodarone therapy.

Pulmonary vein isolation (PVI) A catheter ablation procedure in which the pulmonary veins are electrically isolated from the left atrium to prevent the trigger for atrial fibrillation (which is often within the pulmonary vein itself) from initiating atrial fibrillation.

Pulmonic stenosis Narrowing of the pulmonary valve, which may impair blood flow from the right heart to the lungs, and place increased demand on the right atrium and ventricle.

Purkinje fibers Specialized electrical tissue that helps to conduct electrical signals from the His bundle to the ventricular muscles.

QT dispersion A measurement obtained from a standard ECG that can give useful information related to the risk of developing ventricular tachycardia.

Racial disparities Differences based on race that can influence the type of heart disease people acquire and the healthcare they receive.

Raynaud disease A vascular disorder in which blood flow is impeded as a result of exposure to cold or stress. Fingers, toes, ear lobes, and the nose may turn pale as a result.

Recall The term used when a repetitive problem is identified with a device or one of its components. The specific action taken by the manufacturer, the United States Food and Drug Administration, and doctors will depend on how critical the problem is.

Red yeast rice An over-the-counter supplement that has been shown to lower LDL cholesterol.

ResQPUMP ACD-CPR device A device manufactured by Zoll Medical Corp. (Chelmsford, MA). Used for active compression-decompression CPR. The device was coinvented by this book's author, Dr. Todd Cohen. Also, part of the ResQCPR™ system.

Restrictive cardiomyopathy A form of heart muscle weakness in which the ventricles are stiff and cannot fill properly. Often caused by the buildup of a protein called amyloid. See also *amyloidosis, cardiomyopathy.*

Revascularization therapy Restoration of blood flow to a body part that has suffered from inadequate blood flow (ischemia). It is typically accomplished surgically via vascular bypass or angioplasty.

Rhabdomyolysis The breakdown of damaged muscle in the body. May result in kidney damage. An adverse effect of statin and fibrate therapy.

Rheumatic fever An autoimmune disorder following a streptococcus infection in children, which can adversely affect the valves of the heart later in life.

Rheumatic mitral stenosis Following an infection with streptococci bacteria, the body's immune system may respond with a condition called rheumatic fever, which is inflammation primarily of the heart and joints. The mitral valve is commonly affected and, as a result, may lead to a stenotic mitral valve. See also *streptococci, mitral stenosis*.

Rheumatoid arthritis An acquired autoimmune disease that targets the joints and is characterized by morning stiffness, arthralgias, and arthritis. See also *connective tissue disorder*.

Scleroderma An acquired autoimmune disease involving hardening and tightening of the skin and connective tissues. Scleroderma may be confined to just the skin or may manifest systemically and affect the extremities, digestive system, heart, lungs, or kidneys. See also *connective tissue disorder*.

Scurvy Connective tissue weakness caused by a deficiency of vitamin C. Symptoms include fatigue, weakness, severe joint pain, swollen bleeding gums, red/blue spots on skin, as well as easy bruising. Blood vessels become fragile, and this leads to the visible lesions and rashes. See also *connective tissue disorder*.

Secondary prevention The emphasis of early disease detection and prevention of disease progression in individuals who had a prior heart attack, stroke, arterial bypass, or angioplasty/arterial stenting procedure.

Septal defect Also known as a hole in the heart and is present at birth. May occur in the upper chambers (atrial septal defect or ASD) or may occur in the lower chambers (ventricular septal defect or VSD). See also *atrial septal defect, patent foramen ovale, and ventricular septal defect*.

Septal myotomy-myomectomy A surgical procedure in which a part of the heart muscle is surgically removed to relieve the obstruction that may be found in some forms of hypertrophic cardiomyopathy. See also *hypertrophic cardiomyopathy*.

Signal-averaged ECG (SAECG) A specialized ECG that can give useful information related to the risk of developing ventricular tachycardia.

Simply yoga A smartphone health application that contains premade yoga routines of 20, 40, and 60 min of length.

Sinus node (sinoatrial node, SA node) The start of the electricity in the heart, high up in the right atrium.

Sjogren's syndrome An autoimmune disorder characterized by dysfunction of white blood cells (our immune system), causing them to attack the salivary and lacrimal glands, leading to symptoms of dry eyes and a dry mouth. See also *connective tissue disorder*.

Sleep apnea A potentially serious medical condition where breathing repeatedly stops and starts during sleep.

Sodium glucose transport inhibitors (SGLT2 inhibitors) Antidiabetic drugs used in the treatment of type 2 diabetes that work in the kidneys to allow more sugar to be passed into urine, where it is eliminated from the body. Examples include canagliflozin (Invokana), empagliflozin (Jardiance), and dapagliflozin (Farxiga).

Sotalol A heart rhythm medication useful in treating atrial fibrillation, atrial flutter, ventricular tachycardia, and ventricular fibrillation. This medication can also cause or worsen life-threatening heart rhythm problems such as ventricular tachycardia and ventricular fibrillation (proarrhythmia). See also *proarrhythmia*.

Square breathing A technique to reduce anxiety by breathing in and out in a square pattern.

Stage I hypertension Blood pressure that is repeatedly above 130/80 mmHg. Treated with lifestyle modifications and possibly medications.

Stage II hypertension Blood pressure repeatedly above 140/90 mmHg that usually requires both lifestyle modifications and medications.

Staphylococci Bacteria that can cause endocarditis.

Statins See *HMG-CoA reductase inhibitors*.

Stent A piece of mesh metal deployed inside a coronary artery across a blockage to keep the blockage open. The stent may be made of bare metal or coated with drugs (drug-eluting stents, or DES) to prevent restenosis. The placement of a stent may also be referred to as stenting. See also *angioplasty, percutaneous coronary intervention*.

Streptococci Bacteria that can cause endocarditis.

Stress echocardiogram A form of stress test in which wall-motion abnormalities may be visualized by echocardiogram (indicating a blocked artery or damaged heart muscle) following exercise or drug-induced stress to a patient. See also *echocardiogram*.

Stress test A procedure in which the body is stressed either by exercise or medications to determine how well the heart is functioning. The test is often useful in determining the presence of blocked coronary arteries and whether a person has had a heart attack (myocardial infarction).

Stroke A sudden interruption of blood supply to the brain. May be caused by an abrupt blockage of arteries to the brain (ischemic stroke) by a burst blood vessel in the brain that leads to bleeding into brain tissue. Signs and symptoms include headache, dizziness, vomiting, paralysis or numbness of the face and/or extremities, trouble seeing, trouble speaking and understanding, and trouble walking.

Sudden cardiac arrest The number one killer. It is the collapse of a person's circulatory system and the abrupt loss of heart function. It may come on suddenly and lead to loss of consciousness and absence of a pulse. Immediate recognition by bystanders and subsequent cardiopulmonary resuscitation (CPR) and use of an automated external defibrillator (AED) until EMS arrives increases chances of survival. Usually caused by a rapid heart rhythm from the lower chambers of the heart (ventricles), called ventricular tachycardia or ventricular fibrillation.

Sudden Cardiac Arrest Association A support group for patients and families who have survived sudden cardiac death and/or those who have an implantable defibrillator. See www.suddencardiacarrest.org.

Sulfonylureas An antidiabetic agent used to manage type 2 diabetes that helps with blood sugar control by increasing the output of insulin from the pancreas.

Supraventricular Above the ventricle.

Supraventricular tachycardia (SVT) A rapid heart rhythm occurring above the ventricle (typically in the atria or AV node).

Support groups Organizations that can help you and your family members navigate your heart disease-related problems. This includes the American Heart Association, American College of Cardiology, the American Red Cross, the Sudden Cardiac Death Association, and the Heart Rhythm Society.

Surviving and Thriving Card An important card that is your gift with this book. It allows you to carry your important medical information ("Plan B" side) and track your important health-related numbers ("Know Your Numbers" side) all the time. The card is available in Appendix J in this book and also available via Dr. Cohen's practice's website at www.liheartrhythmcenter.com, where you can create your Surviving and Thriving Card and have it available in multiple places and easily updated.

Syncope Loss of consciousness. See also *presyncope, tilt table test, vasovagal syncope.*

Systemic lupus erythematosus An autoimmune disorder that affects the joints, skin, lungs, kidneys, nervous system, and heart. It may cause myocarditis. See also *myocarditis, connective tissue disorder.*

Systole The phase of the heart cycle when the heart muscle contracts and pumps blood from the chambers into the arteries.

Tachycardia A rapid heart rhythm with rates of 100 beats per minute or more. At rest, tachycardias may be abnormal, depending on the circumstance, when the heart rate exceeds 120 beats per minute.

Telehealth A remote way to monitor and treat patients; also called *telemedicine.*

Telehealth Associates A major provider of telehealth services located on Long Island, New York. www.telehealthassociates.com

TeleFellow™ A dual video platform for providing telehealth to patients and educating fellows.

TeleMedstuden™ A dual video platform for providing telehealth to patients and educating medical students.

Tertiary prevention The improvement of the quality of life of people with an ongoing illness or injury that has lasting effects, thereby softening the impact while also limiting and delaying complications and restoring function.

Tetralogy of Fallot A rare congenital disease that usually requires surgical repair. Its classification led to a new era of cardiac shunts and surgical repairs that are currently used to treat those with congenital heart defects. See also *congenital heart disease.*

The Mindfulness App A smartphone health App that provides users with guided meditations while also incorporating mindfulness reminders and a meditation journal.

Thiazide diuretic Used to treat high blood pressure. May cause hyponatremia, hypercalcemia, hypokalemia, and other electrolyte imbalances. See also *diuretics.*

Thiazolidinediones (glitazones) A class of antidiabetic agents used to treat type 2 diabetes by acting as peroxisome proliferator-activated receptor agonists (PPARs). These medications, rosiglitazone (Avandia) and pioglitazone (Actos), work to lower the production of glucose and increase the way some of our cells react to insulin, thus lowering blood sugars.

Thrombolytics Medication used to break up clots that may be indicated during a heart attack. Dangerous side effects include internal bleeding. See also *myocardial infarction*.

Ticagrelor (Brilinta) An antiplatelet agent used to prevent platelets from forming clots that may cause a heart attack or stroke. Used in conjunction with acetylsalicylic acid (Aspirin) in patients who cannot tolerate clopidogrel (Plavix) following stent placement to prevent reocclusion of the coronary artery.

Tilt table test A simple procedure in which a patient is strapped to a table and then tilted almost upright (typically between 60° and 80°) for up to 45 min to determine the cause of syncope or presyncope. Heart rate and blood pressure are monitored during the procedure, and in some cases, a medication may be infused to facilitate the procedure. See also *presyncope, syncope, vasovagal syncope*.

Torsades de pointes (also called torsade de pointes and torsades des pointes) A serious form of ventricular tachycardia caused by medications that lengthen the QT interval or by the hereditary long QT syndrome. The ventricular tachycardia appears to be turning or twisting about an axis. See also *long QT syndrome*.

Transcatheter aortic valve replacement (TAVR) A minimally invasive procedure performed by an interventional cardiologist and/or surgeon in order to replace a narrowed aortic valve that fails to open properly (aortic stenosis) by guiding a catheter from the leg or chest to the heart. Also known as transcatheter aortic valve implantation (TAVI).

Transcatheter mitral valve repair (TMVr) A minimally invasive procedure performed by an interventional cardiologist and/or surgeon in order to repair/replace a leaky mitral valve (treat significant mitral regurgitation).

Transesophageal echocardiogram A procedure in which a tube containing an echo probe is inserted down the esophagus to view specific structures in and around the heart. It is particularly useful in defining the presence of blood clots in the left atrial appendage (a spot not well seen by a standard echocardiogram). This procedure is frequently performed prior to cardioverting atrial fibrillation, especially if the patient has been in atrial fibrillation for some time and has not been well-anticoagulated. See also *echocardiogram*.

Transseptal procedure A procedure that uses a needle to puncture the tissue that separates the right and left atrium (atrial septum) to advance a catheter from the right side of the heart into the left side (left atrium or ventricle). This procedure is a standard part of a routine atrial fibrillation procedure, such as pulmonary vein isolation.

Transthoracic echocardiogram A noninvasive ultrasound that creates a moving picture of your heart through the chest wall. Allows for the evaluation of valves and chambers of the heart, in addition to the heart's ability to pump blood.

Tricuspid valve The valve that directs blood flow from the right upper chamber (atrium) to the right lower chamber (ventricle).

Triglycerides A type of fat found in blood. If a person eats more calories than they burn, the extra calories are converted to triglycerides. Triglycerides are stored in fat cells, and during periods of fasting, the body will begin to use triglycerides for energy, typically after available carbohydrates that are stored in the liver and muscles are utilized. A value <150 mg/dl is considered a healthy range for blood triglycerides. Triglycerides are different from cholesterol in that they store unused calories, and cholesterol is used to build cells and hormones. See also *cholesterol.*

Trypanosoma cruzi The parasitic cause of Chagas disease.

T-wave Alternans (TWA) A test to help determine a patient's risk for sudden death. This test is often performed with a special computer during a stress test.

Universal protocol The Joint Commission on Accreditation of Healthcare Organizations national patient safety goals in order to prevent wrong patient, wrong site, and wrong surgery procedures. The process includes a preprocedure verification, including double identification to determine the correct patient, marking of the procedural site by a licensed practitioner, and the performance of a "time-out" immediately before initiating the procedure. The time-out allows all parties to review that the patient, procedure, and procedural site are correct and that all important documents and equipment are in place prior to initiating the procedure.

Valvuloplasty A procedure to repair a narrowed (stenotic) heart valve.

Vasculitis Inflammation of the blood vessels where the body's immune systems attack blood vessels. There are many different forms of vasculitis and precipitating factors, though the reasons are not always clear.

Vasovagal syncope (neurocardiogenic syncope) A common type of fainting, or syncope (loss of consciousness), often triggered by standing for a long period, in which the blood pressure (and possibly the heart rate) drops precipitously.

Ventricular fibrillation (VF) A very rapid and irregular rhythm from the lower chamber or chambers of the heart (ventricles), which may cause sudden cardiac arrest. If this rhythm problem is not immediately terminated, sudden death may result.

Ventricular septal defect (VSD) A hole in the ventricular septum, which can lead to deoxygenated blood traveling to the body and brain (turning blue or cyanosis). May need to be surgically repaired.

Ventricular tachycardia (VT) A rapid rhythm from the lower chamber or chambers of the heart (ventricles), which may cause sudden cardiac arrest.

Verapamil A calcium channel blocker that works specifically at the heart because of its interactions with different calcium channel receptors (referred to as a non-dihydropyridine agent). Works to slow down the heart's force as well as rhythm and thus should be used with caution in patients with heart failure or certain arrhythmias. Used particularly for treatment of angina; also can be used to treat supraventricular tachycardias (SVT) and treat high blood pressure. Because of its specific non-dihydropyridine effects, it has less of an effect on blood vessels than other calcium channel blockers and thus causes fewer related adverse effects such as headache, flushing, and peripheral edema. See also *calcium chan-nel blocker, diltiazem, arrhythmia, angina.*

Vital signs The first tests performed when visiting a doctor including your tem-perature, blood pressure, heart rate, and respirations.

Warfarin (Coumadin) A medication used to prevent the formation of blood clots in the heart and to prevent stroke in patients with conditions such as atrial fibril-lation and atrial flutter. Warfarin can also be used to treat clots in other blood vessels and in the lungs and to prevent clotting in people with mechanical heart valves. This medication must be carefully monitored by a blood test called an INR. The major side effect is increased bleeding tendency. See also *INR.*

Watchman™ (device) A permanent heart implant that acts as an alternative to life-long warfarin use for people with nonvalvular atrial fibrillation and effectively functions to reduce the risk of stroke. This device eliminates the risk of bleeding and the need for regular blood tests and food-and-drink restrictions that come with long-term use of warfarin.

Waterlogged A smartphone health App that can help keep you hydrated by setting goals and sending reminders to drink water.

White coat syndrome Occurs when the blood pressure readings in the office are higher than they are in other settings, usually due to feelings of anxiety in a medi-cal environment.

Wolff-Parkinson-White (WPW) syndrome A condition in which there is an extra connection between the upper and lower chambers of the heart (called an acces-sory pathway). Patients with this condition often have a specific ECG finding called a delta wave and are symptomatic with palpitations, lightheadedness and dizziness, or loss of consciousness. This condition can be readily treated by cath-eter ablation.

You are your own gym A smartphone health application that provides bodyweight exercise routines that can be done at home.

Zio Patch A patch containing heart rhythm recording circuitry that can be worn to record your ECG over a number of days and weeks. Manufactured by iRhythm™.

Bibliography

Abdelrahman M, Subzposh FA, Beer D, et al. Clinical outcomes of his bundle pacing compared to right ventricular pacing. J Am Coll Cardiol. 2018;71:2319–30.

Abovich A, Matasic DS, Cardoso R, Ndumele CE, Blumenthal RS, Blankstein R, Gulati M. The AHA/ACC/HFSA 2022 heart failure guidelines: changing the focus to heart failure prevention. Am J Prevent Cardiol. 2023;15:100527.

Apple heart study identifies AFib in small group of Apple watch wearers. American College of Cardiology, 16 Mar. 2019, www.acc.org/latest-in-cardiology/articles/2019/03/08/15/32/sat-9am-apple-heart-study-acc-2019.

Al-Khatib SM, Stevenson WG, Ackerman MJ, et al. 2017 AHA/ACC/HRS guideline for management of patients with ventricular arrhythmias and the prevention of sudden cardiac death: executive summary: a report of the American College of Cardiology/American Heart Association Task Force on Clinical Practice Guidelines and the Heart Rhythm Society. J Am Coll Cardiol. 2018;72:1677–749.

Alam M, Dokainish H, Lakkis N. Alcohol septal ablation for hypertrophic obstructive cardiomyopathy: a systematic review of published studies. J Interv Cardiol. 2006;19(4):319–27. https://doi.org/10.1111/j.1540-8183.2006.00153.x.

Alexander JH, Smith PK. Coronary-artery bypass grafting. N Engl J Med. 2016;374(20):1954–64. https://doi.org/10.1056/NEJMra1406944.

Alexandrescu DT, Levi M. The vascular purpuras. In: Kaushansky K, Lichtman MA, Prchal JT, Levi MM, Press OW, Burns LJ, Caligiuri M, editors. Williams hematology. 9th ed. New York: McGraw-Hill; 2016. p. 2097–112.

Alexandrescu DT, Levi M. The vascular purpuras. In: Kaushansky K, Lichtman MA, Prchal JT, Levi MM, Press OW, Burns LJ, Caligiuri M, editors. Williams hematology. 9th ed. New York: McGraw-Hill. http://accessmedicine.mhmedical.com.arktos.nyit.edu/content.aspx?bookid=1581&sectionid=108082497.

Anjum I, Sohail W, Hatipoglu B, Wilson R. Postural orthostatic tachycardia syndrome and its unusual presenting complaints in women: a literature minireview. Cureus. 2018;10(4):e2435. https://doi.org/10.7759/cureus.2435.

Aranki S, Cutlip D. Operative mortality after coronary artery bypass graft surgery. In: Aldea GS, Verrier E, Gersh BJ, Saperia GM, editors. UpToDate. Waltham: UpToDate, Inc.; 2018. https://www.uptodate.com/contents/operative-mortality-after-coronary-artery-bypass-graft-surgery?topicRef=1627&source=see_link#H1.

Arbustini E, Serio A, Favalli V, Dec G, Narula J. Dilated cardiomyopathy. In: Fuster V, Harrington RA, Narula J, Eapen ZJ, editors. Hurst's the heart. 14th ed. New York: McGraw-Hill. http://accessmedicine.mhmedical.com.arktos.nyit.edu/content.aspx?bookid=2046&sectionid=176571642.

T. J. Cohen, R. S. Blumenthal (eds.), *Surviving and Thriving With Heart Disease*, Contemporary Cardiology, https://doi.org/10.1007/978-3-032-00579-3

Armstrong EJ, Foster E. Transcatheter mitral valve repair. In: Gaash WH, Yeon SB, editors. UpToDate. Waltham: UpToDate, Inc.; 2020. https://www.uptodate.com/contents/transcatheter-mitral-valve-repair?search=transcatheter%20mitral%20valve%20repair&source=search_result&selectedTitle=1~31&usage_type=default&display_rank=1.

Arnett DK, Blumenthal RS, Albert MA, et al. ACC/AHA Guideline on the Primary Prevention of Cardiovascular Disease: Executive Summary: A Report of the American College of Cardiology/American Heart Association Task Force on Clinical Practice Guidelines [published correction appears in Circulation. 2019 Sep 10;140(11):e647-e648] [published correction appears in Circulation. 2020 Jan 28;141(4):e59] [published correction appears in Circulation. 2020 Apr 21;141(16):e773]. Circulation. 2019;140(11):e563–95. https://doi.org/10.1161/CIR.0000000000000677.

Barouch, L.. Heart disease gender differences: Johns Hopkins Women's Cardiovascular Health Center. 2020. Retrieved September 11, 2020, from https://www.hopkinsmedicine.org/heart_vascular_institute/centers_excellence/women_cardiovascular_health_center/patient_information/health_topics/heart_disease_gender_differences.html.

Bhatt DL, Miller M, Brinton EA, et al. REDUCE-IT USA. Circulation. 2020;141(5):367–75. Published online 2019 Nov 11. https://doi.org/10.1161/CIRCULATIONAHA.119.044440.

Bisignani A, De Bonis S, Mancuso L, Ceravolo G, Bisignani G. Implantable loop recorder in clinical practice. J Arrhythm. 2018;35(1):25–32. https://doi.org/10.1002/joa3.12142.

Blumenthal RS, Alfaddagh A. The ABCDE'S of primary prevention of cardiovascular disease. Trans Am Clin Climatogical Assoc. 2022;132:135–54.

Blumenthal RS, Grant J, Whelton SP. Incidental coronary artery calcium: nothing is more expensive than a missed opportunity. J Am Coll Cardiol. 2023;82(12):1203–5.

Blumenthal RS, Leucker TM. Disruptive innovation in CVD primary prevention: assessing the equivalency for secondary prevention strategies. J Am Coll Cardiol Img. 2023;16(9):1190–2.

Brugada J, Campuzano O, Arbelo E, Sarquella-Brugada G, Brugada R. Present status of Brugada syndrome: JACC state-of-the-art review. J Am Coll Cardiol. 2018;72:1046–59.

Burke MV, Hays JT, Ebbert JO. Varenicline for smoking cessation: a narrative review of efficacy, adverse effects, use in at-risk populations, and adherence. Patient Prefer Adherence. 2016;10:435–41. https://doi.org/10.2147/PPA.S83469.

Carlson MD, Wilkoff BL, Maisel WH, et al. Recommendations from the Heart Rhythm Society Task Force on device performance policies and guidelines endorsed by the American College of Cardiology Foundation (ACCF) and the American Heart Association (AHA) and the International Coalition of Pacing and Electrophysiology Organizations (COPE). Heart Rhythm. 2006;3(10):1250–73. https://doi.org/10.1016/j.hrthm.2006.08.029.

Castori M, Tinkle B, Levy H, Grahame R, Malfait F, Hakim A. A framework for the classification of joint hypermobility and related conditions. Am J Med Genet C Semin Med Genet. 2017;175(1):148–57. https://doi.org/10.1002/ajmg.c.31539.

Chambers JB, Bridgewater B. Epidemiology of valvular heart disease. In: Otto CM, Bonow RO, editors. Valvular heart disease: a companion to Braunwald's heart disease. 4th ed. Philadelphia: Elsevier; 2014. p. 1–13.

Chauvet-Gelinier JC, Bonin B. Stress, anxiety and depression in heart disease patients: a major challenge for cardiac rehabilitation. Ann Phys Rehabil Med. 2017;60(1):6–12. https://doi.org/10.1016/j.rehab.2016.09.002.

Cheitlin MD, Armstrong WF, Aurigemma GP, et al. ACC/AHA/ASE 2003 guideline update for the clinical application of echocardiography: summary article. A report of the American College of Cardiology/American Heart Association Task Force on practice guidelines (ACC/AHA/ASE Committee to update the 1997 guidelines for the clinical application of echocardiography). J Am Soc Echocardiogr. 2003;16(10):1091–110. https://doi.org/10.1016/S0894-7317(03)00685-0.

Chikwe J, Castillo JG. Prosthetic heart valves. In: Fuster V, Harrington RA, Narula J, Eapen ZJ, editors. Hurst's the heart. 14th ed. New York: McGraw-Hill; 2017. http://accessmedicine.mhmedical.com.arktos.nyit.edu/content.aspx?bookid=2046&sectionid=176558021.

Cohen TJ. A patient's guide to heart rhythm problems. Baltimore: Johns Hopkins University Press; 2010.

Cohen TJ. Practical electrophysiology. 3rd ed. Malvern: HMP Communications; 2016.

Cohen TJ, Liem LB. A hemodynamically responsive antitachycardia system; development and basis for design in humans. Circulation. 1990;82(2):394–406. (PMID: 2372890)

Cohen TJ, Goldner BG, Maccaro PC, Ardito AP, Trazzera S, Cohen MB, Dibs SR. Comparison of active compression-decompression cardiopulmonary resuscitation with standard cardiopulmonary resuscitation for cardiac arrests occurring in the hospital. N Engl J Med. 1993;329(26):1918–21. (PMID: 8018138).

Cohen TJ, Tucker KJ, Lurie KG, Chin MC, Redberg RF, Schiller NB, Callaham M and the Cardiopulmonary Resuscitation Working Group. Active compression-decompression (ACD); a new method of cardiopulmonary resuscitation. JAMA. 1992;267(21):2916–23. (PMID: 1583761).

Crawford MH. Aortic regurgitation. In: Crawford MH, editor. Current diagnosis & treatment: cardiology. 5th ed. New York: McGraw-Hill; 2017a. p. 237–45.

Crawford MH. Chronic ischemic heart disease. In: Crawford MH, editor. Current diagnosis & treatment: cardiology. 5th ed. New York: McGraw-Hill; 2017b. p. 59–70.

Crawford MH. Mitral regurgitation. In: Crawford MH, editor. Current diagnosis & treatment: cardiology. 5th ed. New York: McGraw-Hill; 2017c. p. 262–70.

Cronin EM, Bogun FM, Maury P, et al. 2019 HRS/EHRA/APHRS/LAHRS expert consensus statement on catheter ablation of ventricular arrhythmias. Heart Rhythm. 2020;17:e2–e154.

Curi ACC, Maior Alves AS, Silva JG. Cardiac autonomic response after cranial technique of the fourth ventricle (cv4) compression in systemic hypertensive subjects. J Bodyw Mov Ther. 2018;22(3):666–72. https://doi.org/10.1016/j.jbmt.2017.11.013.

El Sabbagh A, Reddy YNV, Nishimura RA. Mitral valve regurgitation in the contemporary era: insights into diagnosis, management, and future directions. JACC Cardiovasc Imaging. 2018;11(4):628–43. https://doi.org/10.1016/j.jcmg.2018.01.009.

Epstein AE, DiMarco JP, Ellenbogen KA, et al. American College of Cardiology Foundation, American Heart Association Task Force on Practice Guidelines, Heart Rhythm Society. 2012 ACCF/AHA/HRS focused update incorporated into the ACCF/AHA/HRS 2008 guidelines for device-based therapy of cardiac rhythm abnormalities: a report of the American College of Cardiology Foundation/American Heart Association Task Force on Practice Guidelines and the Heart Rhythm Society. J Am Coll Cardiol. 2013;61:e6–75.

Farkouh ME, Sharma SK, Tomey MI, Puskas J, Fuster V. Coronary artery bypass grafting and percutaneous interventions in stable ischemic heart disease. In: Fuster V, Harrington RA, Narula J, Eapen ZJ, editors. Hurst's the heart. 14th ed. New York: McGraw-Hill; 2017. http://accessmedicine.mhmedical.com.arktos.nyit.edu/content.aspx?bookid=2046&sectionid=176557150.

Faxon DP, Bhatt DL. Percutaneous coronary interventions and other interventional procedures. In: Jameson J, Fauci AS, Kasper DL, Hauser SL, Longo DL, Loscalzo J, editors. Harrison's principles of internal medicine. 20th ed. McGraw-Hill; 2020. https://accessmedicine-mhmedical-com.arktos.nyit.edu/content.aspx?bookid=2129&sectionid=192030175. Accessed 7 Sept 2020.

Feldman AM, Kersten DJ, Chung JA, Asheld WJ, Germano J, Islam S, Cohen TJ. Gender-related and age-related differences in implantable defibrillator recipients: results from the pacemaker and implantable defibrillator leads survival study ("PAIDLESS"). J Invasive Cardiol. 2015;27(12):530–4. (PMID: 26630641)

Fletcher GF, Ades PA, Kligfield P, et al. Exercise standards for testing and training: a scientific statement from the American Heart Association. Circulation. 2013;128(8):873–934. https://doi.org/10.1161/CIR.0b013e31829b5b44.

Galindez-Ibarbengoetxea X, Setuain I, Andersen LL, et al. Effects of cervical high-velocity low-amplitude techniques on range of motion, strength performance, and cardiovascular outcomes: a review. J Altern Complement Med. 2017;23(9):667–75. https://doi.org/10.1089/acm.2017.0002.

Gami A, Everitt I, Blumenthal RS, Newby LK, Virani SS, Kohli P. Applying the ABCs of cardiovascular disease prevention to the 2023 AHA/ACC multisociety chronic coronary disease guidelines. Am J Med. 2024;137:85–91.

Gershman ML, Needelman BS, Schwarzwald SN, Cohen TJ. The development of innovative hand-held devices to augment cardiopulmonary resuscitation therapy and external cardioversion and defibrillation. J Innov Cardiac Rhythm Manage. 2017:2930–8.

Geva T, Martins JD, Wald RM. Atrial septal defects. Lancet. 2014;383(9932):1921–32. https://doi.org/10.1016/S0140-6736(13)62145-5.

Giles PD, Hensel KL, Pacchia CF, Smith ML. Suboccipital decompression enhances heart rate variability indices of cardiac control in healthy subjects. J Altern Complement Med. 2013;19(2):92–6. https://doi.org/10.1089/acm.2011.0031.

Gillis AM, Russo AM, Ellenbogen KA, et al. HRS/ACCF expert consensus statement on pace-maker device and mode selection. Developed in partnership between the Heart Rhythm Society (HRS) and the American College of Cardiology Foundation (ACCF) and in collabora-tion with the Society of Thoracic Surgeons. Heart Rhythm. 2012;9(8):1344–65. https://doi.org/10.1016/j.hrthm.2012.06.026.

Grady KL, Wang E, Higgins R, et al. Symptom frequency and distress from 5 to 10 years after heart transplantation. J Heart Lung Transplant. 2009;28(8):759–68.

Grundy SM, Stone NJ, Bailey AL, et al. 2018 AHA/ACC/AACVPR/AAPA/ABC/ACPM/ADA/AGS/APhA/ASPC/NLA/PCNA guideline on the Management of Blood Cholesterol: a report of the American College of Cardiology/American Heart Association task force on clinical practice guidelines [published correction appears in Circulation. 2019 Jun 18;139(25):e1182-e1186]. Circulation. 2019;139(25):e1082–143. https://doi.org/10.1161/CIR.0000000000000625.

Gupta K, Kakar TS, Jain V, Bupta M, Al Rifai M, Slipczuk L, Nambi V, Bittner V, Blumenthal RS, Stone NJ, Lavie CJ, Virani SS. Comparing eligibility for statin therapy for primary pre-vention under 2022 USPSTF recommendations and the 2018 AHA/ACC/Multi-society guide-line recommendations: from National Health and Nutrition Examination Survey. Progress in Cardiovascular Diseases. 2022;75:78–82.

Gupta DK, Lewis CE, Varady KA, et al. Effect of dietary sodium on blood pressure: a crossover trial. JAMA. 2023;330(23):2258–66. https://doi.org/10.1001/jama.2023.23651.

Hahn B. Systemic lupus erythematosus. In: Jameson J, Fauci AS, Kasper DL, Hauser SL, Longo DL, Loscalzo J, editors. Harrison's principles of internal medicine, 20th ed. McGraw-Hill; 2020. https://accessmedicine-mhmedical-com.arktos.nyit.edu/content.aspx?bookid=2129&sectionid=192284866. Accessed 7 Sept 2020

Haller JD, Olearchyk AS. Cardiology's 10 greatest discoveries. Tex Heart Inst J. 2002;29:342–4.

Hampl JS, Taylor CA, Johnston CS. Vitamin C deficiency and depletion in the United States: the third national health and nutrition examination survey, 1988 to 1994. Am J Public Health. 2004;94(5):870–5. https://doi.org/10.2105/ajph.94.5.870.

Han JJ, Acker MA, Atluri P. Left ventricular assist devices. Circulation. 2018;138(24):2841–51. https://doi.org/10.1161/CIRCULATIONAHA.118.035566.

Hartmann M, Bäzner E, Wild B, Eisler I, Herzog W. Effects of interventions involving the family in the treatment of adult patients with chronic physical diseases: a meta-analysis. Psychother Psychosom. 2010;79:136–48. https://doi.org/10.1159/000286958.

Hillis LD, Smith PK, Anderson JL, et al. 2011 ACCF/AHA guideline for coronary artery bypass graft surgery: a report of the American College of Cardiology Foundation/American Heart Association task force on practice guidelines [published correction appears in Circulation. 2011 Dec 20;124(25):e957]. Circulation. 2011;124(23):e652–735. https://doi.org/10.1161/CIR.0b013e31823c074e.

Hoit BD. Tricuspid & pulmonic valve disease. In: Crawford MH, editor. Current diagnosis & treat-ment: cardiology. 5th ed. New York: McGraw-Hill; 2017. p. 271–83.

Intuitive Surgical Corporation. 2020. Retrieved from https://www.intuitive.com/en-us/products-and-services/da-vinci#.

January CT, Wann LS, Calkins H, et al. AHA/ACC/HRS Focused Update of the 2014 AHA/ACC/HRS Guideline for the Management of Patients With Atrial Fibrillation: A Report of the American College of Cardiology/American Heart Association Task Force on Clinical Practice Guidelines and the Heart Rhythm Society in Collaboration With the Society of Thoracic

Surgeons [published correction appears in Circulation. 2019 Aug 6;140(6):e285]. Circulation. 2019;140(2):e125–51. https://doi.org/10.1161/CIR.0000000000000665.

Jensen MD, Ryan DH, Apovian CM, et al. 2013 AHA/ACC/TOS guideline for the management of overweight and obesity in adults: a report of the American College of Cardiology/ American Heart Association Task Force on Practice Guidelines and The Obesity Society [published correction appears in Circulation. 2014 Jun 24;129(25 Suppl 2):S139-40]. Circulation. 2014;129(25 Suppl 2):S102–38. https://doi.org/10.1161/01.cir.0000437739.71477.ee.

Jessup M, Drazner MH, Book W, et al. ACC/AHA/HFSA/ISHLT/ACP advanced training statement on advanced heart failure and transplant cardiology (revision of the ACCF/AHA/ACP/ HFSA/ISHLT 2010 clinical competence statement on management of patients with advanced heart failure and cardiac transplant): a report of the ACC competency management committee [published correction appears in Circ Heart Fail. 2018 May;11(5):e000028]. Circ Heart Fail. 2017;10(6):e000021. https://doi.org/10.1161/HHF.0000000000000021.

Khan SU, Khan MU, Riaz H, et al. Effects of nutritional supplements and dietary interventions on cardiovascular outcomes: an umbrella review and evidence map [published correction appears in Ann Intern Med. 2020 Jan 7;172(1):75–76]. Ann Intern Med. 2019;171(3):190–8. https:// doi.org/10.7326/M19-0341.

Khush KK, Cherikh WS, Chambers DC, et al. The International Thoracic Organ Transplant Registry of the International Society for Heart and Lung Transplantation: Thirty-sixth adult heart transplantation report – 2019; focus theme: donor and recipient size match [published correction appears in J Heart Lung Transplant. 2020 Jan;39(1):91]. J Heart Lung Transplant 2019;38(10):1056–1066. doi:https://doi.org/10.1016/j.healun.2019.08.004.

Kilgore T, Malia M, Di Giacinto B, Minter S, Samies J. Adjuvant lymphatic osteopathic manipulative treatment in patients with lower-extremity ulcers: effects on wound healing and edema. J Am Osteopath Assoc. 2018;118(12):798–805. https://doi.org/10.7556/jaoa.2018.172.

Kittleson MM, Patel JK, Kobashigawa JA. Cardiac transplantation. In: Fuster V, Harrington RA, Narula J, Eapen ZJ, editors. Hurst's the heart, 14th ed. McGraw-Hill; 2020. https:// accessmedicine-mhmedical-com.arktos.nyit.edu/content.aspx?bookid=2046&sectio nid=176562189. Accessed 13 June 2020.

Koyawal N, Mathews LM, Marvel FA, Martin SS, Blumenthal RS, Sharma G. A clinician's guide to addressing cardiovascular health based on a revised AHA framework. Am J Cardiovasc Dis. 2023;13(2):52–8.

Kusumoto FM, Schoenfeld MH, Wilkoff BL, et al. 2017 HRS expert consensus statement on cardiovascular implantable electronic device lead management and extraction. Heart Rhythm. 2017;14(12):e503–51. https://doi.org/10.1016/j.hrthm.2017.09.001.

Kusumoto FM, Schoenfeld MH, Barrett C, et al. 2018 ACC/AHA/HRS guideline on the evaluation and management of patients with bradycardia and cardiac conduction delay: a report of the American College of Cardiology/American Heart Association Task Force on Clinical Practice Guidelines and the Heart Rhythm Society. J Am Coll Cardiol. 2019;74:e51–e156.

Le D. Mitral stenosis. In: Crawford MH, editor. Current diagnosis & treatment: cardiology. 5th ed. New York: McGraw-Hill; 2017. p. 246–61.

Leong MC, Uebing A, Gatzoulis MA. Percutaneous patent foramen ovale occlusion: current evidence and evolving clinical practice. Int J Cardiol. 2013;169(4):238–43. https://doi. org/10.1016/j.ijcard.2013.08.095.

Lester SJ, Abbas AE. Aortic stenosis. In: Crawford MH, editor. Current diagnosis & treatment: cardiology. 5th ed. New York: McGraw-Hill; 2017. p. 224–36.

Levine GN, Bates ER, Blankenship JC, et al. 2011 ACCF/AHA/SCAI guideline for percutaneous coronary intervention: a report of the American College of Cardiology Foundation/American Heart Association Task Force on Practice Guidelines and the Society for Cardiovascular Angiography and Interventions [published correction appears in Circulation. 2012 Feb 28;125(8):e412. Dosage error in article text]. Circulation. 2011;124(23):e574–651. https://doi. org/10.1161/CIR.0b013e31823ba622.

Lim DS, et al. 5-year durability results of transcatheter mitral valve repair with the MitraClip™ system in patients with severe degenerative mitral regurgitation and prohibitive surgical risk. J Am Coll Cardiol. 71(11 Supplement):A1262. https://doi.org/10.1016/So735-1097(18)31803-5.

Lombardini R, Marchesi S, Collebrusco L, et al. The use of osteopathic manipulative treatment as adjuvant therapy in patients with peripheral arterial disease. Man Ther. 2009;14(4):439–43. https://doi.org/10.1016/j.math.2008.08.002.

Lund LH, Edwards LB, Kucheryavaya AY, et al. The Registry of the International Society for Heart and Lung Transplantation: thirty-second official adult heart transplantation report--2015; focus theme: early graft failure. J Heart Lung Transplant. 2015;34(10):1244–54. https://doi.org/10.1016/j.healun.2015.08.003.

Mahmaljy H, Tawney A, Young M. Transcatheter Aortic Valve Replacement (TAVR/TAVI, Percutaneous Replacement) [Updated 2019 Dec 20]. In: StatPearls [Internet]. Treasure Island: StatPearls Publishing; 2020. Available from: https://www.ncbi.nlm.nih.gov/books/NBK431075/.

Malfait F, Francomano C, Byers P, et al. The 2017 international classification of the Ehlers-Danlos syndromes. Am J Med Genet C Semin Med Genet. 2017;175(1):8–26. https://doi.org/10.1002/ajmg.c.31552.

Mas JL, Derumeaux G, Guillon B, et al. Patent foramen ovale closure or anticoagulation vs. antiplatelets after stroke. N Engl J Med. 2017;377(11):1011–21. https://doi.org/10.1056/NEJMoa1705915.

McLaughlin TJ, Aupont O, Bambauer KZ, et al. Improving psychologic adjustment to chronic illness in cardiac patients. J Gen Intern Med. 2005;20:1084–90. https://doi.org/10.1111/j.1525-1497.2005.00256.x.

Meshoyrer, D. I.. The utility of Beta-blockers immediately prior to alcohol consumption in order to prevent atrial fibrillation. 2019. Retrieved September 11, 2020, from https://www.eplabdigest.com/utility-beta-blockers-immediately-prior-alcohol-consumption-order-prevent-atrial-fibrillation

Miranda B, Fonseca AC, Ferro JM. Patent foramen ovale and stroke. J Neurol. 2018;265(8):1943–9. https://doi.org/10.1007/s00415-018-8865-0.

Mojadidi MK, Roberts SC, Winoker JS, et al. Accuracy of transcranial Doppler for the diagnosis of intracardiac right-to-left shunt: a bivariate meta-analysis of prospective studies. JACC Cardiovasc Imaging. 2014;7(3):236–50. https://doi.org/10.1016/j.jcmg.2013.12.011.

Mortensen SA, Rosenfeldt F, Jumar A, et al. The effect of coenzyme Q10 on morbidity and mortality in chronic heart failure: results from Q-SYMBIO: a randomized double –blind trial. J Am Coll Cardiol Heart Fail. 2014;2(6):641–9. https://doi.org/10.1016/j.jchf.2014.06.008.

Ndumele CE, Rangaswami J, Chow SL, et al. Cardiovascular-kidney-metabolic health: a presidential advisory from the American Heart Association. Circulation. 2023;148(20):1606–35.

Nakamura T, Schaeffer B, Tanigawa S, et al. Catheter ablation of polymorphic ventricular tachycardia/fibrillation in patients with and without structural heart disease. Heart Rhythm. 2019;16:1021–7.

Nishimura RA, Otto CM, Bonow RO, et al. AHA/ACC guideline for the management of patients with valvular heart disease: a report of the American College of Cardiology/American Heart Association Task Force on Practice Guidelines [published correction appears in J Am Coll Cardiol. 2014 Jun 10;63(22):2489. Dosage error in article text]. J Am Coll Cardiol. 2014;63(22):e57–e185. https://doi.org/10.1016/j.jacc.2014.02.536.

Nishimura RA, Seggewiss H, Schaff HV. Hypertrophic obstructive cardiomyopathy: surgical myectomy and septal ablation. Circ Res. 2017;121(7):771–83. https://doi.org/10.1161/CIRCRESAHA.116.309348.

Nishimura RA, et al. Faculty opinions recommendation of 2017 AHA/ACC focused update of the 2014 AHA/ACC guideline for the Management of Patients with Valvular heart disease: a report of the American College of Cardiology/American Heart Association task force on clinical practice guidelines. Faculty Opinions—Post-Publication Peer Review of the Biomedical Literature. 2017c;135(25):e1159–95. https://doi.org/10.3410/f.727426955.793533368.

Nobuyoshi M, Arita T, Shirai S, et al. Percutaneous balloon mitral valvuloplasty: a review. Circulation. 2009;119(8):e211–9. https://doi.org/10.1161/CIRCULATIONAHA.108.792952.

Nuño V, Siu A, Deol N, Juster RP. Osteopathic manipulative treatment for allostatic load lowering. J Am Osteopath Assoc. 2019;119(10):646–54. https://doi.org/10.7556/jaoa.2019.112.

Obeyesekere MN, Antzelevitch C, Krahn AD. Management of ventricular arrhythmias in suspected channelopathies. Circ Arrhythm Electrophysiol. 2015;8:221–31.

Ockene IS, Miller NH. Cigarette smoking, cardiovascular disease, and stroke. Circulation. 1997;96(9):3243–7. https://doi.org/10.1161/01.CIR.96.9.3243.

Over 182,000 Heart Valve Replacements per Year in the United States. iDataResearch website. https://idataresearch.com/over-182000-heart-valve-replacements-per-year-in-the-united-states/. Published June 13, 2018. Accessed September 7, 2020.

Page RL, Joglar JA, Caldwell MA, et al. 2015 ACC/AHA/HRS guideline for the management of adult patients with supraventricular tachycardia: a report of the American College of Cardiology/American Heart Association Task Force on Clinical Practice Guidelines and the Heart Rhythm Society [published correction appears in Circulation. 2016 Sep 13;134(11):e234–5]. Circulation. 2016;133(14):e506–74. https://doi.org/10.1161/CIR.0000000000000311.

Panaich S, Holmes DR. Left atrial appendage occlusion. American College of Cardiology website January 31, 2017. https://www.acc.org/latest-in-cardiology/articles/2017/01/31/13/08/left-atrial-appendage-occlusion. Accessed 7 Sept 2020.

Panchal AR, Berg KM, Hirsch KG, et al. 2019 American Heart Association focused update on advanced cardiovascular life support: use of advanced airways, vasopressors, and extracorporeal cardiopulmonary resuscitation during cardiac arrest: an update to the American Heart Association guidelines for cardiopulmonary resuscitation and emergency cardiovascular care. Circulation. 2019;140(24):e881–94. https://doi.org/10.1161/CIR.0000000000000732.

Pedersen CT, Kay GN, Kalman J, et al.; EP-Europace, UK. EHRA/HRS/APHRS expert consensus on ventricular arrhythmias. Heart Rhythm 2014;11:e166–e196.

Prendergast BD, Redwood SR. Transcatheter aortic valve replacement. Circulation. 2019;139(24):2724–7. https://doi.org/10.1161/CIRCULATIONAHA.119.040016.

Priori SG, Wilde AA, Horie M, et al. HRS/EHRA/APHRS expert consensus statement on the diagnosis and management of patients with inherited primary arrhythmia syndromes: document endorsed by HRS, EHRA, and APHRS in May 2013 and by ACCF, AHA, PACES, and AEPC in June 2013. Heart Rhythm. 2013;10:1932–63.

Racca V, Bordoni B, Castiglioni P, Modica M, Ferratini M. Osteopathic manipulative treatment improves heart surgery outcomes: a randomized controlled trial. Ann Thorac Surg. 2017;104(1):145–52. https://doi.org/10.1016/j.athoracsur.2016.09.110.

Rechberger V, Biberschick M, Porthun J. Effectiveness of an osteopathic treatment on the autonomic nervous system: a systematic review of the literature. Eur J Med Res. 2019;24(1):36. https://doi.org/10.1186/s40001-019-0394-5.

Riley B. The many facets of hypermobile Ehlers-Danlos syndrome. J Am Osteopath Assoc. 2020;120(1):30–2. https://doi.org/10.7556/jaoa.2020.012.

Riley B, Bombei B. The Ehlers–Danlos syndromes. Osteopathic Family Phys. 2020;12(1):26–9. https://doi.org/10.33181/12013.

Rogers FJ. The muscle hypothesis: a model of chronic heart failure appropriate for osteopathic medicine. J Am Osteopath Assoc. 2001;101(10):576–83.

Rogers JG, Patel CB, Milano CA. Mechanically assisted circulation. In: Fuster V, Harrington RA, Narula J, Eapen ZJ, editors. Hurst's the heart, 14th ed. McGraw-Hill; 2020. https://accessmedicine-mhmedical-com.arktos.nyit.edu/content.aspx?bookid=2046&sectionid=176562373. Accessed 7 Sept 2020.

Roldan CA. Connective tissue diseases & the heart. In: Crawford MH, editor. Current diagnosis & treatment: cardiology. 5th ed. New York: McGraw-Hill; 2017. p. 533–62. http://accessmedicine.mhmedical.com.arktos.nyit.edu/content.aspx?bookid=2040&sectionid=152997983.

Romero J, Cerrud-Rodriguez RC, Di Biase L, et al. Combined endocardial-epicardial versus endocardial catheter ablation alone for ventricular tachycardia in structural heart disease: a systematic review and meta-analysis. JACC Clin Electrophysiol. 2019;5:13–24.

Russo AM, Stainback RF, Bailey SR, et al. ACCF/HRS/AHA/ASE/HFSA/SCAI/SCCT/SCMR 2013 appropriate use criteria for implantable cardioverter-defibrillators and cardiac resynchronization therapy: a report of the American College of Cardiology Foundation appropriate use criteria task force, Heart Rhythm Society, American Heart Association, American Society of Echocardiography, Heart Failure Society of America, Society for Cardiovascular Angiography and Interventions, Society of Cardiovascular Computed Tomography, and Society for Cardiovascular Magnetic Resonance. Heart Rhythm. 2013;10(4):e11–58. https://doi.org/10.1016/j.hrthm.2013.01.008.

Sacher F, Lim HS, Derval N, et al. Substrate mapping and ablation for ventricular tachycardia: the LAVA approach. J Cardiovasc Electrophysiol. 2015;26:464–71.

Schill MR, Khiabani AJ, Kachroo P, Damiano RJ Jr. Acquired heart disease. In: Brunicardi F, Andersen DK, Billiar TR, Dunn DL, Kao LS, Hunter JG, Matthews JB, Pollock RE, editors. Schwartz's principles of surgery. 11th ed. New York: McGraw-Hill; 2019. p. 801–52.

Seffinger M. Foundations of osteopathic medicine: philosophy, science, clinical applications, and research. 4th ed. Philadelphia: Wolter Kluwer; 2019.

Shahani R. Coronary Artery Bypass Grafting. Medscape. https://emedicine.medscape.com/article/1893992. Updated December 4, 2019.

Shaikh ZA, Eilenberg MF, Cohen TJ. The amigo™ remote catheter system: from concept to bedside. J Innov Cardiac Rhythm Manage. 2017;2017:2795–802.

Shen WK, Sheldon RS, Benditt DG, et al. 2017 ACC/AHA/HRS guideline for the evaluation and management of patients with syncope: a report of the American College of Cardiology/American Heart Association Task Force on Clinical Practice Guidelines and the Heart Rhythm Society [published correction appears in Circulation. 2017 Oct 17;136(16):e271–e272]. Circulation. 2017;136(5):e60–e122. https://doi.org/10.1161/CIR.0000000000000499.

Shibayama K, Harada K, Berdejo J, et al. Effect of transcatheter aortic valve replacement on the mitral valve apparatus and mitral regurgitation: real-time three-dimensional transesophageal echocardiography study. Circ Cardiovasc Imaging. 2014;7(2):344–51. https://doi.org/10.1161/CIRCIMAGING.113.000942.

Silvestry FE. Postoperative complications among patients undergoing cardiac surgery. In: Manaker S, King TE, Finlay G, editors. UpToDate. Waltham: UpToDate Inc.; 2019. https://www.uptodate.com/contents/postoperative-complications-among-patients-undergoing-cardiac-surgery#H547631153.

Slotwiner D, Varma N, Akar JG, et al. HRS expert consensus statement on remote interrogation and monitoring for cardiovascular implantable electronic devices. Heart Rhythm. 2015;12:e69–100.

Soar J, Maconochie I, Wyckoff MH, et al. 2019 international consensus on cardiopulmonary resuscitation and emergency cardiovascular care science with treatment recommendations: summary from the basic life support; advanced life support; pediatric life support; neonatal life support; education, implementation, and teams; and first aid task forces. Circulation. 2019;140(24):e826–80. https://doi.org/10.1161/CIR.0000000000000734.

Sorajja P, Valeti U, Nishimura RA, et al. Outcome of alcohol septal ablation for obstructive hypertrophic cardiomyopathy. Circulation. 2008;118(2):131–9. https://doi.org/10.1161/CIRCULATIONAHA.107.738740.

Steinwender C, Khelae SK, Garweg C, et al. Atrioventricular synchronous pacing using a leadless ventricular pacemaker: results from the MARVEL 2 study. JACC Clin Electrophysiol. 2020;6:94–106.

Stone GW, Lindenfeld JA, Abraham WT, et al. Transcatheter mitral-valve repair in patients with heart failure. N Engl J Med. 2018;379(24):2307–18.

Tan A, Ashrafian H, Scott A, Mason S, Harling L, Athanasiou T, Darzi A. Robotic surgery: disruptive innovation or unfulfilled promise? A systematic review and meta-analysis of the first 30 years. Surg Endosc. 2016;30:4330–52.

The Marfans Foundation. https://www.marfan.org/about/marfan. Assessed March 29, 2020.

Thomaz SR, Teixeira FA, de Lima ACGB, Cipriano Júnior G, Formiga MF, Cahalin LP. Osteopathic manual therapy in heart failure patients: a randomized clinical trial. J Bodyw Mov Ther. 2018;22(2):293–9. https://doi.org/10.1016/j.jbmt.2017.07.011.

Tracy CM, Epstein AE, Darbar D, et al. 2012 ACCF/AHA/HRS focused update of the 2008 guidelines for device-based therapy of cardiac rhythm abnormalities: a report of the American

College of Cardiology Foundation/American Heart Association Task Force on Practice Guidelines. J Am Coll Cardiol. 2012;60:1297–313.

Ungprasert P, Wannarong T, Panichsillapakit T, et al. Cardiac involvement in mixed connective tissue disease: a systematic review. Int J Cardiol. 2014;171(3):326–30. https://doi.org/10.1016/j.ijcard.2013.12.079.

Valvular Heart Disease. Centers for Disease Control and Prevention website. https://www.cdc.gov/heartdisease/valvular_disease.htm. Updated December 9, 2019.

Varshney R, Budoff MJ. Garlic and heart disease. J Nutr. 2016;146(2):416S–21S. https://doi.org/10.3945/jn.114.202333.

Vassiliou VA, Moyssakis I, Boki KA, Moutsopoulos HM. Is the heart affected in primary Sjögren's syndrome? An echocardiographic study. Clin Exp Rheumatol. 2008;26(1):109–12.

Veselka J, Anavekar NS, Charron P. Hypertrophic obstructive cardiomyopathy [published correction appears in Lancet. 2017 Mar 25;389(10075):1194]. Lancet. 2017;389(10075):1253–67. https://doi.org/10.1016/S0140-6736(16)31321-6.

Wieting JM, Beal C, Roth GL, et al. The effect of osteopathic manipulative treatment on postoperative medical and functional recovery of coronary artery bypass graft patients. J Am Osteopath Assoc. 2013;113(5):384–93.

Wróblewska-Kałuzewska M, Ozimek W, Pleskot M, Jedrasik P. Rodzinna kardiomiopatia przerostowa [Familial hypertrophic cardiomyopathy]. Pol Merkur Lekarski. 1997a;2(8):129–31.

Wróblewska-Kałuzewska M, Ozimek W, Pleskot M, Jedrasik P. Familial hypertrophic cardiomyopathy. Polski Merkuriusz Lekarski: Organ Polskiego Towarzystwa Lekarskiego; 1997b. https://doi.org/10.1161/circresaha.113.301406.

Song Y, Lindquist R, Windenburg D, Cairns B, Thakur A. Review of outcomes of cardiac support groups after cardiac events. West J Nurs Res. 2011;33(2):224–46. https://doi.org/10.1177/0193945910371481.

Zhang S, Zhou X, Gold MR. Left bundle branch pacing: JACC review topic of the week. J Am Coll Cardiol. 2019;74:3039–49.

Zipes DP, Calkins H, Daubert JP, et al. 2015 ACC/AHA/HRS advanced training statement on clinical cardiac electrophysiology (a revision of the ACC/AHA 2006 update of the clinical competence statement on invasive electrophysiology studies, catheter ablation, and cardioversion). Heart Rhythm. 2016;13(1):e3–e37. https://doi.org/10.1016/j.hrthm.2015.09.014.

Index

© The Editor(s) (if applicable) and The Author(s), under exclusive license to Springer Nature Switzerland AG 2025
T. J. Cohen, R. S. Blumenthal (eds.), *Surviving and Thriving With Heart Disease*, Contemporary Cardiology, https://doi.org/10.1007/978-3-032-00579-3